Whole Grains and Health

Whole Grains and Health

Edited by Len Marquart, David R. Jacobs, Jr.,
Graeme H. McIntosh, Kaisa Poutanen, Marla Reicks

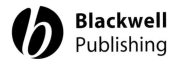

©2007 Blackwell Publishing
All rights reserved

Blackwell Publishing Professional
2121 State Avenue, Ames, Iowa 50014, USA

Orders: **1-800-862-6657**
Office: **1-515-292-0140**
Fax: **1-515-292-3348**
Web site: **www.blackwellprofessional.com**

Blackwell Publishing Ltd
9600 Garsington Road, Oxford OX4 2DQ, UK
Tel.: +44 (0)1865 776868

Blackwell Publishing Asia
550 Swanston Street, Carlton, Victoria 3053, Australia
Tel.: +61 (0)3 8359 1011

First edition, 2007

Library of Congress Cataloging-in-Publication Data

Whole grains and health / edited by Len Marquart—1st ed.
     p. ; cm.
   Includes bibliographical references.
   ISBN-13: 978-0-8138-0777-5 (alk. paper)
   ISBN-10: 0-8138-0777-8 (alk. paper)
  1. Health. 2. Grain—Therapeutic use. 3. Grain in human nutrition. I. Marquart, Len.
   [DNLM: 1. Cereals. 2. Diet—standards. 3. Health Promotion. 4. Nutrition. WB 431
W6285 2007]

RA776.W4556 2007
613—dc22

                                                            2006014421

The last digit is the print number: 9 8 7 6 5 4 3 2 1

Table of Contents

Foreword

The current worldwide interest in whole grains has gained momentum in the past decade, based on scientific studies linking whole grain consumption to improved health. So widespread is the interest that national and international conferences have been convened to bring interested parties together to further the learning about whole grains. Recommendations in the United States encourage consumption of at least three one-ounce servings of whole grain daily, yet the average intake is less than one serving per day. Furthermore, it is estimated that less than 10% of the United States population consumes three servings of whole grains daily. Estimates for Europe and other nations is no better, with 30% of United Kingdom adults failing to consume whole grain foods at all during a week and more than 97% failing to meet the United States recommendation of three servings daily. Explanations for the shortfalls are many, but their continued existence is puzzling when the links between whole grain consumption and good health are undisputed and continue to make research and news headlines.

The 2003 World Health Organization report on Diet, Nutrition, and Prevention of Chronic Diseases lists whole grains among the recommended ways to increase fiber consumption. The 2005 Dietary Guidelines for Americans, a rigorous review of the scientific literature presented in a United States government report and accompanying documents, concluded that consuming at least three one-ounce servings of whole grain per day can reduce the risk of diabetes and coronary heart disease and can assist with weight maintenance. Likewise, the United States food guidance system, now called MyPyramid, also recommends three servings of whole grains daily as part of recommendations for grain intake overall.

More specifically, whole grain intake has been associated with a reduction in the risk of coronary heart disease among both men and women. Taken collectively, the studies strongly suggest as much as a 30% decrease in risk of coronary heart disease with three or more servings of whole grain foods daily. The Nurses' Health Study showed that women who ate the highest level of whole grains daily had half the relative risk of developing coronary heart disease than did those who ate the fewest whole grains.

Several major epidemiological studies showed an inverse relationship between whole grain consumption and the risk of developing type 2 diabetes—the more whole grain consumed, the less the risk of developing diabetes. Risk of diabetes was reduced in those eating the highest level of whole grains and was reduced further—by at least 30% among those eating the highest level of cereal-fiber—compared to the lowest level of whole-grain intake.

In the area of weight maintenance, when comparing consumption of whole grains, a recent study showed that women who ate at least three servings of whole grains gained significantly less weight than did counterparts who ate only refined grains made from white flour. Other studies suggest that because whole grain foods typically contain more fiber, there is a link with fiber intake and health as well. Fiber tends to fill us up, often helping to decrease the number of calories we consume. Over time, consumption of more whole grains, more fiber, and fewer calories can lead to weight loss and can help with longer-term weight maintenance—certainly relevant to the growing levels of obesity plaguing the United States. Consumption of more whole grain foods offers a viable solution to reduce global obesity trends.

Why a gap exists between recommendations for whole grain consumption and actual behavior is not clear. Research is needed to explore potential barriers and motivators to whole grain consumption among adults and children worldwide. Improving the brownish appearance and hearty texture and finding ways to expose whole grains to consumers at earlier ages may help consumers to be more amenable to whole grain acceptance. An understanding of the best ways to communicate the health benefits of whole grains in different languages and among diverse cultures is missing from the literature. Also needed is a global investment in technological development and innovation—from plant breeding to milling and processing—to deliver more of the health potential of the whole grain to consumers.

What is clear is that efforts on the whole grain front cannot operate in isolation. A collaborative effort among scientists, industry, academia, government, educators, farmers, community agencies, food service personnel, and health-related organizations around the world is needed to move whole grains from field to fork and fill the consumption gap. With increasingly more epidemiological data about the health benefits of whole grain intake, an international consensus about recommendations to increase the intake of whole grain foods would be beneficial.

A list of recommendations for advancing whole grain research efforts and encouraging greater use and consumption has been developed and shared at such meetings of the minds as the successful Whole Grains & Health: A Global Summit held in Minneapolis, Minnesota in May 2005. Based on key learnings, continuing dialogue, and shared insights of more than 400 attendees from various areas of discipline and many parts of the world, the list, contained in this book *Whole Grains and Health*, reflects a collaboration of sorts, highlighting three key areas of focus: biological science and health, consumer research and education, and grain science and technology. In addition, this text captures the novel work of leading experts in the whole grain field, much of which was presented at the meeting. Continuing efforts and sharing, such as the publishing of this book, *Whole Grains and Health*, is critical to keeping whole grains in the forefront of global contemporary science.

Sincerely,
Allen S. Levine, PhD
Professor and Department Head
Department of Food Science and Nutrition
University of Minnesota, St. Paul, MN

Gilbert A. Leveille, PhD
Advisory Chair
Department of Food Science and Nutrition
University of Minnesota, St. Paul, MN

Acknowledgments

We would like to express our deepest appreciation to the Organizing Committee: Ed Welsch, Lori Engstrom, Allen Levine, and Gary Fulcher for their dedication in the planning and flawless execution of Whole Grains & Health: A Global Summit. A special thanks to co-chair Julie Miller Jones, Fred Hegele, Gil Leveille, and Bill Atwell for their wisdom and expertise in our selection of conference goals, objectives, and outcomes. We commend Hal Schroer for his leadership and expertise in the process evaluation and summary of conference research priorities. We would like to thank our session chairs, speakers, and authors for their excellent presentations and articulate book chapters.

We are grateful to the University of Minnesota Department of Food Science and Nutrition faculty Dan Gallaher, Mindy Kurzer, Bill Schafer, Cindy Gallaher, and Elizabeth Parks for their concerted efforts in their facilitation and artful summation of session research priorities. The conference comments were carefully collected and compiled by Department of Food Science and Nutrition graduate students Dave Pascoe, Kristen Schmitz, Renee Rosen, Hing wan Chan, Teri Burgess Champoux, Joanne Delk, Leila Sadeghi, Sara Sjoberg, Alyssa Bakke, and Lindsey Orr. A special thanks to the stakeholder team who assisted with the prioritization of research issues: Julie Miller Jones, David Jacobs, Jr., Marla Reicks, Mark Kantor, David Klurfeld, Sylvia Rowe, and Van Hubbard.

We extend our appreciation to Kay Behall, Gary Fulcher, Lore Kolberg, and Elyse Cohen for their contributions in organizing and conducting the highly successful pre-conference session, The Future of Barley.

We thank Steve McCarthy and his graphics design students for their expertise in the design and development of the conference program, signs, and PowerPoint slides, and Bill Kauffman for his expertise in designing the grain carousels for the conference dinner. We are appreciative of Sue Winkelman for her administrative support in corresponding with authors, Alison Grabau for her fine editorial work, and Raechel Bosch and Sam Hanson for the compilation and organization of conference materials.

We are in deep gratitude to Paul Lynch, executive chef for Radisson and the Fire Lake Restaurant, for his delicious whole grain meals, snacks, and desserts throughout the conference. A special thanks to Syb Woutat for her planning and organization of the awards ceremony at the Mill City Museum, Marcus Buggs and Carol Lund for their administration and organization of conference registration, Sue Viker for her administrative support, and Sue Moores for her development of the initial Whole Grains and Health book proposal.

A heartfelt thanks and deep appreciation to Mary Grabau for her unending support and dedication during the planning, organizing, and execution of Whole Grains & Health: A Global Summit.

Contributing Authors

Chapter 1

Len Marquart, University of Minnesota, U.S.A.
Julie Miller Jones, The College of St. Catherine, U.S.A.
Elyse A. Cohen, Cohen Health and Nutrition Communications, U.S.A.
Kaisa Poutanen, V.T.T. Biotechnology and University of Kuopio, Finland

Chapter 2

Jeffery Sobal, Cornell University, U.S.A.

Chapter 3

James W. Anderson, University of Kentucky, U.S.A.
Shannon B. Conley, University of Kentucky, U.S.A.

Chapter 4

Nicola McKeown, U.S. Department of Agriculture and Tufts University, U.S.A.
Mary Serdula, Centers for Disease Control and Prevention and Harvard University, U.S.A.
Simin Liu, University of California at Los Angeles, U.S.A.

Chapter 5

Joanne Slavin, University of Minnesota, U.S.A.

Chapter 6

Graeme H. McIntosh, University of Adelaide, Australia

Chapter 7

Joel J. Pins, University of Minnesota, U.S.A.
Harminder Kaur, University of Minnesota, U.S.A.
Ellen Dodds, University of Minnesota, U.S.A.
Joseph M. Keenan, University of Minnesota, U.S.A.

Chapter 8

David A Pascoe, University of Minnesota, U.S.A.
R. Gary Fulcher, University of Manitoba, Canada

Chapter 9

Karin Autio, V.T.T. Biotechnology, Finland
Kirsi-Helena Liukkonen, V.T.T. Biotechnology, Finland
Hannu Mykkänen, University of Kuopio, Finland
Irene Katina, V.T.T. Biotechnology, Finland
Katariina Roininen, V.T.T. Biotechnology, Finland
Kaisa Poutanen, V.T.T. Biotechnology and University of Kuopio, Finland

Chapter 10

Bill Atwell, Cargill, Incorporated, U.S.A.
Walter von Reding, Buhler A.G., Switzerland
Jessica Earling, Cargill, Incorporated, U.S.A.
Mitch Kanter, Cargill, Incorporated, U.S.A.
Kim Snow, Cargill Incorporated, U.S.A.

Chapter 11

Susan Cho, NutriSuccess, L.L.C., U.S.A.
Carol J. Pratt, Kellogg Company, U.S.A.

Chapter 12

Scott R. Frazer, Cargill, Incorporated, U.S.A

Chapter 13

Isabel Trogh, Katholieke Universiteit Leuven, Belgium
Christophe Courtin, Katholieke Universiteit Leuven, Belgium
Jan Delcour, Katholieke Universiteit Leuven, Belgium

Chapter 14

Inger Björck, Lund University, Sweden
Elin Östman, Lund University, Sweden
Anne Nilsson, Lund University, Sweden

Chapter 15

Rui Hai Liu, Cornell University, U.S.A.
Kafui Kwami Adom, Cornell University, U.S.A.

Chapter 16

Per Åman, Swedish University of Agricultural Sciences, Sweden
Alastair B. Ross, Nestle Research Center, Switzerland
Rikard Landberg, Swedish University of Agricultural Sciences, Sweden
Afaf Kamal-Eldin, Swedish University of Agricultural Sciences, Sweden

Chapter 17

David Topping, C.S.I.R.O. Human Nutrition, Australia
Anthony Bird, C.S.I.R.O. Human Nutrition, Australia
Shusuke Toden, C.S.I.R.O. Human Nutrition, University of Adelaide, Australia
Michael Conlon, C.S.I.R.O. Human Nutrition, Australia
Manny Noakes, C.S.I.R.O. Human Nutrition, Australia
Roger King, C.S.I.R.O. Human Nutrition, Australia
Gulay Mann, C.S.I.R.O. Human Nutrition, Australia
Zhong Yi Li, C.S.I.R.O. Human Nutrition, Australia
Matthew Morell, C.S.I.R.O. Human Nutrition, Australia

Chapter 18

Kirsi-Helena Liukkonen, V.T.T. Biotechnology, Finland
Kati Katina, V.T.T. Biotechnology, Finland
Anu Kaukovirta-Norja, V.T.T. Biotechnology, Finland
Anna-Maija Lampi, University of Helsinki, Finland
Susanna Kariluoto, University of Helsinki, Finland
Vieno Piironen, University of Helsinki, Finland
Satu-Maarit Heinonen, University of Helsinki, Finland
Herman Adlercreutz, University of Helsinki, Finland
Anna Nurmi, University of Helsinki, Finland
Juha-Matti Pihlava, M.T.T. AgriFood Finland, Finland
Kaisa Poutanen, V.T.T. Biotechnology and University of Kuopio, Finland

Chapter 19

Chris J. Seal, University of Newcastle, U.K.
Angela R. Jones, University of Newcastle, U.K.

Chapter 20

Alyssa Bakke, University of Minnesota, U.S.A.
Zata Vickers, University of Minnesota, U.S.A.
Len Marquart, University of Minnesota, U.S.A.
Sara Sjoberg, University of Minnesota, U.S.A.

Chapter 21

Jeff Dahlberg, The Whole Grains Council, U.S.A.
K. Dun Gifford, Oldways Preservation Trust, U.S.A.
Cynthia W. Harriman, Oldways Preservation Trust, U.S.A.

Chapter 22

Mary Ann Johnson, University of Georgia, U.S.A.
Teri Burgess-Champoux, University of Minnesota, U.S.A.
Mark A. Kantor, University of Maryland, U.S.A.
Marla Reicks, University of Minnesota, U.S.A.

Chapter 23

Judi Adams, Grain Foods Foundation, U.S.A.

Chapter 24

Trish Griffiths, B.R.I. Australia Ltd., Australia

Chapter 25

Mindy Hermann, The Hermann Group, U.S.A.

Chapter 26

Kristen Schmitz, University of Minnesota, U.S.A.
Nils-Georg Asp, Lund University/Lund Institute of Technology, and Swedish Nutrition
  Foundation, Sweden
David Richardson, D.P.R. Nutrition Limited, U.K.
Len Marquart, University of Minnesota, U.S.A.

Part I

Introduction to Whole Grains and Health

1   The Future of Whole Grains

Len Marquart, Julie Miller Jones, Elyse A. Cohen, and Kaisa Poutanen

Introduction

Current recommendations in the United States encourage at least three servings of whole grains daily, yet the average intake is less than one serving per day, and it is estimated that less than 10% of the U.S. population consumes three servings daily. Clearly, a collaborative effort among scientists, industry, government, educators, farmers, and health-related organizations is needed to move whole grains from the field to the fork and fill the consumption gap. With the increasing epidemiological data about the health benefits of whole grain intake, it would also be useful to have international consensus about recommendations to increase the intake of whole grain foods.

Basic Whole Grains

Whole grains have been part of the human diet for centuries. Commonly consumed whole grains in Western nations are wheat, oats, corn, rye and barley, but recently a variety of other grains are being selected more frequently. Table 1.1 lists the types of whole grains used in

Table 1.1.   Whole grains consumed in the U.S.

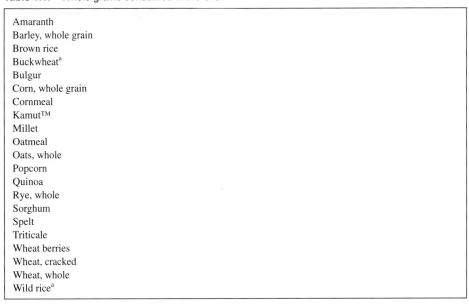

Amaranth
Barley, whole grain
Brown rice
Buckwheat[a]
Bulgur
Corn, whole grain
Cornmeal
Kamut™
Millet
Oatmeal
Oats, whole
Popcorn
Quinoa
Rye, whole
Sorghum
Spelt
Triticale
Wheat berries
Wheat, cracked
Wheat, whole
Wild rice[a]

[a] Not strictly a grain but has similar whole-grain makeup and is consumed as a grain.
Adapted from U.S.D.A./H.H.S. (2005a) and WGC (2004).

the United States. It also includes buckwheat and wild rice, which botanically are not true cereal grains. These pseudo grains offer nutritional compositions similar to whole grains and are used in many foods similarly to how whole grains are used.

Grains are made up of three main parts (Figure 1.1): the germ, which contains the plant embryo or seed; the endosperm, which provides food for the growing seed; and the outer hull, which contains the aleurone that protects the grain from bacteria, molds, insects, and severe weather (Fulcher and Rooney-Duke 2002). According to the current definitions, all three parts of the grain must be included for the food to be a whole grain product.

The endosperm is mainly starch and protein, whereas the aleurone and germ contain the dietary fiber and most of the biologically active components. They include traditional nutrients,

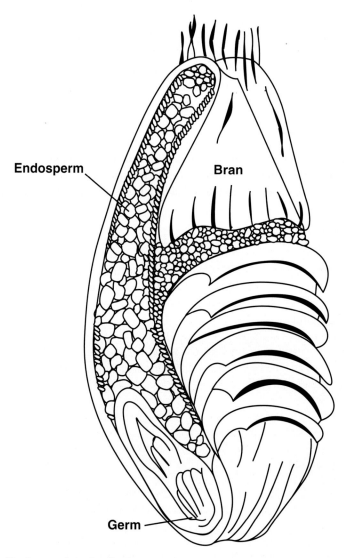

Figure 1.1.   The three main parts of grain.

namely protein and amino acids, essential fatty acids, B vitamins (thiamin, riboflavin, niacin, vitamin B_6, folate, and pantothenic acid); vitamin E, and minerals (calcium, magnesium, phosphorus, potassium, sodium, zinc, and iron). Whole grains also contain phytochemicals—plant components such as phytates, lignans, phenolic acids, and polyphenols—which show antioxidant, phytoestrogen, and other bioactivities that may offer health benefits.

Peasant diets of old times included whole grains in their entirety. While it was common practice to grind the grain, it was a lengthy and difficult process to manually separate the bran from the endosperm and germ. Modern roller milling enabled the easy separation of whole grains into their different parts, making refined products readily available. Refined flour with the outer bran layer and most of the germ removed became the most widely consumed flour. Removal of the outer portions of the grain helped resultant products to yield textures and flavors in baking that had wide appeal. On the downside, milling caused nutritional losses of much of the dietary fiber and many of the vitamins, minerals, and phytonutrients. Enrichment programs have attempted to rectify the nutrient losses by mandating the addition of some of the B vitamins and iron lost in the refining process. However, the end products still fail to deliver all the nutritional benefits of whole grain. In contrast, whole grain flours such as whole wheat flour retain the nutrients and all three parts found in the native grain—hence the name whole grain.

Today we often define whole grains as "foods made from the entire grain seed, usually called the kernel, which consists of the bran, germ, and endosperm. If the kernel has been cracked, crushed or flaked, it must retain nearly the same relative proportions of bran, germ, and endosperm as the original grain in order to be called whole grain." This definition was developed by the U.S. Whole Grains Council (2004) and was adapted from an earlier definition developed by the American Association of Cereal Chemists International (2000).

Global Interest in Whole Grains

The current interest in whole grains has gained momentum in the past ten to fifteen years. The first Whole Grain Conference, an effort to help build interest and more closely examine whole grains and possible links to better health, was a joint effort sponsored by U.S. Department of Agriculture (U.S.D.A.), General Mills, and the American Dietetic Association in 1993 in Washington, D.C. This collaborative effort led to the development of the phrase "3 are key" referring to the daily recommendation of three servings of whole grains. As data continued to emphasize the health importance of whole grains, more national and international meetings sponsored by different organizations were convened to further whole grain learning and interest.

The first symposium was the European Whole Grain Meeting in Paris in 1997. It was followed by a series of annual sessions at the American Dietetic Association meetings (1998, 1999, 2000, 2001) and American Association of Cereal Chemists meetings (1999, 2002, 2005). Whole grain sharing also occurred at the Vahouny Fiber Conferences in Washington, D.C., (2000) and Edinburgh, Scotland (2002). The Whole Grains and Health International Conference in Porvoo, Finland (2001) was devoted completely to discussing the science underlying the health effects of grains. It was followed by Grains for the Health of It, in Minneapolis, Minnesota, (2001) and Experimental Biology in San Diego, California. (2003). Most recently, the largest meeting, Whole Grains & Health: A Global Summit, was convened in Minneapolis, Minnesota (2005).

Connecting Whole Grains to Health

Based on rising interest and mounting evidence worldwide, scientists continued to link increased whole grain consumption and reduced risk of disease, namely cardiovascular disease, diabetes, and assistance with weight maintenance.

Cardiovascular Disease

Cardiovascular disease (C.V.D.) and diabetes are among the top causes of death for both men and women in the U.S. and around the world. Epidemiological data show a strong association between whole grain intake and a reduction in risk of coronary heart disease (C.H.D.) among both men and women (Anderson et al. 2000; Erkkilä et al. 2005; Jacobs et al. 1998, 1999; Jensen et al. 2004; Liu et al. 1999; Rimm et al. 1996; Steffen et al. 2003). Together, these studies show a strong inverse association with a risk of C.H.D. for those who ate three or more servings of whole grain foods daily. C.H.D. risks might be reduced by as much as 30%. In the Nurses' Health Study, Liu et al. (1999) showed that women who ate the highest level of whole grains daily had half the relative risk of developing C.H.D. than did those who ate the fewest whole grains.

Diabetes

As for C.H.D., the development of type 2 diabetes is affected by diet, in addition to other lifestyle factors. Sedentary lifestyle and obesity are important risk factors, contributing to the rapidly increasing epidemic of type 2 diabetes. Several epidemiological studies (Fung et al. 2002; Liu et al. 2000; Montonen et al. 2003; Salmeron et al. 1997a, b) showed an inverse relationship between whole grain consumption and the risk of developing type 2 diabetes. There appeared to be a dose response relationship—that means the risk of developing diabetes decreased as the amount of whole grain in the diet increased. There is also recent evidence about whole grain intake as a protective factor against metabolic syndrome (Esmaillzadeth et al. 2005, McKeown et al. 2004).

Weight Management

When comparing whole grain consumption over a twelve-year period, Liu et al. (2003) found that women who ate at least three servings of whole grain foods daily gained significantly less weight than women who ate only foods made from refined white flour.

Because whole grain foods typically contain more fiber, other studies suggest there also may be a link between fiber intake and health. A growing body of evidence suggests that soluble fiber such as β-glucan from oats and barley plays a role in the management of body weight, blood pressure, and blood cholesterol (F.D.A. 2003a, Brown et al. 1999). Ludwig et al. (1999) showed that over a prolonged period of time, as more fiber is consumed, less weight is gained—saving about 8 pounds of weight gain in ten years.

Additional studies suggest that when whole grain intake is increased, body mass index (BMI), a standard measure for weight-to-height appropriateness, decreases—indicating a healthier body proportion among eaters of whole grain foods (Koh-Banerjee et al. 2004, Ludwig et al. 1999). Fiber may act in a number of ways to help fight weight gain, such as the extra chewing often required with high-fiber foods. Another way is the greater feeling of satiety resulting from fiber intake. Consuming more fiber, more whole grains, and fewer calories, over time, can lead to weight loss or long-term weight maintenance, which is relevant to the growing levels of global obesity.

Dietary Recommendations and Consumer Communication

The mounting positive evidence about whole grains fueled initiatives by the U.S. government to improve the dietary status of whole grains. The 1995 Dietary Guidelines for Americans included recommendations for whole grain consumption. Healthy People 2010, from the U.S. Department of Health and Human Services, recommended increases in whole grain intake. In 2003, the World Health Organization report on Diet, Nutrition and Prevention of Chronic Diseases listed whole grain foods, together with fruit and vegetables, as the preferred source of dietary fiber, and evaluated whole grains as a probable protective factor against cardiovascular disease. In 2005, both the Dietary Guidelines for Americans and the revised Food Guide Pyramid called MyPyramid.gov specifically recommend whole grain consumption. Based on the substantial scientific evidence from numerous studies, the 2005 Dietary Guidelines for Americans concluded that consuming at least three 1-ounce servings of whole grain daily can reduce the risk of diabetes and coronary heart disease and can assist with weight maintenance.

While there is worldwide agreement that whole grains have positive health effects, there is not one uniformly agreed upon definition for what constitutes a whole grain. Having different descriptions for whole grain is confusing. Being able to increase whole grain consumption, in part, depends upon the ability of government agencies to create a standard for whole grain food. A determination of appropriate portion sizes also is needed. These actions will help expedite uniform labeling and promotion of whole grain foods.

Consistent whole grain messaging and labeling is crucial to increasing consumer consumption. In the United States, a health claim was approved in 1999 by the Food and Drug Administration (F.D.A.): "In a low-fat diet, whole grain foods like (name food) may reduce the risks of heart disease and some cancers." The increase in whole grain consumption following the institution of the claim demonstrated the impact of a consistent message. Despite the hesitancy on the part of some consumers, others are embracing whole grain foods.

Increased consumer interest and the availability of a health claim is reflected by the large number of new whole grain product introductions in the United States in 2005. Figure 1.2 shows that more than 650 new Universal Product Codes (U.P.C.s) were introduced for whole grain foods in the past year in the United States (A.C. Nielsen, 2005). A.C. Nielsen (2005) reports that sales of whole grain pastas and whole grain crackers have increased by 34% and 10%, respectively, compared to 2004. U.S. bread manufacturers have reformulated products to include more whole grain or whole wheat offerings. Sales of whole grain breads have increased by 18%, the equivalent of $1.1 billion U.S. dollars, compared to last year. Many national efforts include advertising, bold package graphics and descriptive copy.

Two European countries have accepted health claims on whole grain foods: the United Kingdom (2002) and Sweden (2003). Although these claims have slightly different wording, the U.S., U.K., and Swedish claims refer to the association between whole grain foods and heart disease. More whole grain labeling standards should follow and work toward consistency. Additional consumer communication is also necessary to educate consumers about the health benefits of whole grain foods, and a few national campaigns have already begun in Europe.

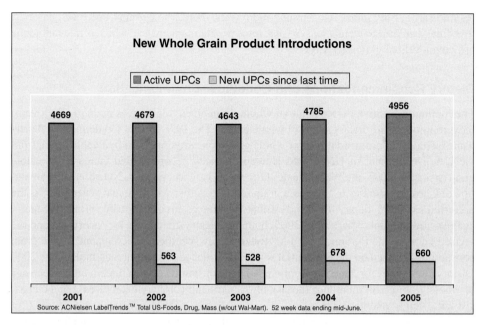

Figure 1.2.   New whole grain product introductions.

The European Union, however, is waiting for the common regulation on nutrition and health claims to be accepted. Currently each of the twenty-five member countries has their own regulations and claim acceptance procedures. A process for the assessment of scientific support for claims in foods, however, has been worked out in a consensus panel (Aggett et al. 2005).

Health claims contribute not only to consumer communication but indirectly to the availability of whole grain foods as well. The availability of a claim also encourages the food industry to develop whole grain foods, because the possibility to communicate the value added is foreseen. The U.S. example described above shows the importance of interactions of different stakeholders: government recommendations and education programs combined with a health claim and labels has led to increased consumer demand and new whole grain products.

Barriers to Adequate Consumption

Despite recommendations to consume at least three servings of whole grains daily, the average intake of whole grains in the United States is less than one serving daily, and it is estimated that less than 10% of the U.S. population consumes three servings per day (Cleveland et al. 2000). About 30% of U.K. adults did not consume whole grain foods during a one-week survey period and more than 97% did not meet the U.S. recommendation of three servings per day (Lang and Jebb 2003). Some researchers suggest that consumers often find it difficult to identify whole grain foods. People may also believe that they do not have the necessary skills to prepare and cook whole grain foods, while others think whole grain foods may not taste good (Lang and Jebb 2003). A recent study from the United Kingdom shows that the mean whole grain intake of young British people is 13 g/day, and 27% consumed no whole grain at all (Thane et al. 2005).

Why this gap exists may be answered by learning more about consumer perceptions, motivations, and barriers to whole grain consumption. Focus group studies indicate that consumers don't like the brown appearance, taste, texture, and potential differences in cost or convenience of whole grain foods. Research is needed to further clarify the barriers and to see if products can be developed to meet consumer expectations while delivering the important nutritional benefits of whole grains.

One possible reason for the lack of whole grain acceptance is the lack of exposure in the typical product categories consumed, particularly among the young. Recent studies (Chan et al. 2005) showed that pizza made with a 50/50 mixture of ConAgra Foods' Ultragrain™ white whole-wheat flour and refined wheat flour was accepted by elementary school children. No differences were noted in consumption or plate waste between the pizza made with the mixture and pizza made with only refined wheat flour. The idea that whole grain consumption can be increased among children is promising.

Increasing children's acceptance of whole grains through early introduction is just one strategy to increase whole grain intake. Research also is needed to determine how to communicate the health benefits of whole grains to consumers, such as which messages positively influence public interest, understanding, and purchase. Messages must be tested to ensure that they speak to a diverse audience of health professionals and consumers. Broad scale collaborative programs by academics, government, and community agencies are needed to pilot whole grain food usage and messaging in schools, restaurants, other food service environments, and retail markets.

Food service and restaurant channels are other ways to help increase whole grain consumption. Of the one serving of whole grain consumed per day, only 15% is eaten away from home and only 6% comes from whole grain foods consumed in restaurants (Kantor et al. 2001). That suggests an opportunity to work with restaurants, chefs, and the food service industry to help boost whole grain consumption.

Regular surveillance systems are needed in various countries to document whole grain intake among different population groups. Establishing a current benchmark will ease our ability to chart progress toward greater whole grain consumption in the future. Incorporating whole grain data into nutrient databases such as the University of Minnesota's Nutrition Data System/Nutrition Coordinating Center (www.ncc.umn.edu/) and the U.S.D.A. National Nutrient Database for Standard Reference (www.nal.USda.gov/fnic/foodcomp/search/) is important as well. Developing biomarkers such as alkyl resorcinol for specific grains and grain components is another way to assess grain intake. As a next step, the systems may need to link the intake of whole grain foods to long-term health outcomes such as obesity, diabetes, and C.V.D.

Technology and Innovation

To narrow the gap between whole grain recommendations and consumption, Marquart et al. (2005) suggest six potential ways to gradually introduce foods containing whole grains into diets of disbelieving consumers:

1. Use white whole wheat instead of red whole wheat to mask the brown appearance.
2. Make changes slowly. Gradually increase the amount of whole grain into bread recipes and other formulations. This will allow consumers to adapt to changes in palatability.
3. Use fine-particle-size flour to minimize texture changes.

4. Create more 100% whole grain food options.
5. Vary the grains—blend white wheat, red wheat, oats, barley, and other grains to improve flavor and whole grain goodness.
6. Develop novel products containing whole grains in foods other than grains (e.g. dairy, meats).

It has taken about one hundred years to develop the current grain refining and processing technologies, including the baking methodology, of white wheat flour. Now, if we invest a small portion of those efforts to develop technologies to use all or more of the grain, we can improve grain foods by combining nutritional and sensory assets. The whole grain chain—starting from trait selection and breeding, through grain handling, milling, and processing—can be fine-tuned to deliver more of the health potential of the grain. Scientifically, a key question lies in understanding the mechanisms by which the grains deliver health benefits. The majority of the evidence currently originates from epidemiological studies, where the estimates on type of grain food consumed are based on dietary questionnaires.

Several efforts to develop new tools for better uses of grain reflect great interest in the potential to improve cereal food quality. From 2005 through 2010, the European Union is undertaking an integrated project: "Exploiting Bioactivity of European Cereal Grains for Improved Nutrition and Health Benefits," or HEALTHGRAIN (www.healthgrain.org/pub/). This project aims to improve the well-being and reduce the prevalence of insulin resistance syndrome in the European population by increasing the intake of protective whole grain components. HEALTHGRAIN develops a technology and nutritional expertise base to identify health-relevant cereal food quality criteria and enable production of foods tailored to contain health-promoting grain constituents such as dietary fiber, oligosaccharides, and phytochemicals. HEALTHGRAIN has forty-three research and development partners, and forty additional companies already have joined the industrial platform to participate in the dissemination and communication program.

In Australia, the Grain Foods Cooperative Research Centre (www.grainfoodscrc.com.au/) has been established to act as a collaboration forum between academia, government, and industry, and to assist in developing healthy, consumer-friendly grain foods.

Overall Recommendations for the Future

A list of recommendations was developed for advancing whole grain research efforts and encouraging greater use and consumption during the May 2005 Whole Grains & Health: A Global Summit in Minneapolis. It was based on key learnings, continuing dialogue, and shared insights of the 400 attendees. The following list represents the recommendations for each of the three key areas of focus as developed by experts from various disciplines during the conference.

  I. **Recommendations for Biological Science and Health**
   - **Establish the long-term effects of increasing whole grain intake on the risk of developing chronic diseases, such as cardiovascular disease, diabetes, and cancer.**
     - Delineate the health effects attributed to whole grains from confounding lifestyle factors that correlate with whole grain intake.

- Conduct clinical trials to:
  - Measure the effect of whole grain intake on long-term health outcomes, including obesity, diabetes, cardiovascular disease, and cancer in a long-term, large-scale, multi-center study.
  - Determine whole grain intake of healthy and diseased people (with conditions such as diabetes and gastro-intestinal inflammation).
  - Understand the impact of grain foods on glycemic response.
- Create more sensitive and simplified in-vitro and animal models for assessing the health effects of whole grains.
- **Evaluate the parts/single components of whole grains to determine which improve health and work well in product development.**
  - Examine the bioactive components of whole grains and their bioavailability.
  - Elucidate the function of whole grain endosperm in overall health.
  - Explore endosperm modification to reduce caloric density without compromising product acceptability/health benefits to help with global obesity.
  - Examine specific extracts of whole grains and the feasibility of their use in foods other than grains, e.g. extracted barley β-glucan in beverages.
- **Develop biomarkers for specific grains and grain components to assess wheat and rye intake, e.g. alkyl resorcinol.**
- **Monitor the whole grain products on the market and intake by consumers. Attempt to link the intake of whole grain foods to positive long-term health outcomes such as obesity, diabetes, cardiovascular disease, and cancer.**

II. **Recommendations for Consumer Research and Education**
- **Develop international regulatory and policy standards for whole grains.**
  - Create one international definition for whole grains by committee involvement.
  - Build international whole grain food labeling standards and eliminate confusing terminology.
  - Explore fortification of whole grains with nutrients low or deficient in the population, e.g. folic acid, phytonutrients.
  - Educate the public about what constitutes whole grain foods and where to find them in the marketplace.
  - Create meaningful and easy-to-understand portion size descriptions.
- **Evaluate perceptions, motivations, and barriers to whole grain consumption; develop key messages that speak to health professionals and consumers.**
  - Assess consumer perceptions and unlock the barriers to consumption (availability, cost, taste perceptions, texture, convenience, and appearance).
  - Determine key messages that positively influence public interest, understanding, and purchase decisions surrounding whole grain foods.
  - Conduct a large-scale public/private marketing campaign/health promotion initiative to increase whole grain food consumption.
  - Pilot an approach for incorporating whole grains into schools, retail markets, and restaurant environments (e.g. use products made with different proportions of white, red, and whole wheat flour to assess usage, palatability).
  - Test new materials and programs to educate health professionals about whole grains and health and how to promote consumption.
- **Investigate and monitor marketplace changes.**

- Add whole grain information to nutrient databases such as the National Nutrient Database for Standard Reference.
- Monitor intake of whole grain foods to evaluate the effectiveness of consumer education and note market changes.

III. Recommendations for Grain Science and Technology

- **Identify, characterize, and determine bioavailability of bioactive components within whole grains.**
  - Improve analytical methods for measuring whole grain components and forms within food matrices.
  - Understand the effect of processing on bioavailability; explore the physical interactions and synergies between whole grain components in foods and apply that knowledge to processing and product development.
- **Upgrade grain technology to better determine the effects of grain structure on sensory properties and digestibility.**
  - Use new technologies that allow industry/science to tailor the levels and bioavailability of beneficial substances in whole grains to optimize sensory and nutritional properties.
  - Conduct commercial and academic seed hybrid development to achieve grain varieties that provide improved characteristics, e.g. lighter color, softer texture, and reduced bitterness.
  - Develop whole grain products that supply dietary fiber, a low glycemic response, and resistant starch.
  - Improve food processing and storage technology; optimize grains to improve processing and storage characteristics.
- **Create new market-friendly whole-grain foods.**
  - Broaden the range of whole grain options available to consumers. Explore nontraditional whole grain products, e.g. beverages, whole grain extracts for soups, and whole-grain powders for salads.
  - Use baking and other technologies that produce whole grain products with wide consumer acceptability and improved convenience.
  - Assess characteristics of whole wheat bread, e.g. taste and color, that impact preferences and acceptance by children and determine whether modified formulas increase their acceptance.
- **Investigate and monitor production of whole grain foods and bioactive components.**

Working Together

As the whole grain conversation continues, experts from each area of practice (Figure 1.3)—biological science and health, consumer research and education, and grain science and technology—must set priorities within their own areas and look to others to determine the path to achieving the recommendations coming from Whole Grains & Health: A Global Summit.

A volume of epidemiological data exists, yet there is little published clinical data on the effect of whole grain intake on long-term health outcomes, including obesity, diabetes, and cardiovascular disease. Furthermore, the epidemiological research has many confounders. Those in the upper quartiles or quintiles of whole grain intake also have other stellar health

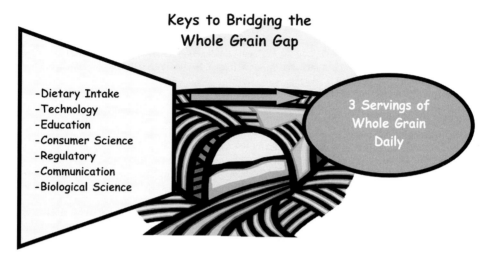

Keys to Bridging the Whole Grain Gap

-Dietary Intake
-Technology
-Education
-Consumer Science
-Regulatory
-Communication
-Biological Science

3 Servings of Whole Grain Daily

Figure 1.3. Experts from all areas must work together to increase the consumption of whole grains.

habits that lead to confounding. Whole grain eaters tend to eat less fat and red meat and eat more fruits and vegetables; they smoke less and exercise more. Thus, additional research is needed to specifically tease out the attributes of whole grains from the confounding lifestyle factors identified in existing studies.

Clinical research studies must be conducted to document the beneficial effects of whole grain foods. A pipeline of published studies helps keep whole grains on the minds of research scientists, government groups, industry leaders, educators, and consumers. Consumers want to rely on sound data rather than a generalized belief that whole grains are good for you. A whole grain food standard and consistent labeling and messaging are still needed for effective communication, marketing, and sales of whole grain products to consumers.

Whole grain product innovation must incorporate taste, texture, color, and other sensory properties that will allow a majority of refined-grain eaters to gradually adapt to more consistent whole grain consumption—close to three servings per day. We must evaluate grains, other than wheat, and oats for biologically active components to incorporate a greater variety of grains into the diet. It is also critical to look for ways to include grain components in foods that are not grain-based to determine their effects on risk factors and disease.

Collaboration among scientists, industry, government, educators, farmers, and organizations is also needed. Relevant organizations include the heart, cancer and diabetes associations and other health promotion agencies. A campaign for whole grains, similar to the successful 5 A Day for Better Health program (www.5aday.gov), which includes a "5 A Day" seal and promotion for fruits and vegetables in grocery stores and on restaurant menus, would help keep whole grains more visible to consumers. It also is important to include recommendations for whole grain intake in dietary guidelines on the international level.

When we speak with a common voice and mission to provide practical solutions, we will begin to narrow the whole-grain-intake gap. Together we can combine our strengths so that whole-grain consumption will meet and exceed the three servings per day that have been shown to be beneficial to human health.

References

A.C. Nielsen. 2005. A.C. Nielsen Label Trends. Reported in *Milling and Baking News*, Aug. 30.

Aggett, P.J.; Antoine, J.-M.; Asp, N.-G.; Bellisle, F.; Contor, L.; Cummings, J.; Howlett, J.; Muller, D.J.G.; Persin, C.; Pijls, L.T.J.; Rechkemmer, G.; Tuijtelaars, S.; and Verhagen, H. 2005. PASSCLAIM: consensus on criteria. *Eur. J. Nutr.* 44 (Suppl.1):15–30.

American Association of Cereal Chemists. 2000. Whole grain definition. A.A.C.C., International. *Cereal Foods World* 45(2):45–88.

Anderson, J.W.; Hanna, T.J.; Peng, X.; and Kryscio, R.J. 2000. Whole grain foods and heart disease risk. *J. Am. Coll. Nutr.* 19:291S–299S.

Brown, L.; Rosner, B.; Willett, W.W.; and Sacks, F.M. 1999. Cholesterol-lowering effects of dietary fiber: A meta-analysis. *Am. J. Clin. Nutr.* 69(1):30–42.

Chan, H.-W.; Burgess Champoux, T.; Rosen, R.; Sadeghi, L.; Reicks, M.; and Marquart, L. 2005. Incorporating white whole wheat flour into traditional grain foods in an elementary school cafeteria. Presented at Whole Grains & Health: A Global Summit, Minneapolis, Minn., May 18–20.

Cleveland, L.E.; Moshfegh, A.J.; Albertson, A.M.; and Goldman, J.D. 2000. Dietary intake of whole grains. *J. Am. Coll. Nutr.* 19:331S–338S.

Erkkilä, A.T.; Herrington, D.M.; Mozaffarian, D.; and Lichtenstein, A.H. 2005. Cereal fiber and whole-grain intake are associated with reduced progression of coronary-artery atherosclerosis in postmenopausal women with coronary artery disease. *Am. Heart J.* 150:94–101.

Esmaillzadeh, A.; Mirmiran, P.; and Azizi, F. 2005. Whole-grain consumption and the metabolic syndrome: a favorable association in Tehranian adults. 59:353–362.

Food and Drug Administration. 1999. Whole grain foods authoritative statement claim notification. Docket 99P–2209, Food and Drug Administration, Washington, D.C., July 8.

Food and Drug Administration. 2003. Food labeling: Health claims; soluble dietary fiber from certain foods and coronary heart disease. Final rule. Docket 2001Q–0313, Food and Drug Administration, Washington, D.C., July 28.

Food and Drug Administration. 2004. Citizen petition filed by General Mills, Inc. Food labeling standard for whole grain. Docket 2004P–0223, Food and Drug Administration, Washington, D.C., May 11.

Fulcher, R.G. and Rooney-Duke, T.K. 2002. Whole grain structure and organization: Implications for nutritionists and processors. Ch. 2 in *"Whole Grains in Health and Disease,"* ed. L. Marquart, J. Slavin, and G. Fulcher, pp. 9–46. American Association of Cereal Chemists, Intl., St. Paul, Minn.

Fung, T.T.; Hu, F.B.; Pereira, M.A.; Liu, S.; Stampfer, M.J.; Colditz, G.A.; and Willet, W.C. 2002. Whole-grain intake and the risk of type 2 diabetes: a prospective study in men. *Am. J. Clin. Nutr.* 76:535–540.

Jacobs, D.R.J; Meyer, K.A.; Kushi, L.H.; and Folsom, A.R. 1998. Whole grain intake may reduce the risk of ischemic heart disease death in postmenopausal women: The Iowa Women's Health Study. *Am. J. Clin. Nutr.* 68:248-257.

Jacobs, D.R.J; Meyer, K.A.; Kushi, L.H.; and Folsom, A.R. 1999. Is whole grain intake associated with reduced total and cause-specific death rates in older women? The Iowa Women's Health Study. *Am. J. Pub. Health.* 89:322–332.

Jensen, M.K.; Koh-Banerjee, P.; Hu, F.B.; Franz, M.; Sampson, L.; Gronbaek, M.; and Rimm, E.B. 2004. Intakes of whole grains, bran, and germ and the risk of coronary heart disease in men. *Am. J. Clin. Nutr.* 80:1492–1499.

Kantor, L.; Variyam, J.; Allshouse, J.; Putnam, J.; and Biing-Hwan, L. 2001. Choose a variety of grains daily, especially whole grains: A challenge for consumers. *J. Nutr.* 131:473S–486S.

Koh-Banerjee, P.; Franz, M.; Sampson, L.; Liu, S.; Jacobs, D.; Spiegelman, D.; Willett, W.C.; and Rimm, E.B. 2004. Changes in whole grain, bran, and cereal fiber consumption in relation to 8-year weight gain among men. *Am. J. Clin. Nutr.* 80(5):1237–1245.

Lang, K. and Jebb, S. 2003. Who consumes whole grains, and how much? *Proc. Nutr. Society* 62:123–27.

Liu, S.M.; Stampfer, M.J.; Hu, F.B.; Giovannucci, E.; Rimm, E.; Manson, J.E.; Hennekens, C.H.; and Willett, W.C. 1999. Whole grain consumption and risk of coronary heart disease: Results from the Nurses' Health Study. *Am. J. Clin. Nutr.* 70:412–419.

Liu, S.; Manson, J.A.; Stampfer, M.; Hu, F.; Giovannucci, E.; Colditz, G.; Hennekens, C.; and Willett, W. 2000. A prospective study of whole-grain intake and risk of type 2 diabetes mellitus in U.S. women. *Am. J. Public Health.* 90:1409–1415.

Liu, S.; Willett, W.C.; Manson, J.E.; Hu, F.B.; Rosner, B.; and Colditz, G.A. 2003. Relation between changes in intakes of dietary fiber and grain products and changes in weight and development of obesity among middle-aged women. *J. Am. Coll. Nutr.* 78:920–927.

Lorenzo, C.; Okoloise, M.; Williams, K.; Stern, M.P.; and Haffner, S.M. 2003. The metabolic syndrome as predictor of type 2 diabetes: The San Antonio Heart Study. *Diab. Care* 26:3153–3159.

Ludwig, D.S.; Pereira, M.A.; Kroenke, C.H.; Hilner, J.E.; Van Horn, L.; Slattery, M.L.; and Jacobs, D.R. 1999. Dietary fiber, weight gain, and cardiovascular disease risk factors in young adults. *J.A.M.A.* 282:1539–1546.

Marquart, L.; Chan, H-W.; and Jacobs, D.R. 2005. A theoretical model for incorporating whole grain flour into traditional grain foods. Presented at Whole Grains & Health: A Global Summit, Minneapolis, Minn., May 18–20.

McKeown, N.M.; Meigs, J.B.; Liu, S.; Saltzman, E.; Wilson, P.W.F.; and Jacques, P.F. 2004. Carbohydrate nutrition, insulin resistance, and the prevalence of the metabolic syndrome in the Framingham Offspring Cohort. *Diab. Care.* 27:538–546.

Montonen, J.; Knekt, P.; Jarvinen, R.; Aromaa, A.; and Reunanen, A. 2003. Whole-grain and fiber intake and the incidence of type 2 diabetes, *Am. J. Clin. Nutr.* 77:622–629

Rimm, E.B.; Ascherio, A.; Giovannucci, E.; Spiegelman, D.; Stampfer, M.J.; and Willett, W.C. 1996. Vegetable, fruit, and cereal fiber intake and risk of coronary heart disease among men. *J.A.M.A.* 275:447–451.

Salmeron, J.; Ascherio, A.; Rimm, E.B.; Colditz, G.A.; Spiegelman, D.; Jenkins, D.J.; Stampfer, M.J.; Wing, A.L.; and Willett, W.C. 1997a. Dietary fiber, glycemic load, and risk of NIDDM in men. *Diab. Care* 20:545–550.

Salmeron, J.; Manson, J.E.; Stampfer, M.J.; Colditz, G.A.; Wing, A.L.; and Willett, W.C. 1997b. Dietary fiber, glycemic load, and risk of non-insulin-dependent diabetes mellitus in women. *J.A.M.A.* 277:472–477.

Steffen, L.M.; Jacobs, D.R.J; and Stevens, J. 2003. Associations of whole grain, refined-grain, and fruit and vegetable consumption with risks of all-cause mortality and incident coronary artery disease and ischemic stroke: the Atherosclerosis Risk in Communities (A.R.I.C.) Study. *Am. J. Clin. Nutr.* 78:383–390.

Thane, C.W.; Jones, A.R.; Stephen A.M.; Ceal, C.J.; and Jubb, S.A. 2005. Whole-grain intake of British young adults aged 14–18 years. *Brit. J. Nutr.* 94:825–831.

Third Report of the National Cholesterol Education Program (NCEP) Expert Panel on Detection, Evaluation, and Treatment of High Blood Cholesterol in Adults (Adult Treatment Panel III) final report. 2002. Circulation. 106(25):3143–3421. December 17.

U.S. Department of Agriculture/U.S. Department of Health and Human Services. 2005a. Nutrition and Your Health: Dietary Guidelines for Americans. What Are the Relationships between Whole Grain Intake and Health? U.S. Dept. of Agriculture and U.S. Dept. of Health and Human Services, Washington, D.C. www.health.gov/dietaryguidelines/dga2005/report/html/d6_selectedfood.htm. Accessed on 9/16/05.

U.S. Department of Agriculture/U.S. Department of Health and Human Services. 2005b. Mypyramid.gov. U.S. Dept. of Health and Human Services, Washington, D.C. www.mypyramid.gov/pyramid/grains_why.html. Accessed on 9/30/05.U.S. Department of Health and Human Services. 2000. Healthy People 2010: Volumes I and II. Public Health Service. Office of Disease Prevention and Health Promotion, U.S. Dept. of Health and Human Services, Washington, D.C.

Whole Grains Council. 2004. Definition of whole grain. Whole Grains Council, Boston, Mass. www.wholegrainscouncil.org/consumerdef.html. Accessed on 10/15/05.

Whole Grains Council. 2005. Whole grain stamp. Whole Grains Council, Boston, Mass. www.wholegrainscouncil.org/wholegrainstamp.html. Accessed on 11/2/05.

2 Using a Model of the Food and Nutrition System for Examining Whole Grain Foods from Agriculture to Health

Jeffery Sobal

Each whole grain, like all other human foods and beverages, takes complex paths between initial production and final use (Wrigley et al. 2004). This chapter presents a conceptual model of the food and nutrition system, and describes how "systems thinking" can be used to consider whole grains as they move from agriculture to health and beyond. Food and nutrition systems thinking offers a way of linking a wide variety of disciplines, fields, professions, and occupations involved in whole grains.

A food and nutrition system can be defined as the "set of operations and processes involved in transforming raw materials into foods, and transforming nutrients into health outcomes, all functioning as an integrated system within biophysical and sociocultural contexts" (Sobal et al. 1998). Food and nutrition system thinking takes a broad perspective that shows linkages, interdependencies, and dynamics both within the system and between the system and its contexts (Sobal 1999, 2004; Sobal et al. 1998).

The concept of a "food system" is widely used in agriculture, food processing, food distribution, and consumer studies (Jones and Street 1990, Rizzo 1975, Spedding 1990), but less often in nutrition and medicine. Food systems are discussed in many fields and professions as holistic ways of tracing transformations of particular foods (Sobal et al. 1998). The concept of a food and nutrition system offers an even broader scope than considering only the food system alone; it offers a more comprehensive examination of the links between agriculture, health, environment, and society (Heywood and Lund-Adams 1991, Sobal et al. 1998).

A Model of the Food and Nutrition System

Systems theory suggests that entities such as foods and nutrients are parts of holistic, contextual, dynamic relationships (Bertalanffy 1968, Boulding 1985, Midgley 2003, Miller 1978). Systems are sets of interdependent elements that are greater than the sum of their parts, and have patterns and processes that emerge as the system is identified and examined. Systems thinking emphasizes a process perspective, considering relationships of parts treated in the context of the whole. Systems often include subsystems, which are components of the larger system.

Boundaries separate a system from its environments. Systems with permeable boundaries are termed "open systems" and those with less permeable boundaries are termed "closed systems." Systems are embedded within larger contexts that include other systems. These concepts in systems thinking reveal intermediate processes linking agriculture and health.

Materials, information, and energy flow through systems and in open systems are exchanged between the system and its environment. Multiple pathways exist in complex systems, with different initial conditions leading to similar effects, and similar initial conditions also leading to different outcomes. Food chain models focus on the movement of these elements through the system, such as following whole grains from food industries to the household and into the body.

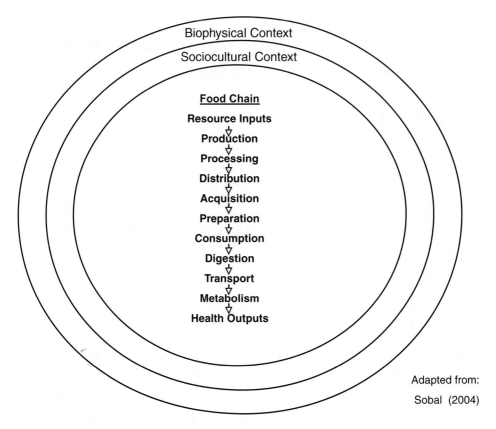

Figure 2.1.   A model of a food chain.

Communication as feedback and feedforward occur between parts of a system in interdependent processes among a system's elements. Complex systems seek and maintain homeostasis and equilibrium. Food web models focus on the reciprocal, cybernetic feedback between diverse and interrelated parts of a system.

These systems theory concepts were used to develop an integrated model of the food and nutrition system (Sobal et al. 1998). A diagram representing the food and nutrition chain in this model is presented in Figure 2.1. This model describes how foods and beverages move through a food chain that includes series of nine stages in three subsystems, all operating within two major types of system context. The model can operate as a map of the system that can be used for many purposes. This chapter uses the model to consider the ways whole grains progress through the system, first focusing on the subsystems and stages delineated in this model and then discussing food webs and food contexts.

Resource Inputs

Whole grains require a variety of resource inputs. The key biological input is the germplasm in seeds that is necessary for growing each particular whole grain cultivar and variety. Considerable plant breeding work has gone into and continues to be invested in particular grain crops (Wrigley et al. 2004). Other resource inputs are physical (land, water, chemicals, etc.) and sociocultural (economic capital, human capital, policies, etc.), which are similar for whole grains and refined grains.

Producer Subsystem

Food producers transform raw materials into foodstuffs for sale to consumers and provide foods for self-consumption. The producer subsystem of the larger food and nutrition system involves three ordered and interlinked stages that involve input, throughput, and output: production, processing, and distribution.

Production

Production converts resources into crops and commodities. Agronomy involves tilling, sowing, crop nutrition, pest and weed management, irrigation, and harvesting of whole grains as field crops using the raw materials described in the previous section. The majority of the whole grain crops in Western societies is currently propagated using industrialized agricultural techniques on large corporate farms, although small-scale production also occurs. In general, grains are staple crops for most societies; wheat, rice, and maize (corn) are the three top world crops. However, most of this production uses crop varieties and procedures for producing refined grain products rather than whole grain products, although commercial whole grain production is increasing.

Processing

Processing transforms harvested crops into foodstuffs and foods (Sobal 1999). Crude processing involves preliminary cleaning, drying, grading and sorting/separating, while further refined processing typically involves manufacturing into final products ready for consumers and transport to wholesale and retail outlets (Wrigley et al. 2004). While the hallmark of whole grains is that they are subject to less processing than refined grains, they generally are not consumed without some processing to make them more durable and stable and to enhance their sensory appeal to consumers (Slavin et al. 2000).

Processing whole grains may involve wet or dry milling, fractionation, mixing, baking, extrusion, and/or brewing, with specific processing techniques for the characteristics of each particular whole grain product (Slavin et al. 2000, Wrigley et al. 2004). Processing is a crucial stage in the food and nutrition system, where treatment of crops establishes different pathways into whole grain and refined grain foods channels downstream in the system.

Distribution

Ingredients, foodstuffs, and foods are channeled to wholesale and retail sites that make food products available to consumers, creating an evolving "foodscape" of potential sources for whole grains (Guptill and Wilkins 2002). Many types of food distribution "nodes" exist as transfer points in the system, and the majority can be classified as grocery or foodservice outlets. Retail groceries are a major distribution point for whole grain products, especially specialty distributors such as health food stores, consumer food cooperatives, and supermarkets that stock whole grain foods. Whole grain products are less prevalent in discount and warehouse food stores. Supermarket sales of whole grain products are lower than for refined grain products, but are increasing (Kantor et al. 2001). Foodservice is an important and growing portion of the food distribution stage, although whole grain products are not prevalent in most family restaurants, fast food outlets, or catering, vending, delivery, and take-out foodservice operations (Reicks 2001). Specialty and alternative grocery and foodservice nodes may offer whole grain foods in their product mix and on their menus, but often whole grain foods have limited availability in mainstream food distribution sources.

Consumer Subsystem

Food consumers obtain and transform foodstuffs and foods into meals and snacks that they consume themselves and serve to others. The consumer subsystem of the larger food and nutrition system includes three sequential and coupled stages that accomplish input, throughput, and output: acquisition, preparation, and consumption.

Acquisition

Acquisition occurs as individuals and households procure foodstuffs and foods. It is a transfer point between food producers and food consumers, and food choice at the point of acquisition is a complex and multifaceted process (Furst et al. 1996). Consumer tradeoffs in food choice typically favor taste and convenience over health (Connors et al. 2001), which commonly leads to the purchase of refined grain products instead of whole grain products. Acquisition of whole grain products is constrained among many consumers by higher prices of whole grain foods (Drenowski and Darmon 2005, Kantor et al. 2001), lack of awareness of whole grain foods (Adams et al. 2002), reluctance to try new or different whole grain foods due to food neophobia (Pliner and Hobden 1992), and taste preferences for refined rather than whole grains (Reicks 2001).

Preparation

Preparation involves diverse activities broadly labeled as "cooking" that transform raw foodstuffs into consumable foods by making physical, chemical, and water content changes, including various forms of heating and cooling, and combining various ingredients. Cooking increases the digestibility of many foods, and makes some nutrients more or less available for digestion. Whole grain foods may require more cooking time than refined grain foods, creating greater "time cost" and less convenience for food preparers. Preparation transforms foodstuffs into foods in accordance with the rules of a particular cuisine that include specific ingredients, flavorings, cooking procedures, and forms of serving that are appropriate to a certain food culture (Rozin 1983). Whole grain foods may or may not be included in or substitutable into some specific cuisines.

Consumption

Consumption is the selection and eating of foods, which occurs as meals and snacks in accordance with individual preferences and cultural norms. Consumption is performed in eating episodes, in which bites and swallows of foods are ingested. Breads, cereals, and pastas/

noodles are the major forms in which whole grains are consumed in most Western societies (Smith et al. 2003), but the intake of whole grain foods is low, averaging less than one serving per person per day in the U.S. (Adams and Engstrom 2000, Kantor et al. 2001). Food consumption links the consumer and nutrition subsystems, and is a crucial transfer point of foods such as whole grains that have important health consequences.

Nutrition Subsystem

Human bodies transform foods into nutrients that are used in a variety of physiological functions. The nutrition subsystem of the larger food and nutrition includes three progressive stages that function in input, throughput, and output: digestion, transport, and use.

Digestion

Digestion is the breakdown of foods and absorption of nutrients into the body. Digestion begins with mastication and salivary action. The unrefined components of whole grains need more chewing than refined grains, so they require additional time and effort to consume whole grain foods by both healthy individuals and those with chewing limitations. Whole grains also have other dental considerations, including unrefined components lodging between teeth and gums. Digestion proceeds with swallowing and movement through the gastrointestinal track. Whole grain foods produce greater sensations of satiety and fullness once they are ingested, compared with refined grains which have less bulk and fiber. Whole grains and the foods they are eaten with pass more rapidly through the intestines because of the bulky fiber. Whole grain foods produce considerably greater volumes of feces because of this indigestible fiber from bran and other unrefined portions of the grain.

Transport

Transport of nutrients throughout the body occurs after absorption in the intestines. Nutrients are differentiated according to the amounts required by the body, and commonly designated as macronutrients (carbohydrates, proteins, fats, alcohol), micronutrients (vitamins, minerals, etc.), and other substances (fiber, water, etc.). Some nutrients are converted into other forms for transportation and storage. Whole grains typically have a greater variety of essential nutrients than refined grains because of nutrient losses in milling and other refining processes. Once nutrients reach the appropriate anatomical sites, they are stored or used.

Use

Nutrient use occurs in a huge variety of biological processes in sites throughout the body, including energy metabolism, tissue growth and repair, and other essential physiological activities. Several types of nutrients that are not refined out of whole grain foods serve important physiological functions in the body, including prevention of a variety of diseases (Marquart et al. 2002). Among those nutrients are carbohydrates, fiber, vitamins, minerals, antioxidants, and phytochemicals. Refining grains may remove essential nutrients and lead to deficiency diseases, such as thiamin deficiencies that cause Beriberi among consumers of high volumes of refined white rice (Carpenter 2000).

Outputs

Several outputs occur for foods in the food and nutrition system, including whole grains. Two major outputs are health and waste.

Health

Health is proper functioning of the body and mind, which is more than just the absence of diseases. Whole grains contribute to well-being in many forms, including the prevention and treatment of diseases (Marquart et al. 2002 Gordon and Wrigley 2004). In contemporary post-industrial Western societies, chronic diseases are the major causes of morbidity and mortality. Whole grains reduce the risk of many of the most prevalent chronic diseases, including heart disease, type 2 diabetes, some cancers, and obesity, plus all-cause mortality (Marquart et al 2002). Fortification reduces some micronutrient deficiencies for some refined grain foods (Rosell 2004).

Waste

Whole grains contain considerably more undigestible fiber than processed grains. As a result, they have a faster transit time through the digestive system and also produce stools that are larger in volume and weight. Stool weights vary from 72 to 470 grams per person per day (Cummings 1993), and higher whole grain consumption increases stool weights. Stools comprise the major component of sanitary waste disposal systems, and population level increases in whole grain consumption have important implications for sewage treatment system capacities. It is important to consider human waste in the full pathway of whole grains from field to feces.

Food Webs

Food webs are networks of nodes in the food and nutrition system, and are comprised of interrelationships between diverse individuals and organizations that shape and control the system (Sobal 2004, Sobal et al. 1998). A diagram of a food and nutrition system web is presented in Figure 2.2. The whole grain food web encompasses many roles and relationships, including suppliers, producers, millers, manufacturers, bakers, wholesalers, buyers, restaurateurs, grocers, shoppers, cooks, consumers, health professionals, waste treatment professionals, and many others.

People in various roles in the food and nutrition web tend to trace substances differently through food and nutrition chains. For example, workers in the producer subsystem tend to trace commodity chains downstream in the system, from farm to table. In contrast, workers in the nutrition subsystem tend to trace health recommendations upstream, from diseases to eating. Looking at the whole grain food and nutrition system from opposite ends can lead to conflicts rather than cooperation, unless both groups realize their interconnectedness in the full food and nutrition system.

Food web thinking can permit individuals to locate themselves in the larger flow of whole grain foods through the system, and to situate themselves with respect to others in the web who have important information and materials to exchange.

As the food and nutrition system grew and globalized (Sobal 1999), its size and scope became so large that various sectors and stages became increasingly specialized and distant

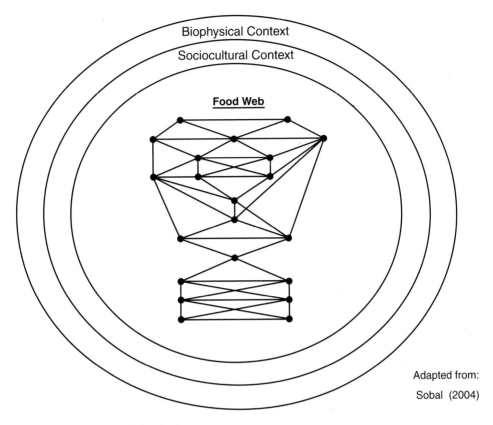

Figure 2.2. A model of a food web.

from other actors in the web. This can be seen in the different focal points of individuals in each subsystem in the food web. Producers focus on the profits and costs involved in whole grains as commodities. Consumers focus on the taste and convenience of whole grains as foods. Nutritionists focus on the health and diseases of whole grains as sources of nutrients. The value of food webs is to show how all of these interests are inextricably woven together and dependent upon the actions of individuals located far from them in the food and nutrition system. Physicians are linked with farmers, dietitians with millers, and shoppers with seed suppliers.

Contexts

Food and nutrition system contexts are the environments within which food systems operate. The food and nutrition system is an open system, with permeable boundaries that permit exchange of materials, energy, and information with its environment. Two major types of contexts exist: biophysical and sociocultural (Sobal et al. 1998).

Biophysical contexts of food and nutrition systems include geology, climate, ecosystems, and other features of the world (Sobal et al. 1998). Biophysical systems, such as the hydrological, meteorological, evolutionary, and others interact with food and nutrition systems to provide inputs and receive outputs. Biophysical systems may limit food and nutrition systems, such as when soil and climate influence which grains and particular cultivars can be grown in a particular place.

Sociocultural contexts of food and nutrition systems include cultural, economic, political, demographic, and other aspects of the social world that provide important inputs and receive outputs (Sobal et al. 1998). Sociocultural systems may control food and nutrition systems, such as when food cultures emphasize refined grains rather than whole grains or governmental bodies develop regulations about whole grain health claims (Gordon and Wrigley 2004).

Conclusions

Conceptualizing whole grains as part of a food and nutrition system offers a holistic and dynamic perspective that is not apparent in thinking that focuses on only a narrow piece of the system. Food and nutrition systems thinking extends far beyond commodity chain analyses (Raikes et al. 2000; Talbot 2002), examining the entire product life cycle rather than just the commercial segment of the pathway. Whole grains are more than products, being embedded in processes that have impacts both upstream and downstream, as well as far from any particular point in the food and nutrition system. Similarly, food webs reveal important activities far beyond the farming, milling, sales, shopping, cooking, eating, and diseases that have often been the focus of whole grain discussions.

Systems exhibit adaptation and homeostasis, changing in response to internal shifts and environmental influences. Whole system thinking about whole grains identifies areas for potential change, both intended and unintended. Whole system perspectives also offer insights about identifying potential effects of changes in the system, perhaps stimulating identification of consequences of changes that would be otherwise unanticipated.

Food and nutrition system thinking offers insights about whole grains as they move from agriculture to health. A holistic systems perspective seeks to be extensive and inclusive, not limited and reductionist. Systems thinking attempts to integrate disparate participants in food webs, and to trace causes and effects as far as possible in the system. A food and nutrition system model was applied here as a food analysis (whole grains), as it has been applied in the examination of a specific health condition such as obesity (Sobal 2001) and the characterization of food and nutrition systems in a particular place (Sobal and Lee 2003).

This food and nutrition system model articulates linkages between diverse parts of the system, both those that are tightly bound such as food processors and grocers, and those that are more remotely connected such as farmers and physicians. Identifying such ties can contribute to integration and understanding that overcomes disciplinary divisions between diverse parts of the food and nutrition system in a chain of activities and web of relationships between all people involved with whole grain foods.

References

Adams, J.F. and Engstrom, A. 2000. Helping consumers achieve recommended intakes of whole grain foods. *Journal of the American College of Nutrition* 19(3):339S–344S.

Adams, J.F.; Griffiths, P.; and Reicks, M. 2002. The consumer and whole grain foods. In: Marquart, L.; Slavin, J.L.; and Fulcher, F.G. (eds). *Whole grain foods in health and disease*. St. Paul, Minn.: American Association of Cereal Chemists. pp 341–358.

Bertalanffy, L. 1968. *General systems theory: Foundations, development, applications*. New York: George Braziller.

Boulding, K.E. 1985. *The world as a total system*. Beverly Hills, Calif.: Sage.

Carpenter, K.J. 2000. *Beriberi, white rice, and Vitamin B*. Berkeley, Calif: University of California Press.

Connors, M.M.; Bisogni, C.A.; Sobal, J.; Devine, C. 2001. Managing values in personal food systems. *Appetite* 36:189–200.

Cummings, J.H. 1993. The effect of dietary fiber on fecal weight and composition. In: Spiller, G.A. (ed). *CRC Handbook of dietary fiber in human nutrition*. Boca Raton, Fla.: CRC Press. pp 263–333.

Drenowski, A. and Darmon, N. 2005. Food choices and diet costs: An economic analysis. *Journal of Nutrition* 135(4).900–904.

Furst, T.; Connors; M., Bisogni, C.A.; Sobal, J.; and Winter Falk, L. 1996. Food choice: A conceptual model of the process. *Appetite* 26(3):247–65.

Gordon, D.T. and Wrigley, C. 2004. Whole grain versus refined products. In: Wrigley, C.; Corke, H.; and Walker, C.E. (eds). *Encyclopedia of grain science*. New York: Elsevier. pp 424–429.

Guptill, A. and Wilkins, J.L. 2002. Buying into the food system: Trends in food retailing in the U.S. and implications for local foods. *Agriculture and Human Values* 19:39–51.

Heywood, P. and Lund-Adams, M. 1991. The Australian food and nutrition system: A basis for policy formation and analysis. *Australian Journal of Public Health* 15:258–270.

Jones, J.G.W. and Street, P.R. (eds). 1990. *Systems theory applied to agriculture and the food chain*. New York: Elsevier.

Kantor, L.S.; Variyam, J.N.; Allshouse, J.E.; Putnam, J.J.; and Lin, B. 2001. Choose a variety of grains daily, especially whole grains: A challenge for consumers. *Journal of Nutrition* 131:473S–486S.

Marquart, L.; Slavin, J.L.; and Fulcher, F.G. (eds). 2002. *Whole grain foods in health and disease*. St. Paul, Minn.: American Association of Cereal Chemists.

Midgley, G. (ed). 2003. *Systems thinking. Volumes 1–4*. Thousand Oaks, Calif.: Sage.

Miller, J.G. 1978. *Living systems*. New York: McGraw-Hill.

Pliner, P. and Hobden, K. 1992. Development of a scale to measure the trait of food neophobia in humans. *Appetite* 19:105–120.

Raikes, P.; Jensen, M.F.; and Ponte, S. 2000. Global commodity chain analysis and the French filiere approach: Comparison and critique. *Economy and Society* 29(3):390–417.

Reicks, M. 2001. Using behavior theories to increase whole grain intake. *Dietitian's Edge* Jan/Feb:49–52.

Rizzo, N. 1975. General systems theory: Its impact in the health fields. In: Werley, H.; Zurich, A.; Zajkowski, M.; and Zagornik, A. (eds). *Health Research: The systems approach*. New York: Springer Publishing. pp 15–24.

Rosell, C.M. 2004. Fortification of grain based foods. In: Wrigley, C.; Corke, H.; and Walker, C.E. (eds). *Encyclopedia of grain science*. New York: Elsevier. pp 399–405.

Rozin, E. 1983. *Ethnic cuisine: The flavor-principal cookbook*. Brattleboro, Vt.: Stephen Greene Press.

Slavin, J.L.; Jacobs, D.; and Marquart, L. 2000. Grain processing and nutrition. *Critical Reviews in Food Science and Nutrition* 40(4):309–326.

Smith, A.T.; Kuznesof, S.; Richardson, D.P.; and Seal, C.J. 2003. Behavioral, attitudinal, and dietary responses to the consumption of wholegrain food. *Proceedings of the Nutrition Society* 62:455–467.

Sobal, J. 1999. Food System Globalization, Eating Transformations, and Nutrition Transitions. In: Grew, R. (ed). *Food in Global History*. Boulder, Colo.: Westview Press. pp 171–193.

Sobal, J. 2001. Social and Cultural Influences on Obesity. In: Bjorntorp, P. (ed). *International Textbook of Obesity*. London: John Wiley and Sons. pp 305–322.

Sobal, J. 2004. Food and nutrition systems. In: Smith, A. (ed). *The Oxford encyclopedia of food and drink in America*. New York: Oxford University Press. pp 495–498.

Sobal, J.; Khan, L.K.; and Bisogni, C.A. 1998. A conceptual model of the food and nutrition system. *Social Science and Medicine* 47(7):853–63.

Sobal, J. and Lee, S. 2003. A food and nutrition system analysis of South Korea. *Journal of Community Nutrition* 5(4):209–217.

Spedding, C.R.W. 1990. *Systems theory applied to agriculture and the food chain*. New York: Elsevier.

Talbot, J.M. 2002. Tropical commodity chains, forward integration strategies and international inequality: Coffee, cocoa and tea. *Review of International Political Economy* 9(4):701–734.

Wrigley, C.; Corke, H.; and Walker, C.E. (eds). *Encyclopedia of grain science. Volumes 1–3*. New York: Elsevier. 2004.

Part II

Whole Grains, Dietary Fiber, and Chronic Disease

3 Whole Grains and Diabetes

James W. Anderson and Shannon B. Conley

Introduction

Early into the twenty-first century, the diabetes mellitus epidemic is rapidly spreading indiscriminately across age, gender, racial/ethnic, and geographic lines. In terms of health impairment, the impact of type 2 diabetes relates to the fact that, besides being a serious disease in itself, it is a risk for many other diseases, including heart disease, stroke, peripheral vascular disease, hypertension, kidney disease, dyslipidemia, blindness, nerve damage, gastrointestinal problems, and depression. Some of the risk factors for type 2 diabetes are nonmodifiable; these include family history, age, and ethnicity (Murtaugh 2003). However, many factors are modifiable, including obesity (Anderson 2003), central adiposity (Meyer 2000), food choices, and a sedentary lifestyle (Fung 2002).

Parallel increases in diabetes and obesity have appeared worldwide, requiring lifestyle changes for prevention and treatment. Whole grains have a wide range of health-promoting effects, including life extension (Murtaugh 2003). Many of the health benefits of whole grains have been attributed to their rich dietary fiber content (Anderson 2003). However, dietary fiber is only one of many beneficial components of the whole grain package. Whole grains are filled with numerous phytochemicals that have powerful antioxidant properties, as well as essential vitamins and important minerals. Dietary fiber and whole grain consumption have protective and therapeutic effects with respect to diabetes and its co-morbidities, namely metabolic syndrome, obesity, hypertension, dyslipidemia, and atherosclerotic cardiovascular disease (Meyer 2000).

In this chapter, the whole grain story related to diabetes will be systematically reviewed in the following categories: protection from diabetes, treatment of diabetes, protection from other associated diseases, the association between favorable lifestyle practices and whole grain intake, and proposed mechanisms by which whole grains and their specific components affect risk for diabetes and insulin resistance. The highest consumption level of whole grains is associated with a 26% reduction in the risk for development of type 2 diabetes mellitus, while the highest ingestion level of cereal fiber is associated with a 30% reduction in this risk compared to lowest intake. Although there is persuasive epidemiological evidence indicating that whole grain intake has a protective relationship to diabetes, the role of a health-promoting lifestyle for people who consume large amounts of whole grains cannot be excluded (Murtaugh 2003). Proposed mechanisms for these protective effects relate to the fiber or magnesium content of the grain or to associated lifestyle patterns. We will review the data related to incidence of diabetes and whole grain consumption as well as dietary fiber intake from different foods. The implications of lifestyle patterns (physical activity, alcohol use, etc.) will be reviewed as they relate to prevention and management of diabetes.

Whole Grains and Risk for Type 2 Diabetes

Lifestyle modification, particularly nutrition changes, has been at the forefront of type 2 diabetes prevention, protection, and treatment. Weight loss is the most important modifiable risk factor for diabetes (Anderson 2003). However, other dietary measures and their protective contributions are not as widely recognized. In the last five years, five large prospective cohort studies have examined the relationship between whole grain consumption and the risk of type 2 diabetes. These studies consistently indicate an inverse association between whole grain intake and type 2 diabetes. The average relative risk for developing diabetes among individuals consuming the highest level of whole grain was 0.74, indicating a 26% lower risk than for individuals with the lowest level of whole grain intake.

Meyer and colleagues (2000), reporting the Iowa Women's Health Study, were the first to document the specific inverse relationship between whole grain intake and the risk of type 2 diabetes (Table 3.1). This was a prospective cohort study of almost 36,000 women that examined the relationship between the incidence of diabetes over six years and baseline dietary variables. Subjects were mailed a detailed questionnaire, including a 127-item food-frequency questionnaire, at baseline. The incidence of diabetes (1,141 cases) was determined by responses to mailed questionnaires at follow-up surveys. After appropriate adjustments for covariates, the relative risk for diabetes was 0.79 (P = 0.0089 for trend) in the highest quintile for whole grain intake compared to the lowest quintile. Thus, women who consumed an average of 21 servings of whole grains weekly were 21% less likely to develop diabetes than women who consumed only one serving weekly.

In the Health Professionals Follow-up Study, Fung and associates (2002) found a slightly greater reduction in the risk for diabetes for almost 52,000 men who were followed for twelve years. In this prospective cohort study, detailed questionnaires, including a food-frequency questionnaire, were mailed at baseline and follow-up questionnaires were mailed biannually. The development of diabetes (1,197 cases) was identified by mailed questionnaires. After appropriate adjustment for covariates, the relative risk for diabetes was 0.70 (P = 0.0006). Thus, men who consumed an average of 22 servings of whole grains weekly were 30% less likely to develop diabetes than men who consumed only 2.8 servings per week.

In the Nurses' Health Study, Liu and associates (2000) provided further evidence for an inverse relationship between whole grain intake and risk of type 2 diabetes. This prospective cohort study of almost 76,000 women used baseline and follow-up mailed general health and food-frequency questionnaires. The diagnosis of diabetes (1,879 cases) was made by specific follow-up questionnaires. When the highest and lowest quintiles of intake were compared, after adjustment for appropriate covariates, the relative risk for diabetes was 0.73 (P = <.0001). Thus, female nurses who consume approximately twenty-one servings of whole grains per week had a 27% lower risk for diabetes than nurses who consumed less than one serving per week.

The Finnish Mobile Clinic Health Examination Survey reported by Montonen and colleagues (2003) was a prospective cohort of 2,286 men and 2,030 women who completed self-administered detailed questionnaires and had a dietary history interview with a nutrition professional as part of a health examination. During the ten-year follow-up, 156 cases of diabetes were identified from a nationwide register. After adjustment for appropriate covariates, a significant inverse relationship between whole grain intake and risk of type 2 diabetes was reported. Relative risk in the highest quartile of whole grain consumption was 0.65 compared with those in the lowest quartile (P = 0.02). The Finnish people, in general, have much higher intakes of whole grains than reported for U.S. residents, but the Finns, who average approximately ten servings (302 grams) per day, have a 35% lower risk for diabetes than those with less than three servings (79 grams) per day.

The Melbourne Collaborative Cohort Study was a prospective cohort study of almost 37,000 men and women reported by Hodge and colleagues (2004). Baseline data included

Table 3.1. Whole grain or cereal fiber consumption and relative risk (R.R.) and 95%.

Study[1]	No.	Sex[2]	Years	Adjustments[5]	Whole Grains			Cereal Fiber			Reference
					RR	LCI	UCI	RR	LCI	UCI	
HPFS	42,759	M	6	a,b,h,p,s,y				0.7	0.51	0.96	(Salmeron 1997)
NHS	65,173	F	6	a,b,h,p,s,y				0.72	0.58	0.9	(Salmeron 1997)
IWHS	35,988	F	6	a,b,e,k,p,s,y	0.79	0.65	0.96	0.64	0.53	0.79	(Meyer 2000)
				a,b,e,k,p,s,y							
HPFS	51,529	M	12	a,b,h,k,p,s,y	0.7	0.57	0.85				(Fung 2002)
NHS	87,899	F	12	a,b,h,k,p,s,y	0.73	0.63	0.85				(Fung 2002)
ARIC	8,947	M & F[3]	9	b,g,p,s,y				na			(Stevens 2002)
	3,288	M & F[4]		b,g,p,s,y				0.75	0.6	0.92	
								0.86	0.65	1.15	
FMCHES	4,316	M & F	10	b,f,g,k,s,v,y	0.65	0.36	1.18	0.39	0.2	0.77	(Montonen 2003)
MCCS	36,787	M & F	4	a,e,f,k,p,s,y	0.86	0.63	1.18	1.05	0.73	1.52	(Hodge 2004)
NHSII	91,249	F	8	a,b,h,p,s,y				0.63	0.47	0.85	(Schulze 2004)

Confidence Intervals (Lower, LCI; Upper, UCI) for diabetes.
Abbreviations: [1], HPFS, Health Professionals Follow-up Study; NHS, Nurses' Health Study; IWHS, Iowa Women's Health Study; ARIC, Atherosclerosis Risk Intervention Community Study; FMCHES, Finnish Mobile Clinic Health Examination Survey; MCCS, Melbourne Collaborative Cohort Study; NHSII, Nurses' Health Study II. [2], M, male; [3], F, female; [4], white subjects; [5], African-American subjects. a, alcohol intake; b, BMI; e, ethnicity/race; g, gender; h, family history of diabetes; k, kcal (energy intake); p, physical activity; s, smoking; y, years of age.

Table 3.2.   Relative risk (RR) for diabetes associated with consumption of different foods and nutrients.

Parameter	No. of studies	No. of subjects	RR	LCI	UCI
Whole grains	5.0	216,519	0.74	0.68	0.81
Cereal fiber	8.0	288,507	0.69	0.63	0.74
Whole grains and cereal fiber	13.0	427,935	0.71	0.67	0.75
Total dietary fiber	5.0	239,485	0.81	0.7	0.93
Fruit fiber	5.0	239,485	0.95	0.86	1.04
Vegetable fiber	5.0	239,485	1.06	0.95	1.16
Total carbohydrate	4.0	235,169	0.91	0.82	1.0
Refined grain	3.0	175,416	1.02	0.9	1.13
Glycemic index	6.0	247,404	1.02	0.96	1.08
Glycemic load	6.0	247,404	1.02	0.96	1.08
Alcohol	13.0	369,862	0.69	0.58	0.81
Coffee	7.0	181,509	0.65	0.54	0.78

a structured interview, a food-frequency questionnaire, and a plasma glucose measurement. The incidence of diabetes (365 cases) was determined by questionnaire after approximately four years. While total whole grain intake was not reported, those with the highest quartile for whole-meal bread had a non-significantly lower risk for diabetes (0.86, P = 0.8) than those in the lowest quintile. The shorter period of follow-up and lack of total whole grain consumption analyses limits comparison of this study to the other four reports summarized above.

To analyze the reports we used a variance-weighted analysis, as described previously (Anderson 2000), using fixed-effects meta-analysis estimates. The unweighted mean value (a simple average of relative risks (R.R.) from the five studies) was 0.75 (95% confidence intervals [C.I.], 0.67 to 0.83). The variance-weighted R.R. was 0.74 (95% C.I., 0.66 to 0.82). Thus, individuals with whole grain consumption in the highest groups developed diabetes at a 26% lower rate than those with the lowest whole grain intake. (Table 3.2)

Cereal Fiber Intake and Risk for Type 2 Diabetes

While the health benefits of whole grain intake have been recognized for millennia, in 1977 Morris and colleagues (1977) presented scientific data suggesting that the intake of cereal fiber, largely from whole grains, had greater protective effects against coronary heart disease than total dietary fiber or other types of fiber. In the past decade additional studies have clearly supported the hypothesis that cereal fiber is the type of fiber that has the strongest associated protection from coronary heart disease (C.H.D.) (Anderson 2004), stroke (Liu 2000), and diabetes (Liu 2003). Since 1997, seven prospective cohort studies have reported the relative risk for diabetes is approximately 30% lower for persons with the highest consumption of cereal fiber compared to those with the lowest average intake.

Salmeron and colleagues first reported data from the Health Professional Follow-up Study (1997) after six years of follow-up (Table 3.1). They documented 523 cases of diabetes among more than 43,000 men. The relative risk for diabetes, after appropriate adjustment for covariates, was 0.70 (P = 0.007 for trend) for men in the fifth quintile compared to the first quintile. Men who averaged cereal fiber intakes of 10.2 grams/day had a 30% reduction in risk for developing diabetes compared to men consuming only 2.5 grams/day.

For the Nurses Health Study, Salmeron and associates (1997) reported data for more than 65,000 women who were followed for six years. With 915 cases of diabetes, the relative risk for women with the highest quintile of cereal fiber intake was 0.72 (P = 0.001), compared to those in the lowest quintile. Thus, women who consumed an average of 7.5 grams/day of cereal fiber had a 28% lower risk for developing diabetes than women who consumed 2 grams/day.

Meyer and colleagues (2000) also assessed the effects of cereal fiber intake on the incidence of diabetes in the Iowa Women's Health Study. They noted a relative risk for diabetes of 0.64 (P = 0.0001) for women in the highest quintile of cereal fiber consumption compared to the lowest quintile. Women who consumed an average of 9.4 grams/day of cereal fiber had a 36% lower risk of developing diabetes compared to those with intakes of 2.7 grams/day.

Stevens and colleagues (2002) reported the effects of cereal fiber intake in a prospective cohort study of white and African-American men and women who were followed in the multi-center Atherosclerosis Risk in Communities (A.R.I.C.) investigation. Participants were examined in four communities in North Carolina, Mississippi, Minnesota, and Maryland. Baseline dietary intake was assessed by an interviewer-administered, sixty-six-item, semi-quantitative food-frequency questionnaire. Over nine years of follow-up, 1,447 individuals developed diabetes diagnosed by blood glucose measurements in the clinic, received a physician diagnosis of diabetes, or initiated use of anti-diabetes medication. For the more than 8,900 white males and females, the highest quintile of cereal fiber consumption was associated with a significantly lower relative risk for diabetes (0.75) than for the lowest quintile. For the more than 3,200 African-American men and women, the same trend was seen (R.R. = 0.86) but it was not significant. However, cereal fiber intake in this population was lower than in other reports and the range from lowest to highest quintiles for whites was only from 2.7 grams/day to 5.1 grams/day and for African-Americans ranged from 2.8 grams/day to 4.0 grams/day.

Montonen and colleagues (2003) also reported the association between development of diabetes and cereal fiber consumption for the Finnish Mobile Clinic Health Examination Survey. Cereal fiber intake was much higher in the Finnish study than reported from other countries, with average values ranging from 11 grams/day for the lowest quartile to 31 grams/day for the highest quartile. These differences were accompanied by a large reduction in the relative risk for diabetes: 0.39 (P = 0.01).

Hodge and associates (2004) also reported on the association between cereal fiber consumption and diabetes for the Melbourne Collaborative Cohort Study. The range in cereal fiber intake in this study appears to be small and may account for the failure to see a distinct trend in the risk for diabetes. Nevertheless, they reported that the odds ratio for developing diabetes over four years was 0.97 (P = 0.79).

Schulze and colleagues (2004) recently reported the effects of cereal fiber intake on the incidence of diabetes over an eight-year period for more than 90,000 younger and middle-aged women. The Nurses' Health Study II is a prospective cohort study of female nurses in the United States. They calculated cereal fiber intake from responses to general and food-frequency questionnaires returned by mail. The median cereal fiber intake in the highest quintile was 8.8 grams/day compared to 3.1 grams/day in the lowest quintile. After multivariate adjustment (Table 3.1) the relative risk for type 2 diabetes for the group in the highest quintile was 0.70, or 30% lower than for the group in the lowest quintile.

These data for eight comparisons from seven reports are aggregated in Table 3.2. The variance weighted mean relative risk for the highest cereal fiber intake group compared to the lowest intake group for type 2 diabetes was 0.70 (95% C.I., 0.57 to 0.83).

The analysis of thirteen relative risk estimates combining data for whole grain consumption and cereal fiber intake from nine reports can also be aggregated (Table 3.2). The mean relative risk for diabetes for the highest intake of whole grains or cereal fiber compared to the lowest consumption was 0.72 (95% confidence interval, 0.66 to 0.77). Thus, the estimated change in risk for emergence of diabetes over a six-to-twelve-year period for the highest intake compared to the lowest intake can be summarized as follows: whole grain, 26% reduction (five studies); cereal fiber, 30% reduction (eight studies); and either whole grain or cereal fiber consumption, 28% reduction (thirteen estimates from nine studies.)

Other Dietary Fiber and Carbohydrate Intakes and Risk for Type 2 Diabetes

Total dietary fiber (T.D.F.) consumption, as well as insoluble fiber intake, is associated with a lower risk for developing diabetes. Of five studies examining the effects of T.D.F., three reported a significant reduction in diabetes risk with the highest level of T.D.F. consumption (Salmeron 1997, Meyer 2000, Montonen 2003) while two (Salmeron 1997, Schulze 2004) did not; the average relative risk for diabetes was 0.81 (95% C.I., 0.64 to 0.98) for the highest compared to the lowest consumption of T.D.F. (Table 3.2). Both studies (Meyer 2000, Montonen 2003) reporting on insoluble fiber noted a significant negative association and the average RR was 0.61. Five studies (Salmeron 1997, Salmeron 1997, Meyer 2000, Montonen 2003, Schulze 2004) have all concluded that neither fruit fiber (RR 0.96; 95% C.I., 0.84 to 1.08) nor vegetable fiber consumption (RR 1.11; 95% C.I., 1.04 to 1.19) have a significant effect on risk for diabetes. Thus, T.D.F. joins whole grain consumption and cereal fiber intake as a preventive factor for diabetes, with an estimated reduction in risk of approximately 19%.

The role of sugar and starch consumption and risk for diabetes has been debated for centuries. A recent ecological correlation study (Gross 2004) indicated that dietary fiber was associated with a protection from diabetes (p < 0.001) while corn syrup consumption increased risk for diabetes (P = 0.038). One prospective cohort study reported data for various sugars and risk for diabetes, indicating that glucose or fructose consumption significantly increases risk for diabetes while sucrose consumption—the disaccharide containing glucose and fructose—was associated with significant protection from diabetes (Meyer 2000). Several prospective cohort studies have examined the effects of total dietary carbohydrate, refined grains, fruits, vegetables, and potato consumption on risk for diabetes (Table 3.2). In three of four reports (Salmeron 1997, Salmeron 1997, Meyer 2000, Schulze 2004), total carbohydrate intake was associated with a nonsignificant reduction in risk for diabetes with an average RR of 0.91 (95% C.I., 0.81 to 1.01). Three studies have reported nonsignificant effects of refined grain intake on risk for diabetes with an average RR of 1.02. Studies examining the effects of fruit, vegetable, or potato consumption—two reports for each group—did not find a significant association between these foods and risk for diabetes (Meyer 2000, Hodge 2004, Liu 2004). In aggregate, these studies do not indicate that increased carbohydrate consumption increases risk for developing diabetes. When foods containing fiber and carbohydrate are consumed, protection from diabetes is seen.

The effects of the glycemic index (G.I.) or the glycemic load (G.L.) on risk for diabetes also has generated controversy recently. The G.I. reflects the effects of the specific food on post-consumption glycemic excursion while the G.L. represents the product (G.I. times grams of carbohydrate in the food) (Salmeron 1997). Since Jenkins and colleagues (1981) introduced the G.I. concept, the clinical value of this index has been questioned although persuasive data show the health benefits of low G.I. foods (Anderson 2004, Ford 2001). Five recent studies of six groups have evaluated the effects of the G.I. and G.L. on relative risk for diabetes (Salmeron 1997, Salmeron 1997, Meyer 2000, Stevens 2002, Schulze 2004). The reported effects of the G.I. are variable ranging from R.R. for diabetes of 0.89 (P = 0.051) to 1.62 (P = 0.001) with a weighted mean value of 1.17 (95% C.I., 0.96 to 1.38; Table 3.2). These studies, in aggregate, suggest that greater consumption of high GI foods is associated with a slightly, but not significantly, increased risk for development of diabetes. For the G.L., the reported R.R. also shows a range from 0.95 to 1.26 with no significant change in prevalence of diabetes between low and high G.L. intakes. The weighted mean values for R.R. for the association of diabetes and G.L. were 1.06 (95% C.I., 0.97 to 1.15).

Other Nutrition Approaches that Reduce Risk for Diabetes

Alcohol

In a meta-analysis of fifteen prospective cohort studies including approximately 370,000 subjects, Koppes and colleagues (2005) reported approximately 12,000 cases of diabetes identified over a twelve-year period. Compared to non-drinkers, moderate users of alcohol—6 grams/day to 48 grams/day—had a 30% lower risk for developing diabetes (Table 3.2). The lowest risk for diabetes was observed with consumption of 12 grams/day to 24 grams/day with an R.R. of 0.69 (95% C.I., 0.58 to 0.81) but the risk reduction was similar with 6 grams/day to 12 grams/day and 24 grams/day to 48 grams/day. Consumption of more than 48 grams/day did not alter risk for diabetes and the R.R. was 1.04 (95% C.I., 0.84 to 1.29). Additional research suggests that only the amount of alcohol and not the type of alcoholic beverage consumed is the major effector of metabolic parameters (Djousse 2004). While these observations are consistent with other epidemiologic data regarding consumption of one to two servings of alcoholic beverages daily, these benefits and risks of alcohol use are still being debated (Wilson 2003).

Coffee

Van Dam and Hu (Van Dam 2005) recently reported a meta-analysis of nine cohort studies examining the relationship between coffee consumption and development of diabetes (Table 3.2). Persons with the highest consumption had an R.R. for diabetes of 0.65 (95% C.I., 0.54 to 0.78) compared to persons with the lowest intake. Thus, the person who consumes six to seven cups of coffee/day may have a 35% lower risk for diabetes than the person who doesn't drink coffee or does so only occasionally.

Red Meat

Snowdon and Phillips (Snowdon 1985) first noted that Seventh Day Adventists who consumed more red meat than their vegetarian colleagues had a higher risk for diabetes. Because of the other lifestyle practices of this population—e.g., avoidance of tobacco and alcohol products—the broad implications of these observations were uncertain. However, recently three large prospective cohort studies (Van Dam 2002, Song 2004, Schulze 2003) have reported that individuals who consume larger amounts of red meat have a 36% higher risk for diabetes than those with minimal use (Table 3.2). Red meat included these foods: main dish of hamburger, beef, pork or lamb; beef, pork or lamb in a sandwich or mixed dish; and all processed meat (bacon, bologna, hot dogs, salami, and sausage). Song and colleagues (2004) reported that for more than 37,000 women followed for approximately nine years in the Women's Health Study, the highest consumption of red meat was associated with an R.R. for diabetes of 1.24 (95% C.I., 1 to 1.54; $p < 0.005$) compared to the lowest level of intake. Further analyses implicated the protein-rich portion of red meat rather than the saturated fat because the R.R. for diabetes was specifically linked to the animal protein as well as the heme iron intake.

Mineral Intake

Interest in the role of chromium in insulin action as well as prevention and reversal of diabetes has flourished for more than fifty years. Chromium serves as a cofactor for insulin action by mechanisms that are not well understood (Cefalu 2004). When treated by total parenteral nutrition (T.P.N.) without supplemental chromium, some people develop hyperglycemia that is very insulin-resistant but is reversed with chromium supplementation. Chromium supplementation prevents development of diabetes in some experimental models of diabetes (Cefalu 2004). In areas of China where the soil has been depleted of chromium and residents have severe chromium deficiency, diabetes can develop that is reversed with chromium supplementation (Anderson 1997). Based on these and other observations, the theory that chromium will prevent type 2 diabetes and even lead to remission has flourished. In a rigorous review of this area, Cefalu and Hu (Cefalu 2004) conclude that a large body of data support a potential role for chromium in prevention and treatment of type 2 diabetes but randomized, controlled trials are required to carefully assess the safety and efficacy of chromium.

The magnesium story is more compelling than the chromium one. Three prospective cohort studies have noted that higher levels of magnesium consumption are associated with a significant reduction in risk for diabetes (Salmeron 1997, Salmeron 1997, Meyer 2000). The highest levels of magnesium intake are associated with an R.R. for diabetes of 0.67 (95% C.I., 0.61 to 0.73) compared to the lowest group (Table 3.2). Thus, the intake of approximately 400 mg/day of magnesium is associated with a 33% lower risk for diabetes than the intake of approximately 250 mg/day. Vanadium has also attracted attention because of its insulin-like effects (Lukaczer 2004). While administration of fairly large doses—100 mg/day to 125 mg/day—improves insulin sensitivity in humans, these doses have significant side effects. Longer-term clinical trials are required to document the safety and efficacy of vanadium for prevention and treatment of diabetes.

Soy Foods

Soy foods that retain most of the components of the soybean—whole soybeans, soy nuts, green soybeans, tofu, and soy flour—appear to have protective effects related to diabetes (Bhathena 2002, Ali 2004, Jayagopal 2002, Yang 2004, Anderson 2004). These health benefits appear related to the protein, soy peptides, isoflavones, fiber, and other components. Because of the low levels of consumption of soy foods in Western populations it has not been possible to assess the association between soy food use and diabetes. Animal studies indicate that soy protein enhances insulin sensitivity and has favorable effects on glucose metabolism (Iritani 1997, Ishihara 2003). Soy food intake also has protective effects related to the development and management of obesity (Anderson 2004). Whole grains have many constituents, such as fiber, antioxidants, and phytoestrogens, that have similar physiological effects in humans to those of the phytochemicals from whole soybeans.

Herbal Supplements and Other Nutraceuticals

Because diabetes has been recognized as a disabling disease for more than two millennia, many traditional preventive and corrective remedies have been recommended. As new compounds emerge (e.g., stevia) and as traditional foods are further examined (e.g., cinnamon and chocolate), further candidates for diabetes prevention emerge. Only limited evidence supports the protective effects of the following compounds: antioxidant vitamins (Ylönen 2003, Lukaczer 2004), cinnamon (Khan 2003), cyclo(His-Pro) (Song 2001), dark chocolate (Grassi 2005, Grassi 2005), elder (Gray 2000), fenugreek (Sharma 1990), ginseng (Sievenpiper 2004), stevia (Jeppersen 2003), and other phytochemicals (Haddad 2001, Lukaczer 2004). Unidentified phytochemicals from whole grains with similar structures or actions to some of these compounds may contribute to the protective action of whole grains as they relate to diabetes.

Lifestyle and Reduced Risk for Diabetes

The development of type 2 diabetes is multi-factorial in nature. Obesity is a major contributor to the development of diabetes (Anderson 2003). In addition to weight gain, minimal physical activity probably contributes to the emergence of diabetes but this is not well documented. Three persuasive studies (Pan 1997, Tuomilehto 2001, Diabetes Prevention Program Research Group 2002) and other smaller reports (Ericksson 1991, Swinburn 2001, Moore 2000, Resnick 2000, Smith 2005) document that weight loss and increased physical activity decrease development of diabetes in high-risk individuals.

Lifestyle changes for high-risk individuals resulted in a 58% ($p < 0.001$) reduction in the overall incidence of diabetes over a four-year period in the Finnish Diabetes Prevention Study (Tuomilehto 2001). The Diabetes Prevention Program (D.P.P.) was a lifestyle intervention trial of U.S. adults at high risk for diabetes (Diabetes Prevention Program Research Group 2002). Participants in the lifestyle intervention group were educated about achieving a weight reduction of at least 7% of initial body weight with subsequent weight maintenance through a low-calorie, low-fat diet with moderate intensity physical activity for at least 150 minutes per week. Over an average of only 2.8 years the incidence of diabetes was 58% (95% C.I.; 48% to 66%) lower in the intervention group. Thus, the available data indicates that modest weight loss coupled with modest increases in physical activity for people who are at high risk for developing diabetes are accompanied by a 58% reduction in diabetes risk over three years.

People who consume generous amounts of whole grains also are, on average, more physically active and use fewer tobacco products, i.e., they have healthier lifestyles. While these lifestyle variables are evaluated by appropriate statistical adjustments, these analyses may not completely correct for measured and unmeasured lifestyle factors, such as coffee consumption, that may affect risk for diabetes. To better assess differences in lifestyle behaviors in whole grain consumers we evaluated estimates of physical activity, vitamin use, alcohol consumption, and smoking in nine reports. Data from 474,459 individuals were available from these nine studies: Atherosclerosis Risk in Communities (Stevens 2002, Steffen 2003) Cancer Prevention Study II (McCullough 2003), Coronary Artery Risk Development in Young Adults (Pereira 1998), Framingham Offspring Study (McKeown 2002), Health Professionals Follow-up Study (Fung 2002, Koh-Banerjee 2004), Iowa Women's Health Study (Meyer 2000, Jacobs 1998), Physicians' Health Study (Liu 2003), Nurses' Health Study (Liu 2000), and Nurses' Health Study II (Schulze 2004).

In these nine studies, average whole grain consumption in the highest group (quartile or quintile) was 20.2 servings/week compared to 0.9 servings/week in the lowest group. Ratios for highest to lowest whole grain consumers were calculated as follows: if 18% of the highest users smoked cigarettes and 36% of the lowest users were smokers, the ratio was 18 divided by 36, or 0.5. The weighted average was the ratio weighted by the number of participants in each group. Because variances for lifestyle measures were not provided, differences between groups were calculated as paired-T tests comparing average values for the highest and lowest consumers across the nine studies (e.g., 18% smokers vs. 36% smokers).

Whole grain consumption for the highest group was associated with 40% more physical activity (ratio of 1.4, Table 3.3). The generous intake of whole grains was associated with 42% more vitamin use. Alcohol consumption was 25% lower in the highest group for whole grain consumption and current cigarette use was 59% lower than in the lowest whole grain consumers. All of these differences were statistically significant. Thus, people who consume generous amounts of whole grains—three servings/day—appear to have lifestyle practices that are significantly more health-promoting than people who only consume whole grains once weekly. While higher levels of alcohol consumption may protect from diabetes (Table 3.2), higher levels of physical activity (Boule 2005) and vitamin use (Ylönen 2003) may contribute to protection from diabetes.

The American Diabetes Association, the North American Association for the Study of Obesity, and the American Society for Clinical Nutrition released a statement regarding specific recommendations for the prevention and treatment of type 2 diabetes by means of weight management through lifestyle modification (Klein 2004). The first recommendation is weight loss for those individuals with a body mass index (B.M.I.) of 25 kg/m^2 or greater who have or who are at risk for developing type 2 diabetes. Physical activity is an important component in maintaining long-term weight maintenance. The activity should be performed on a regular basis at moderate intensity. Physical activity will not only help with weight loss and maintenance but will also positively effect insulin sensitivity, glycemic control, and certain risk factors for atherosclerotic cardiovascular disease.

Table 3.3. Lifestyle measures comparing highest (20.2 servings/week) with lowest (0.9 serving/week) whole grain consumption reported from nine studies (474,459 participants).

Measure	Ratio: highest to lowest	Lowest 95th CI	Highest 95th CI	P value
Physical activity	1.40	1.18	1.62	0.0004
Vitamin use	1.42	1.25	1.60	0.0084
Alcohol consumption	0.75	0.67	0.83	0.0014
Smoking	0.41	0.36	0.45	<0.0001

Whole Grain Consumption and Diabetes Management

Whole grains rich in soluble fiber—oats and barley—have low glycemic indices and decrease postprandial hyperglycemia in non-diabetic and diabetic subjects (Brand 1991, Kabir 2002). However, increasing dietary fiber intake from a variety of fiber-rich foods, including whole grain wheat products, is associated with improved postprandial glycemia (Anderson 2004). When dietary carbohydrate and fiber intake is increased these values are significantly better than with a moderate-carbohydrate, low-fiber diet: fasting plasma glucose, 14% lower, postprandial plasma glucose, 14% lower, and hemoglobin A_{1c}, 6% lower (Anderson 2004). Based on these observations the international consensus recommendations are that the diabetes diet should provide 50% to 60% carbohydrate with an emphasis on whole grains, legumes, and vegetables (Anderson 2004).

As documented elsewhere (Pereira 2002, Liese 2003), whole grain intake is associated with enhanced insulin sensitivity. Clinical research with arabinoxylan (A.X.), the major component of dietary fiber present in many cereal grains, indicates that consuming bread containing 6 grams/meal of A.X. was associated with significant reductions in postprandial glucose and insulin excursions (Lu 2000). These improvements in postprandial glycemia with A.X. are similar to those seen with the consumption of the soluble fiber psyllium (Anderson 1999).

Whole grain consumption improves or ameliorates many of the fellow-travelers with diabetes, including: overweight or obesity, risk for atherosclerotic cardiovascular disease, hypertension, dyslipidemia, gastrointestinal dysfunction, and renal disease. Because authors in other chapters address the association between whole grain consumption and the risk for obesity (Chapter 4) and coronary heart disease (Chapter 5), we will only examine the role of whole grain intake and clinical management of obesity, hypertension, and dyslipidemia.

Obesity

About 75% of type 2 diabetic individuals in the United States are obese; obesity is a major contributor to the development and maintenance of the diabetic state (Anderson 2003). Extensive research over twenty years documents the benefits of increased consumption of high fiber foods, such as whole grains, for weight management of diabetic (Anderson 1985) and non-diabetic individuals (Howarth 2001). The value of whole grain and other ready-to-eat cereals for weight management are under investigation and appear to be an effective tool for facilitating modest weight loss (Waller 2004). Blood pressure levels also decrease with increased dietary fiber consumption (Anderson 1983, Anderson 2002, Anderson 1994, Appel 1997) and recent studies document the value of whole grain intake for blood pressure reduction (Saltzman 2001, Keenan 2002, He 2004).

Dyslipidemia

Most people with diabetes have one or more distinct lipoprotein abnormalities. The most common pattern includes elevated fasting serum triglyceride values, low H.D.L.-cholesterol values, a predominance of small dense L.D.L. particles (Krauss 2004), and dysfunctional H.D.L. particles (Gowri 1999). These abnormalities can be related to insulin resistance, poor glycemic control, obesity, nutritional habits, and suboptimal physical activity (Krauss 2004,

Anderson 2005). Whole grain consumption addresses all of these abnormalities except physical activity. The hypocholesterolemic effects of whole oats have been appreciated for many years (deGroot 1963). Whole grain barley also has significant cholesterol-lowering properties (Newman 1989). Extensive studies with oat bran (Kirby 1981, Anderson 1990, Ripsin 1992, Everson 1992) extended understanding of the effectiveness and mechanisms of action of oat foods. The β-glucan from oats and barley exert the predominant cholesterol-lowering effects, and significant reductions in serum L.D.L.-cholesterol is seen with the intake of three grams/day of β-glucan, either as a purified extract or in the whole grain (Behall 2004). Furthermore, recent work indicates that oat cereal consumption significantly lowered the small, dense L.D.L. cholesterol (Davy 2002).

Hypertriglyceridemia can result from a diet high in carbohydrates and low in dietary fiber—so-called "carbohydrate-induced hypertriglyceridemia" (Park 2000). The triglyceride abnormality can be further aggravated by poor glycemic control because adequate plasma insulin levels are required to facilitate lipoprotein lipase activity (Krauss 2004). Our observations, however, indicated that diets high in whole grains and dietary fiber systematically decreased fasting serum triglyceride values (Anderson 1986, Anderson 1980). A detailed meta-analysis of published reports also indicated that high-carbohydrate, high-fiber (H.C.H.F.) diets were associated with significantly lower triglyceride values in non-diabetic and diabetic subjects than high-carbohydrate, low-fiber (H.C.L.F.) diets (Anderson 2000). Further review of twelve clinical trials for diabetic subjects revealed that H.C.H.F. diets were associated with 12.8% (95% C.I., 4.3% to 21.2%) lower fasting serum triglyceride values than H.C.L.F. diets. The observations in non-diabetic and diabetic individuals indicate that whole grain consumption can be strongly encouraged for diabetic individuals without concern about baseline levels of triglycerides.

Abnormally low H.D.L.-cholesterol levels present a challenge for many non-diabetic and diabetic individuals. Treatment approaches include increased exercise, smoking cessation, weight loss, and pharmacotherapy (Rubins 1999, Krauss 2004). Improving glycemic control and lowering serum triglycerides lead to increased H.D.L.-cholesterol values in diabetic subjects. Whole grain consumption also can contribute to increases in H.D.L.-cholesterol. Oat and oat bran consumption for several months is accompanied by an increase in H.D.L.-cholesterol, as is an intake of low glycemic foods (Frost 1999). Schaefer (2002), in an authoritative analysis and expert review, recommends that nutritional prevention of C.H.D. includes sparing use of these products: animal, dairy, and hydrogenated fats; tropical oils; egg yolks; and sugar. He recommends the generous consumption of vegetables, fruits, and whole grains. These recommendations are consistent with the international consensus recommendations for nutrition management of diabetes (Anderson 2004).

Proposed Mechanisms of Whole Grains for Protection from Diabetes

Dietary fiber seems to be the strongest candidate for the role of major effector of diabetes risk associated with whole grains. Cereal fiber consumption is associated with a slightly but not significantly greater reduction in diabetes risk than whole grains (Table 3.2). Total dietary fiber intake also has a significant protective effect. Dietary fiber, especially the soluble component, may contribute to a lower glycemic index that would tend to reduce risk for diabetes. Dietary fiber intake also is associated with lower body weight (Howarth 2001), another protector from diabetes (Anderson 2003). Whole grains are rich sources of magnesium, a mineral that has a significant negative association with risk for diabetes. As Pereira (1998) suggests, the generous intake of magnesium and other minerals from whole grains may contribute to the protection from diabetes. Whole grains bring a wide variety of antioxidants to the table. The natural antioxidants contained in whole grains as well as the vitamins added to enrich the products may also contribute to the protective effects. The lignans from whole grains are converted to enterolactone and enterodione by intestinal flora (Slavin 2004); like the isoflavones from soybeans, these phytoestrogens have effects on insulin sensitivity, glucose, and lipid metabolism that may protect from diabetes (Bhathena 2002). The litany of other whole grain phytochemicals that may provide protection from diabetes and other diseases are enumerated by Slavin (Slavin 2004).

Conclusion

Whole grain consumption has many health-promoting effects, including a prolonged life and protection from common Western diseases. Recent prospective cohort studies clearly indicate that higher levels of whole grain intake are associated with a significantly lower risk for development of type 2 diabetes than lower intakes. People who consume approximately twenty servings of whole grains weekly develop diabetes at a 26% lower rate than people who consume an average of less than one serving per week. From five studies the variance-adjusted relative risk for high consumers of whole grains is 0.74 (95% C.I., 0.68 to 0.81) compared to infrequent consumption. Cereal fiber intake is a surrogate measure of whole grain consumption and the relative risk reported from eight studies is 0.69 (95% C.I., 0.63 to 0.74) for high vs. low intakes. Total dietary fiber intake also is associated with a significant reduction in risk of 19% for high vs. low intakes. In this analysis, fruit fiber, vegetable fiber, total carbohydrate, glycemic index, and glycemic load did not significantly affect estimated risk for type 2 diabetes. While generous intakes of red meat appear to increase risk for diabetes, moderate alcohol consumption and higher levels of coffee or magnesium intake lower diabetes risk. These observations from prospective cohort studies are persuasive but need to be confirmed by randomized clinical trials. Nevertheless, the health benefits and diabetes protective effects provide a platform to promote a generous intake of whole grains for the general population.

References

Ali, A.A.; Velasquez, M.T.; Hansen, C.T.; Mohamed, A.I.; and Bhathena, S.J. 2004. Effects of soybean isoflavones, probiotics, and their interaction on lipid metabolism and endocrine system in an animal model of obesity and diabetes. *Journal of Nutritional Biochemistry* 15:583–590.

Anderson, J.W. 1983. Plant fiber and blood pressure. *Annals of Internal Medicine* 98:842–846.

Anderson, J.W. 1985. High-fiber diets for obese diabetic men on insulin therapy: short-term and long-term effects. In *Dietary Fiber and Obesity*, edited by Vahouny, G. V., pp. 49–68. New York: Alan R. Liss Inc.

Anderson, J.W. 2000. Dietary fiber prevents carbohydrate-induced hypertriglyceridemia. *Current Atherosclerosis Reports* 2:536–541.

Anderson, J.W. 2002. Whole-grains intake and risk for coronary heart disease. In *Whole grains in health and disease*, edited by Marquart, L.; Slavin, J. L.; and Fulcher, G., pp. 100–114. St. Paul, Minn.: American Association of Cereal Chemists.

Anderson, J.W. 2004. Soy protein and its role in obesity management. *SCAN's Pulse* 23:8–9.

Anderson, J.W. 2004. Whole grains and coronary heart disease: the whole kernel of truth. *American Journal of Clinical Nutrition* 80. In press (Dec.).

Anderson, J.W. 2005. Nutrition management of diabetes mellitus. In *Modern Nutrition in Health and Disease*, edited by Shils, M. E. and Olson, J. A., pp. 1365–1394. Philadelphia: Lea & Febiger.

Anderson, J.W.; Allgood, L.D.; Turner, C.; Oelgten, P.R.; and Daggy, B.P. 1999. Effects of psyllium on glucose and serum lipid responses in men with type 2 diabetes and hypercholesterolemia. *American Journal of Clinical Nutrition* 70:466–473.

Anderson, J.W.; Chen, W.J.L.; and Sieling, B. 1980. Hypolipidemic effects of high-carbohydrate, high-fiber diets. *Metabolism* 29:551–558.

Anderson, J.W.; Hanna, T.J.; Peng, X.; and Kryscio, R.J. 2000. Whole grain foods and heart disease risk. *Journal of the American College of Nutrition* 19(suppl 3):291S–299S.

Anderson, J.W.; Kendall, C.W.C.; and Jenkins, D.J.A. 2003. Importance of weight management in type 2 diabetes: review with meta-analysis of clinical studies. *Journal of the American College of Nutrition* 22:331–339.

Anderson, J.W.; Randles, K.M.; Kendall, C.W.C.; and Jenkins, D.J.A. 2004. Carbohydrate and fiber recommendations for individuals with diabetes: a quantitative assessment and meta-analysis of the evidence. *Journal of the American College of Nutrition* 235:1–17.

Anderson, J.W.; Smith, B.M.; and Gustafson, N.J. 1994. Health benefits and practical aspects of high-fiber diets. *American Journal of Clinical Nutrition* 59(Suppl):1242S–1247S.

Anderson, J.W.; Spencer, D.B.; Hamilton, C.C.; Smith, S.F.; Tietyen, J.; Bryant, C.A.; and Oeltgen, P.R. 1990. Oat-bran cereal lowers serum total and LDL cholesterol in hypercholesterolemic men. *American Journal of Clinical Nutrition* 52:495–499.

Anderson, J.W. and Tietyen-Clark, J. 1986. Dietary fiber, hyperlipidemia, hypertension, and coronary heart disease. *American Journal of Gastroenterology* 81:907–919.

Anderson, R.A.; Cheng, N.; Bryden, N.A.; Polansky, M.M.; Cheng, N.; Chi, J.; and Feng, J. 1997. Elevated intakes of supplemental chromium improve glucose and insulin variables in individuals with type 2 diabetes. *Diabetes* 46:1786-1791.

Appel, L.J.; Moore, T.J.; Obarzanek, E.; Vollmer, W.M.; Svetkey, L.P.; Sacks, F.M.; Bray, G.A.; Vogt, T.M.; Cutler, J.A.; Windhauser, M.M.; Lin, P.H.; and Karanja, N. 1997. A clinical trial of the effects of dietary patterns on blood pressure. DASH Collaborative Research Group. *New England Journal of Medicine* 336: 1117–1124.

Behall, K.M.; Scholfield, D.J.; and Hallfrisch, J. 2004. Diets containing barley significantly reduce lipids in mildly hypercholesterolemic men and women. *American Journal of Clinical Nutrition* 80:1185–1193.

Bhathena, S.J. and Velasquez, M.T. 2002. Beneficial role of dietary phytoestrogens in obesity and diabetes. *American Journal of Clinical Nutrition* 76:1191–1201.

Boule, N.G.; Weisnagel, S.J.; Lakka, T.A.; Tremblay, A.; Rankinen, T.; Leon, A.S.; Skinner, J.S.; Wilmore, J.H.; Rao, D.C.; and Bouchard, C. 2005. Effects of exercise-training on glucose homeostasis. *Diabetes Care* 28:120–126.

Brand, J.C.; Colagiuri, S.; Crossman, S.; Allen, A.; Roberts, D. C.; and Truswell, A.S. 1991. Low-glycemic index foods improve long-term glycemic control in NIDDM. *Diabetes Care* 14(2):95–101.

Cefalu, W.T. and Hu, F.B. 2004. Role of chromium in human health and diabetes. *Diabetes Care* 27:2741–2751.

Davy, B.M.; Davy, K.P.; Ho, R.C.; Beske, S.D.; Davrath, L.R.; and Melby, C.L. 2002. High-fiber oat cereal compared with wheat cereal consumption favorably alters LDL-cholesterol subclass and particle numbers in middle-aged and older men. *American Journal of Clinical Nutrition* 76:341–359.

deGroot, A.P.; Luyken, R.; and Pikaar, N.A. 1963. Cholesterol-lowering effects of rolled oats. *Lancet* 2:203–204.

Diabetes Prevention Program Research Group. 2002. Reduction in the incidence of type 2 diabetes with lifestyle intervention or metformin. *New England Journal of Medicine* 346:393–403.

Djousse, L.; Arnett, D.K.; Eckfeldt, J.H.; Province, M.A.; Singer, M.R.; and Ellison, R.C. 2004. Alcohol consumption and metabolic syndrome: does the type of beverage matter? *Obesity Research* 12:1375–1385.

Eriksson, K.F. and Lingarde, F. 1991. Prevention of type 2 (non-insulin-dependent) diabetes mellitus by diet and physical exercise. *Diabetologia* 34:891–898.

Everson, G.T.; Daggy, B.P.; McKinley, C.; and Story, J.A. 1992. Effects of psyllium hydrophilic mucilloid on LDL-cholesterol and bile acid synthesis in hypercholesterolemic men. *Journal of Lipid Research* 33:1183–1192.

Ford, E.S. and Liu, S. 2001. Glycemic index and serum high-density lipoprotein cholesterol concentration among U.S. adults. *Archives of Internal Medicine* 161:572–576.

Frost, G.; Leeds, A.A.; Dore, C.J.; Madeiros, S.; Brading, S.; and Dornhorst, A. 1999. Glycaemic index as a determinant of serum HDL-cholesterol concentration. *Lancet* 353:1045–1048.

Fung, T.T.; Hu, F.B.; Pereira, M.A.; Liu, S.; Stampfer, M.J.; Colditz, G.A.; and Willett, W.C. 2002. Whole-grain intake and the risk of type 2 diabetes: a prospective study in men. *American Journal of Clinical Nutrition* 76: 535–540.

Gowri, M.S.; Van der Westhuyzen, D.R.; Bridges, S.R.; and Anderson, J.W. 1999. Decreased protection by HDL from poorly controlled type 2 diabetic subjects against LDL oxidation may be due to the abnormal composition of HDL. *Arteriosclerosis Thrombosis and Vascular Biology* 9:2226–2233.

Grassi, D.; Lippi, C.; Necozione, S. and et al. 2005. Short-term administration of dark chocolate is followed by a significant increase in insulin sensitivity and a decrease in blood pressure in healthy persons. *American Journal of Clinical Nutrition* 81:611–614.

Grassi, D.; Necozione, S.; Lippi, C.; Croce, G.; Valeri, L.; Pasqualetti, P.; Desideri, G.; Blumberg, J. B.; and Ferri, C. 2005. Cocoa reduces blood pressure and insulin resistance and improves endothelium-dependent vasodilitation in hypertensives. *Hypertension* 46:398–405.

Gray, A.M.; Abdel-Wahab, H.A.; and Flatt, P.R. 2000. The traditional plant treatment, Sambucus nigra (elder), exhibits insulin-like and insulin-releasing actions in vitro. *Journal of Nutrition* 130:15–20.

Gross, L.S.; Li, L.; Ford, E.S.; and Liu, S. 2004. Increased consumption of refined carbohydrates and the epidemic of type 2 diabetes in the United States: an ecologic assessment. *American Journal of Clinical Nutrition* 79:774–779.

Haddad, P.S.; Depot, M.; Settaf, A.; and Cherrah, Y. 2001. Use of antidiabetic plants in Morocco and Quebec. *Diabetes Care* 24:608–609.

He, J.; Streiffer, R.H.; Munter, P.; Krousel-Wood, M.A.; and Whelton, P.K. 2004. Effect of dietary fiber intake on blood pressure: a randomized, double-blind, placebo-controlled, trial. *Journal of Hypertension* 22:73–80.

Hodge, A.; English, D.R.; O'Dea, K.; and Giles, G.G. 2004. Glycemic index and dietary fiber and the risk of type 2 diabetes. *Diabetes Care* 27:2701–2706.

Howarth, N.C.; Saltzman, E.; and Roberts, S.B. 2001. Dietary fiber and weight regulation. *Nutrition Reviews* 59: 129–139.

Iritani, N.; Sugimoto, T.; Fukuda, H.; Komiya, M.; and Ikeda, H. 1997. Dietary soybean protein increases insulin receptor gene expression in Wistar fatty rats when dietary polyunsaturated fatty acid level is low. *Journal of Nutrition* 127:1077–1083.

Ishihara, K.; Oyaizu, S.; Fukuchi, Y.; Mizunoya, W.; Segawa, K.; Takahashi, M.; Mita, Y.; Fukuya, Y.; Fushiki, T.; and Yasumoto, K. 2003. A soybean peptide isolate diet promotes postprandial carbohydrate oxidation and energy expenditure in type II diabetic mice. *Journal of Nutrition* 133:752–757.

Jacobs, D.R.; Meyer, K.A.; Kushi, L.H.; and Folsom, A.R. 1998. Whole-grain intake may reduce the risk of ischemic heart disease death in postmenopausal women: the Iowa Women's Health Study. *American Journal of Clinical Nutrition* 68:248–257.

Jayagopal, V.; Albertazzi, P.; Kilpatrick, E.S.; Howarth, E.M.; Jennings, P.E.; Hepburn, D.A.; and Atkin, S.L. 2002. Beneficial effects of soy phytoestrogen intake in postmenopausal women with type 2 diabetes. *Diabetes Care* 25:1709–1714.

Jenkins, D.J.A.; Wolever, T.M.S.; Taylor, R.H.; Barker, H.M.; Fielden, H.; Baldwin, J.M.; Bowling, A.C.; Newman, H.C.; Jenkins, A.L.; and Goff, D.V. 1981. Glycemic index of foods: a physiologic basis for carbohydrate exchange. *American Journal of Clinical Nutrition* 34:362–366.

Jeppersen, P.B.; Gregersen, S.; Rolfsen, S.E.D.; Jepsen, M.; Colombo, M.; Agger, A.; Xiao, J.; Kruhoffer, M.; Orntoft, T.; and Hermansen, K. 2003. Antihyperglycemic and blood-pressure-reducing effects of stevioside in the diabetic Goto-Kakizaki rat. *Metabolism* 52:372–378.

Kabir, M.; Oppert, J-M.; Vidal, H.; Bruzzo, F.; Fiquet, C.; Wursch, P.; Slama, G.; and Rizkalla, S.W. 2002. Four-week low-glycemic index breakfast with a modest amount of soluble fibers in type 2 diabetic men. *Metabolism* 51:819–826.

Keenan, J.M.; Pins, J.J.; Frazel, C.; Moran, A.; and Turnquist, L. 2002. Oat ingestion reduces systolic and diastolic blood pressure in patients with mild or borderline hypertension: a pilot trial. *Journal of Family Practice*

Khan, A.; Safdar, M.; Khan, M.M.A.; Khattak, K.N.; and Anderson, R.A. 2003. Cinnamon improves glucose and lipids of people with type 2 diabetes. *Diabetes Care* 26:3215–3218.

Kirby, R.W.; Anderson, J.W.; Sieling, B.; Rees, E.D.; Chen, W.J.L.; Miller, R.M.; and Kay, R.M. 1981. Oat-bran intake selectively lowers serum low-density lipoprotein cholesterol concentrations of hypercholesterolemic men. *American Journal of Clinical Nutrition* 34:824–829.

Klein, S.; Sheard, N.; Pi-Sunyer, F.X.; Daly, A.; Wylie-Rosett, J.; Kulkarni, K.; and Clark, N. 2004. Weight management through lifestyle modification for the prevention and management of type 2 diabetes: rationale and strategies. *Diabetes Care* 27:2067–2073.

Koh-Banerjee, P.; Franz, M.; Sampson, L.; Jacobs, D.R.; Spiegelman, D.; Willett, W.; and Rimm, E. 2004. Changes in whole-grain, bran, and cereal fiber consumption in relationship to 8-y weight gain among men. *American Journal of Clinical Nutrition* 80:1237–1245.

Koppes, L.; Dekker, J.M.; Hendriks, H.; Bouter, L.; and Heine, R.J. 2005. Moderate alcohol consumption lowers risk of type 2 diabetes. *Diabetes Care* 28:719–725.

Krauss, R.M. 2004. Lipids and lipoproteins in patients with type 2 diabetes. *Diabetes Care* 27:1496–1504.

Liese, A.D.; Roach, A.K.; Sparks, K.C.; Marquart, L.; D'Agostino, R.B.; and Mayer-Davis, E. 2003. Whole-grain intake and insulin sensitivity: the Insulin Resistance Atherosclerosis Study. *American Journal of Clinical Nutrition* 78:965–971.

Liu, S. 2003. Whole-grain foods, dietary fiber, and type 2 diabetes: searching for a kernel of truth. *American Journal of Clinical Nutrition* 77:527–529.

Liu, S.; Manson, J.E.; Stampfer, M.J.; Hu, F.B.; Giovannucci, E.; Colditz, G.A.; Hennekens, C.H.; and Willett, W.C. 2000. A prospective study of whole grain intake and risk of type 2 diabetes mellitus in U.S. women. *American Journal of Public Health* 90:1409–1415.

Liu, S.; Manson, J.E.; Stampfer, M.J.; Rexrode, K.M.; Hu, F.B.; Willett, W.C.; and Willett, W.C. 2000. Whole grain consumption and risk of ischemic stroke in women: a prospective study. *Journal of the American Medical Association* 284:1534–1540.

Liu, S.; Serdula, M.; Janket, S-J.; Cook, N.R.; Sesso, H.D.; Willet, W.C.; Manson, J.E.; and Buring, J.E. 2004. A prospective study of fruit and vegetable intake and the risk of type 2 diabetes in women. *Diabetes Care* 27: 2993–2996.

Liu, S.; Willett, W.C.; Manson, J.E.; Hu, F.B.; Rosner, B.; and Colditz, G. 2003. Relation between changes in intake of dietary fiber and grain products and changes in weight and development of obesity among middle-aged women. *American Journal of Clinical Nutrition* 78:920–927

Lu, Z.X.; Walker, K.Z.; Muir, J.G.; Mascara, T.; and O'Dea, K. 2000. Arabinoxylan fiber, a product of wheat flour processing, reduces the postprandial glucose response in normoglycemic subjects. *American Journal of Clinical Nutrition* 71:1123–1128.

Lukaczer, D. 2004. The dietary solution to diabetes. *Functional Foods & Nutraceuticals* (June):38–46.

McCullough, M.L.; Robertson, A.S.; Chao, A.; Jacobs, E.J.; Stampfer, M.J.; Jacobs, D.R.; Diver, W.R.; Calle, E.E.; and Thun, M.J. 2003. A prospective study of whole grains, fruits, vegetables and colon cancer risk. *Cancer Causes & Control* 14:959–970.

McKeown, N.M.; Meigs, J.B.; Liu, S.; Wilson, P.W.F.; and Jacques, P.F. 2002. Whole-grain intake is favorably associated with metabolic risk factors for type 2 diabetes and cardiovascular disease in the Framingham Offspring Study. *American Journal of Clinical Nutrition* 76:390–398.

Meyer, K.A.; Kushi, L.H.; Jacobs, D.R.; Slavin, J.; Sellers, T.A.; and Folsom, A.R. 2000. Carbohydrates, dietary fiber, and incidence of type 2 diabetes in older women. *American Journal of Clinical Nutrition* 71:921–930.

Montonen, J.; Knekt, P.; Jarvinen, R.; Aromaa, A.; and Reunanen, A. 2003. Whole-grain and fiber intake and the incidence of type 2 diabetes. *American Journal of Clinical Nutrition* 77:622–629.

Moore, L.L.; Visioni, A.J.; Wilson, P.W.F.; Agostino, R.B.; Finkle, W.D.; and Ellison, R.C. 2000. Can sustained weight loss in overweight individuals reduce the risk of diabetes mellitus? *Epidemiology* 11:269–273.

Morris, J.N.; Marr, J.W.; and Clayton, D.G. 1977. Diet and heart: a postscript. *British Medical Journal* 2: 1307–1314.

Murtaugh, M.A.; Jacobs, D.R., Jr.; Jacob, B.; Steffen, L.M.; and Marquart, L. 2003. Epidemiological support for the protection of whole grains against diabetes. *Proc Nutr Soc* 62:143–149.

Newman, R.K.; Lewis, S.E.; and Newman, C.W. 1989. Hypocholesterolemic effect of barley foods on healthy men. *Nutr Rep Internat* 39:749–760.

Pan, X.R.; Li, G.W.; Hu, Y.H. and et al. 1997. Effect of diet and exercise in preventing NIDDM in people with impaired glucose tolerance. *Diabetes Care* 20:537–544.

Park, E.J. and Hellerstein, M.K. 2000. Carbohydrate-induced hypertriacylglycerolemia: historical perspective and review of biological mechanisms. *American Journal of Clinical Nutrition* 71:412–433.

Pereira, M.A.; Jacobs, D.R.; Slattery, M.L. and et al. 1998. The association between whole grain intake and fasting insulin in a bi-racial cohort of young adults: the CARDIA study. *CVD Prev* 1:231–242.

Pereira, M.A.; Jacobs, D.R., Jr.; Pins, J.J.; Raatz, S.K.; Gross, M.D.; Slavin, J.L.; and Seaquist, E.R. 2002. Effect of whole grains on insulin sensitivity in overweight hyperinsulinemic adults. *American Journal of Clinical Nutrition* 75(5):848–855.

Resnick, H.E.; Valsania, P.; Halter, J.B.; and Lin, X. 2000. Relation of weight gain and weight loss on subsequent diabetes risk in overweight adults. *Journal of Epidemiology and Community Health* 54:596–602.

Ripsin, C.M.; Keenan, J.M.; Jacobs, D.R.; Elmer, P.J.; Welch, R.R.; Van Horn, L.; Liu, K.; Turnbull, W.H.; Thye, F.W.; Kestin, M.; Hegsted, M.; Davidson, D.M.; Davidson, M.H.; Dugan, L.D.; Demark-Wahnefried, W.; and Beling, S. 1992. Oat products and lipid lowering. *Journal of the American Medical Association* 267:3317–3325.

Rubins, H.B.; Robins, S.J.; Collins, D.; Fye, C.L.; Anderson, J.W.; Elam, M.B.; Faas, F.H.; Linares, E.; Schaefer, E.J.; Schectman, G.; Wilk, T.J.; and Wittes, J. 1999. Gemfibrozil for the secondary prevention of coronary heart disease in men with low levels of high-density lipoprotein cholesterol. *New England Journal of Medicine* 341:410–418.

Salmeron, J.; Ascherio, A.; Rimm, E.B.; Colditz, G.A.; Spiegelman, D.; Jenkins, D.J.; Stampfer, M.J.; Wing, A.L.; and Willett, W.C. 1997. Dietary fiber, glycemic load, and risk of NIDDM in men. *Diabetes Care* 20:545–550.

Salmeron, J.; Manson, J.E.; Stampfer, M.J.; Coldtiz, G.A.; Wing, A.L.; and Willet, W.C. 1997. Dietary fiber, glycemic load, and risk of non-insulin-dependent diabetes mellitus in women. *J.A.M.A.* 277:472–477.

Saltzman, E.; Das, S.K.; Lichenstein, A.H.; Dallal, G.E.; Corrales, A.; Schaefer, E.J.; Greenberg, A.S.; and Roberts, S.B. 2001. An oat-containing hypocaloric diet reduces systolic blood pressure and improves lipid profile beyond effects of weight loss in men and women. *Journal of Nutrition* (131):1465.

Schaefer, E.J. 2002. Lipoproteins, nutrition, and heart disease. *American Journal of Clinical Nutrition* 75:191–212.

Schulze, M.B.; Liu, S.; Rimm, E.B.; Manson, J.E.; Willett, W.C.; and Hu, F.B. 2004. Glycemic index, glycemic load, and dietary fiber intake and incidence of type 2 diabetes in younger and middle-aged women. *American Journal of Clinical Nutrition* 80:348–356.

Schulze, M.B.; Manson, J.E.; Willett, W.C.; and Hu, F.B. 2003. Processed meat intake and incidence of type 2 diabetes in younger and middle-aged women. *Diabetologia* 46:1465–1473.

Sharma, R.D.; Raghuram, T.C.; and Rao, N.S. 1990. Effect of fenugreek seeds on blood glucose and serum lipids in type I diabetes. *European Journal of Clinical Nutrition* 44:301–306.

Sievenpiper, J.L.; Arnason, J.T.; Leiter, L.A.; and Vuksan, V. 2004. Decreasing null and increasing effects of eight popular types of ginseng on acute postprandial glycemic indices in healthy humans: the role of the ginsenosides. *Journal of the American College of Nutrition* 23:248–258.

Slavin, J. 2004. Whole grains and human health. *Nutrition Research Reviews* 17:99–110.

Smith, G.D.; Bracha, Y.; Svendsen, K.H.; Neaton, J.D.; Haffner, S.M.; and Kuller, L.H. 2005. Incidence of type 2 diabetes in the randomized multiple risk factor intervention trial. *Annals of Internal Medicine* 142:313–322.

Snowdon, D.A. and Phillips, R.L. 1985. Does a vegetarian diet reduce the occurrence of diabetes? *American Journal of Public Health* 75:507–512.

Song, M.K.; Rosenthal, M.J.; Hong, S.; Harris, D.M.; Hwang, I.; Yip, I.; Golub, M.S.; Ament, M.E.; and Go, V.L.W. 2001. Synergistic antidiabetic activities of zinc, cyclo (his-pro), and arachidonic acid. *Metabolism* 50:53–59.

Song, Y.; Manson, J.E.; Buring, J.E.; and Liu, S. 2004. A prospective study of red meat consumption and type 2 diabetes in middle-aged and elderly women: the Women's Health Study. *Diabetes Care* 27:2108–2115.

Steffen, L.M.; Jacobs, D.R., Jr.; Stevens, J.; Shahar, E.; Carithers, T.; and Folsom, A.R. 2003. Associations of whole-grain, refined grain, and fruit and vegetable consumption with risks of all-cause mortality and incident coronary artery disease and ischemic stroke: the Atherosclerosis Risk in Communities (ARIC) Study. *American Journal of Clinical Nutrition* 78:383–390.

Stevens, J.; Ahn, K.; Juhaer, I.; Houston, D.; Steffan, L.; and Couper, D. 2002. Dietary fiber intake and glycemic index and incidence of diabetes in African-American and white adults. *Diabetes Care* 25:1715–1721.

Swinburn, B.A.; Metcalf, P.A.; and Ley, S.J. 2001. Long-term (5-year) effects of a reduced fat diet intervention in individuals with glucose intolerance. *Diabetes Care* 24:619–624.

Tuomilehto, J.; Lindstrom, J.; Ericsson, J.G.; Valle, T.T.; Hamalainen, H.; Iianne-Parikka, P.; Keinanen-Kiukaanniemi, S.; Laakso, M.; Louheranta, A.; Rastas, M.; Salminnen, V.; and Uusitupa, M. 2001. Prevention of type 2 diabetes mellitus by changes in lifestyle among subjects with impaired glucose tolerance. *New England Journal of Medicine* 344:1343–1350.

Van Dam, R.M. and Hu, F.B. 2005. Coffee consumption and risk of type 2 diabetes: a systematic review. *J.A.M.A.* 294:97–104.

Van Dam, R.M.; Willett, W.C.; Rimm, E.B.; Stampfer, M.J.; and Hu, F.B. 2002. Dietary fat and meat intake in relation to risk of type 2 diabetes in men. *Diabetes Care* 25:417–424.

Waller, S.M.; Vander Wal, J.S.; Klurfeld, D.M.; McBurney, M.I.; Cho, S.; Bijlani, S.; and Dhurandhad, N.V. 2004. Evening ready-to-eat cereal consumption contributes to weight management. *Journal of the American College of Nutrition* 23:316–321.

Wilson, J.F. 2003. Should doctors prescribe alcohol to adults? *Annals of Internal Medicine* 139:711–714.

Yang, G.; Shu, X-O.; Jin, F.; Elasy, T.; Li, H-L.; Li, Q.; Huang, F.; Gao, Y-T.; and Zheng, W. 2004. Soyfood consumption and risk of glycosuria: a cross-sectional study within the Shanghai Women's Health Study. *European Journal of Clinical Nutrition* 58:615–620.

Ylönen, K.; Alfthan, G.; Groop, L.; Saloranta, C.; Aro, A.; Virtanen, S.M.; and Botnia Research Group. 2003. Dietary intakes and plasma concentrations of carotenoids and tocopherols in relation to glucose metabolism in subjects at high risk of type 2 diabetes: the Botnia Dietary Study. *American Journal of Clinical Nutrition* 77:1434–1441.

4 Whole Grains and Related Dietary Patterns in Relation to Weight Gain

Nicola McKeown, Mary Serdula, and Simin Liu

Introduction

Obesity rates continue to escalate in the United States (Hedley et al. 2004) and in much of the developing world (Popkin 2001). According to data from the 1999 to 2002 National Health Examination Survey (NHANES), two-thirds of Americans are overweight and about 31% are obese (Hedley et al. 2004). The health burdens associated with obesity are extensive and include increased risk of several chronic diseases such as cardiovascular disease (CVD), type 2 diabetes mellitus (DM), gallbladder disease, and certain cancers (Must et al. 1999).

In fact, obesity is the single most important risk factor for type 2 DM, although other obesity-related factors include increased abdominal fat mass, weight gain since young adulthood, and a sedentary lifestyle (Colditz et al. 1995, Helmrich et al. 1991, Wang et al. 2005). Abdominal obesity is also an important determinant of the metabolic syndrome (Vega 2004), a condition characterized by disturbed glucose and insulin metabolism, obesity, mild dyslipidemia, and hypertension (Reavan 1988). Recently the National Cholesterol Education Program (NCEP 2001) proposed that obesity be a primary target of intervention for this syndrome, which affects an estimated 64 million Americans (Ford et al. 2004).

Although genetic disposition is an underlying risk factor of obesity (Bouchard and Tremblay 1997, Moreno-Aliaga et al. 2005), environmental factors such as diet and physical activity are indisputably the major factors contributing to the obesity epidemic. Weight gain arises as a consequence of positive energy balance, which results from excessive caloric intake and/or reduced physical activity (Swinburn et al. 2004). The percentage of dietary fat has been identified as an important factor in the development of obesity (Bray and Popkin 1998), although some experts disagree (Willett and Leibel 2002). Although evidence from animal studies suggests that overfeeding animals with a large percentage of energy from fat can cause obesity and insulin resistance (Storlien et al. 1986, 1991), the magnitude and long-term significance of the effect of a high-fat diet on obesity in humans remains controversial (Liu and Manson 2001, Willet and Leibel 2002).

Although it appears that the contribution of energy intake derived from dietary fat is decreasing in the United States (Briefel and Johnson 2004), the prevalence of obesity continues to increase (Flegal et al. 2002, Gross et al. 2004). This raises questions as to whether excessive fat intake alone is the main dietary factor to influence caloric consumption and body weight.

The increased contribution of energy from carbohydrates, particularly refined carbohydrates in the form of processed grains, soft drinks, and sugars, is now largely responsible for increases in energy intake (Gross et al. 2004) and for the obesity epidemic. Refined grain products in the diet may be displacing fiber-rich carbohydrate sources such as whole grains. Current dietary recommendations emphasize the benefits of low-fat, high-carbohydrate diets in reducing chronic diseases (DHHS, USDA 2005). However, some experts have expressed concern over these recommendations, arguing that increased carbohydrate intake may adversely affect blood lipid and lipoprotein concentrations and glucose metabolism (Jeppesen et al. 1997, Mittendorfer and Sidossis 2001), thereby predisposing some individuals to develop the metabolic syndrome type 2 DM and CVD.

Over the years, low-carbohydrate, high-protein diets, such as Atkins and the Zone, have gained popularity with respect to weight loss (Westman et al. 2003). Recently, randomized controlled trials compared the effect of low-carbohydrate diets with low-fat diets on body weight in obese adults (Brehm et al. 2003, Foster et al. 2003, Samaha et al. 2003, Stern et al. 2004, Yancy et al. 2004). Although after six months those randomized to the low-carbohydrate diet had greater weight loss than those on the low-fat diet (8.5 kg loss compared to 4 kg loss), after one year the two groups showed no difference in weight loss in two of the trials (Foster et al. 2003, Stern et al. 2004). Thus, for weight loss, the long-term efficacy of low-carbohydrate diets over low-fat diets has yet to be convincingly demonstrated in clinical trials.

Excessive intake of both dietary fats and carbohydrates can contribute to excessive caloric consumption; however, these macronutrients should not be viewed as single entities but rather should be broken down into their sources and types. Dietary carbohydrates traditionally were classified as simple or complex on the basis of the number of simple sugar units per molecule. However, such a classification does not provide a physiological distinction between glucose molecules obtained from starch and those obtained from simple sugars.

Consequently, the glycemic index (GI) was developed as an alternative way of classifying carbohydrates. The GI denotes the blood glucose response to standard amounts of individual foods (containing 50 grams of available carbohydrate) compared with the response to a standard amount of carbohydrate from a control food (glucose or white bread) (Jenkins et al. 1981). In general, refined foods have high GIs, while unprocessed foods such as whole grains, vegetables, legumes, and fruits have lower GIs (Foster-Powell et al. 2002). A related concept, the dietary glycemic load (GL), is the product of the carbohydrate and the GI of a serving of food (Liu et al., 2000c). GL thereby incorporates both quantitative and qualitative effects of carbohydrates on postprandial glycemia.

Recently, Brand-Miller and colleagues (2003) validated this concept by demonstrating that increases in dietary GL predicted stepwise increases in glycemia and insulinemia in a small group of healthy individuals. To date, only a few observational studies have examined the relationship between dietary GI and/or GL and adiposity and weight gain, with inconsistent results (Ma et al. 2005, McKeown et al. 2004b, Sahyoun et al. 2005, Toeller et al. 2001).

In observational studies, carbohydrates have been classified according to their food sources, such as whole or refined grains (Jacobs et al. 1998, Liu et al. 1999) or according to the contribution of dietary fiber from cereals, fruit, vegetables, or legumes (McKeown et al. 2004a, Meyer et al. 2000). Combining these classifications captures several attributes of carbohydrates that may help regulate body weight. Epidemiologic evidence appears to support the hypothesis that diets high in dietary fiber (Koh-Banerjee et al. 2004, Liu et al. 2003, Ludwig et al. 1999b) and whole grain foods (Koh-Banerjee et al. 2003, 2004, Liu et al. 2003) prevent weight gain and obesity, whereas the role of low-GI diets remains inconclusive (Ma et al. 2005, McKeown et al. 2004b, Sahyoun et al. 2005, Toeller et al. 2001).

This chapter emphasizes prospective studies that have examined the relationship between aspects of carbohydrate-related dietary factors and weight gain. The advantage of prospective studies over cross-sectional studies is that dietary data are collected before the outcome data on weight status are collected. Regardless of the study design, however, misclassification of body weight may arise in studies that rely on self-reported rather than measured body weight (Kuczmarski et al. 2001).

In most prospective studies, dietary intake is determined using a food frequency questionnaire (FFQ), an approach that minimizes the day-to-day variation in intake by assessing average long-term dietary intake. Nevertheless, because of the inherent difficulties in assessing dietary intake, misclassification of intake is unavoidable, thereby making the interpretation and comparison of results across studies difficult. Observational studies have attempted to minimize this misclassification by comparing extreme quintiles of dietary intake. The rationale behind this type of analysis is that people with extreme intakes are less likely to be misclassified. In studies of whole-grain intake and body weight, results may be confounded by correlated lifestyle and dietary habits. For instance, individuals who consume more whole grain foods may be more likely to engage in regular physical activity, be less likely to smoke cigarettes, and have a healthier diet (for example lower in fat intake) (Jacobs et al. 1998, Liu et al. 1999). Although prospective studies adjust for potential confounding factors (age, sex, physical activity, smoking, energy intake, and other dietary aspects), unmeasured potential confounders may bias the study findings.

This chapter reviews the epidemiologic evidence linking carbohydrate-related dietary factors, particularly whole grain dietary fiber and related dietary patterns to weight gain and measure of adiposity. These measures include body mass index (BMI), a measure of overall obesity; waist-to-hip ratio, a measure of intra-abdominal obesity; and waist circumference, a measure of visceral and subcutaneous fat.

Whole Grains, Dietary Fiber, and Weight Gain

During the milling process, the bran and germ are removed from the starchy endosperm, resulting in the loss of fiber and several nutrients, thereby interfering with the quality of the carbohydrate (Slavin et al. 2000). For example, processing whole grains into white flour increases caloric density by more than 10%, reduces the amount of dietary fiber by 80%, and reduces the amount of dietary protein by almost 30% (Durtshi 2001). Thus, refined grains are nutritionally inferior to whole grains—lower in fiber, several vitamins and minerals, phenolic compounds, phytoestrogens, and other unmeasured constituents (Slavin et al. 1999). Observational studies have found that diets rich in whole grain foods are related to a lower risk of cardiovascular disease (Jensen et al. 1998, 2004; Liu et al. 2000b, 1999) and type 2 diabetes (Liu et al. 2000a, Meyer et al. 2000), whereas there appear to be no health benefits associated with refined grains.

Until recently, the term "whole grain" was applied uniformly to both foods containing the intact grain and to foods that contain the appropriate proportions of all the milled grain constituents (i.e., bran, endosperm, and germ). However, a recent prospective study classified whole grains by their respective whole grain and non-whole grain ingredients (Jensen et al. 2004, Koh-Banerjee et al. 2004). Emerging evidence suggests that the bran component of whole grain foods may contain the most important bioactive constituents (Anderson 2004). Jensen and colleagues (2004) found that men with the highest intake of added bran had almost a 30% lower risk of CHD compared to men who did not consume bran, independent of dietary fiber.

Few metabolic studies have examined the role of whole grain intake on body composition. One small study found no change in body fat or fat-free mass (determined by underwater weighing) following six weeks on a hypocaloric oat-containing diet (Saltzman et al. 2001). Similarly, a randomized cross-over study of overweight adults found that although body weight was reduced more after six weeks on a whole grain diet than on a refined grain diet, the reduction was not significant (Pereira et al. 2002). In patients with coronary artery disease, replacement of refined white rice with whole grain and legume powder for twelve weeks did not alter BMI (Jang et al. 2001). The short follow-up period (six to twelve weeks) in these studies may have been insufficient to observe significant weight loss in participants.

Although several cross-sectional studies have found that diets high in whole grain are associated with lower body weight (Jacobs et al. 1998, Liu et al. 1999, McKeown et al. 2002, Pereira et al. 1998), only recently have whole grain intake and weight gain been examine in prospective studies (Koh-Banerjee et al. 2003, 20004; Liu et al. 2003). To date, two prospective studies have examined the relationship between changes in grain intake (estimated using FFQs) and weight gain (Koh-Banerjee et al. 2004, Liu et al. 2003). In 74,091 middle-aged women, an increase in whole-grain intake was associated with less weight gain over twelve years of follow-up (Liu et al. 2003). In this cohort, women who increased their intake of whole grain foods gained significantly less weight (1.23 kg compared to 1.52 kg) over a two- to four-year period than did women whose whole-grain intake remained low. These differences in weight gain were independent of changes in intakes of different types of fats and caloric intake. In the same cohort, refined-grain intake was associated with significantly greater weight gain: those who increased their consumption of refined grains gained more weight (1.57 kg compared to 1.14 kg in the highest versus lowest quintile change in refined grain intake) (Liu et al. 2003).

Similarly, Koh-Banerjee and colleagues (2004) examined the changes in whole grain intake and eight-year weight gain in 27,082 healthy middle-aged men. In this cohort, men who increased their intake of whole grain foods gained significantly less weight over eight years than did men with lower changes in intakes of whole grains (1.24 kg compared to 0.75 kg in highest versus lowest quintile change in whole grain intake). After correction for measurement error in estimates of whole-grain intake, the authors estimated that for every 40g increase in whole grain intake, long-term weight gain was reduced by 1.1 kg. Interestingly, increases in added bran (i.e. wheat, corn, rice, or oat bran) intake also predicted less weight gain over eight years. Men in the highest quintile of change (i.e. those increasing their bran intake the most) gained less weight than did men in the lowest quintile. Jensen and colleagues (2004) found that men with the highest intake of added bran had almost a 30% lower risk of coronary heart disease compared to men who did not consume bran, independent of dietary fiber.

Only three prospective studies have investigated dietary fiber and weight gain (Koh-Banerjee et al. 2004, Liu et al. 2003, Ludwig et al. 1999b). In the Coronary Artery Risk Development in Young Adults (CARDIA) study, dietary fiber intake over ten years was inversely associated with body weight in 2,909 young adults (Ludwig et al. 1999b).

Furthermore, Ludwig and colleagues (1999b) reported that individuals who consumed more dietary fiber gained less weight over ten years compared to those eating the least fiber, regardless of the intake of total dietary fat. Liu and colleagues also examined the relationship between dietary fiber intake and weight gain over twelve years in the Nurses Health Study (Liu et al. 2003). In that study, women who increased their intake of dietary fiber over the twelve-year follow-up period gained significantly less weight (3.64 kg compared to 5.16 kg) than did women with the smallest increase in fiber intake. The authors estimated that an increase of 12 grams per day of fiber was associated with approximately 3.5 kg (8 pounds) less weight gain in women, after adjusting for risk factors and correcting for measurement error.

A similar observation was made in middle-aged men participating in the Male Health Professional Study (Koh-Banerjee et al. 2004). In that study, men who increased their intake of dietary fiber over eight years gained significantly less weight (0.39 kg compared to 1.40 kg) than did men with the smallest increase in fiber intake. The authors estimated that long-term weight gain was reduced by 5.5 kg for each 20-gram per day increase in dietary fiber, after adjusting for risk factors and correcting for measurement error.

These findings regarding fiber and weight gain are consistent with the prospective data linking whole-grain intake with less weight gain. In the same study, Koh-Banerjee and colleagues (2004) considered whether the physiologic consequences of a high-fiber diet on weight change depended on the food source of dietary fiber such as fruit, vegetable, or cereal fiber. They found that both fruit and cereal fiber were inversely related in a dose-dependent manner to weight gain in middle-aged men. Thus, there is a need for further prospective studies to evaluate the relationship between fiber source and weight gain.

Only two prospective studies have examined the relationship between dietary fiber and measures of abdominal adiposity (Koh-Banerjee et al. 2003, Ludwig et al. 1999b). In the CARDIA study, dietary fiber was inversely associated with waist-to-hip ratio in young adults (Ludwig et al. 1999b). In a prospective study of middle-aged men, an increase in dietary fiber consumption of 12 grams per day significantly predicted a reduction in waist circumference of 2.21 cm ($P < 0.001$), and this relation was not altered after adjusting for fat sub-types (Koh-Banerjee et al. 2003). A 2.5 cm difference in waist circumference is associated with approximately 20% greater risk for the development of type 2 diabetes (Chan et al. 1994).

Dietary Patterns, Food Groups, and Weight Gain

In recent years, rather than focusing on individual foods and nutrients, observational studies have applied dietary-pattern analysis, such as cluster or factor analysis to capture total diet behavior in relation to weight gain (Newby et al. 2003, 2004; Quatromoni et al. 2002). Cluster analysis separates individuals into mutually exclusive groups on the basis of differences in mean food intakes, thereby grouping individuals with similar dietary characteristics (Romesburg 1984). In contrast, factor analysis reduces the overall diet to a few important food groups on the basis of the correlation between the consumption of specific foods and assigns a score to each of the factors identified (Morrison 1990). The advantage of these techniques is that they capture the complexity of food intake by considering the overall diet rather than individual foods or nutrients.

Prospective studies using dietary patterns have identified carbohydrate-related food patterns that are differentially related to weight gain. Newby and colleagues used both cluster (2003) and factor analysis (2004) to identify food patterns, using data from seven-day diet records, in relation to anthropometric changes in 459 participants in the Baltimore Longitudinal Study of Aging. Using cluster analysis (Newby et al. 2003), five clusters were identified and labeled according to the foods providing the greatest contribution to energy. Energy intakes in the white bread, alcohol, sweets, meats, and potatoes clusters were the greatest from these foods, while the healthy cluster, comprised of foods high in fiber cereals, fruit, vegetables, and reduced fat dairy and low in processed meat, fast food, and soda, had smaller gains in both BMI and waist circumference. The mean annual change in BMI was 0.05 kg/m^2 $\pm$ 0.06 kg/m^2 and 0.43 cm $\pm$ 0.27 cm for waist circumference with the healthy cluster. In contrast, a significant greater gain in waist circumference (1.32 cm/year $\pm$ 0.29 cm/year) was observed with the white bread cluster. In the Framingham Nutrition Study, five dietary patterns identified using cluster analysis did not predict overweight status after twelve years of follow-up in middle-aged men and women (Quatromoni et al. 2002).

Newby and colleagues (2004) confirmed, using factor analysis, that individuals whose diet was high rather than low in reduced-fat dairy products and high-fiber foods had smaller gains in BMI and waist circumference). However, food intake patterns using factor analysis did not predict changes in BMI or development of obesity after five or eleven years of follow-up in Danish middle-aged men and women (Togo et al. 2001). Clearly, the evidence linking dietary patterns to weight gain is inconsistent, which may in part be attributed to different methods used to capture dietary exposures (cluster vs. factor), inadequate control for confounding, or different age groups of populations studied.

Food patterns also have been captured using a novel approach called the reduced rank regression (RRR) (Hoffmann et al. 2004, Kroke 2004). This approach derives dietary patterns using both prior information on nutrient-disease and data from the study, taking into account the correlation structure between foods and nutrients. Schulz and colleagues (2005) used a food pattern score derived from this method to examine whether nutrient density predicted subsequent yearly weight change in 24,958 middle-aged German men and women. They found that a higher food pattern score, characterized by high-fiber and low-fat food choices, predicted less weight gain among older, normal, and overweight adults, but not obese adults. In relation to short-term weight change, a higher intake of cereals predicted greater weight loss ($\leq$ 2kg/year), while higher intakes of meat and fat in women and higher intake of sweets in men predicted weight gain ($\geq$ 2kg/year) (Schulz et al. 2002). In another study, self-reported decreases in fat and fatty foods and increased intake of fruits resulted in the smallest body-weight gain over time in adults (Drapeau et al. 2004), consistent with some prospective studies linking a healthy diet with less body-weight gain over time (Newby et al. 2003, 2004; Schulz et al. 2005). However, the evidence linking dietary patterns or food groups to weight gain is inconsistent. In conclusion, current evidence linking carbohydrate-related dietary patterns to weight gain or weight loss is contradictory, and more prospective studies testing this hypothesis are warranted.

Whole Grains and Body Weight: Potential Mechanisms

There are several potential mechanisms whereby whole-grain foods may prevent weight gain. The low-energy density (i.e. less calories per gram weight of food) or bulk-forming properties of whole-grain foods (attributed to the high dietary fiber and water content) may induce satiety and satiation (Pereira and Pins 2000). Feeding studies have found that increased dietary fiber intake, whether in the form of higher-fiber foods or fiber supplements, appears to increase satiety and/or decrease hunger, thereby facilitating weight loss (Howarth et al. 2001).

Alternatively, enhanced insulin sensitivity, either through the effects of fiber, magnesium, or other attributes (e.g. low GI or particle size) of whole-grain foods, may prevent weight gain. Short-term intervention studies have shown that dietary fiber (Fukagawa et al. 1990, Juntunen et al. 2003) and whole grain diets (Pereira et al. 2002) reduce serum insulin and glucose concentrations and improve insulin sensitivity. In the Framingham Offspring Cohort, fasting insulin concentrations were significantly lower among those consuming more whole-grain foods (McKeown et al. 2002), an observation consistent with other studies (Liese et al. 2003, Steffen et al. 2003). In the same cohort, cereal fiber rather than fiber from other sources (fruit, vegetable, legume) was associated with better insulin sensitivity (determined using the homeostatic model assessment) (McKeown et al. 2004a).

The greater particle size and lower GI of most whole grain foods (compared with refined-grain foods) might favorably affect blood glucose and insulin response. Short-term studies have found that carbohydrates with a high GI increase insulin demand and accentuate hyperinsulinemia (Jenkins et al. 1987, Wolever et al. 1992, Wolever and Mehling 2002). Another possible explanation is that the hormonal changes that occur during the postprandial period after a high-GI meal may stimulate hunger and voluntary food intake (Ludwig et al. 1999a), thereby predisposing a susceptible individual to weight gain.

Single-day feeding studies have demonstrated that low-GI carbohydrate foods enhance satiety and reduce total energy intake at the subsequent meal (Ludwig 2002). However, dietary intervention studies in adults have shown mixed evidence about whether energy-restricted diets based on low-GI foods produce greater weight or body fat loss than do equivalent diets based on high-GI foods. Sloth et al. (2004) investigated the effects of a low-fat, high-carbohydrate diet with either low-GI or high-GI carbohydrates on body weight over ten weeks in healthy overweight adults. Although the reduction in total body fat mass in adults on the low-GI diet was 2.5 times greater than the reduction in adults on the high-GI diet (1.0 compared with 0.4 kg; P = 0.20), this change was not statistically significant. Furthermore, the high-GI and low-GI diet produced no significant differences in trunk fat mass or waist circumference in these adults (Sloth et al. 2005).

In type 2 diabetic patients, no change in fat or lean body mass distribution was observed as determined by dual X-ray absorptiometry (DEXA) after four weeks on a low-GI diet compared to the high-GI diet (Rizkalla et al. 2004). In contrast, one randomized cross-over study observed a 0.7 kg decrease in total fat mass in eleven obese men after five weeks on an energy- and nutrient-controlled low- versus high-GI diet (Bouche et al. 2002). Interestingly, this decrease in fat mass was mostly abdominal (p < 0.001) and occurred in the absence of weight loss. A pilot, randomized controlled trial comparing the effects on CVD risk of a low-GL diet (emphasizing low-GI sources of carbohydrate) with a low-fat diet in a small group of obese young adults found no differences in body weight, percentage fat mass, or lean body mass after twelve months (Ebbeling et al. 2005). Inconsistencies between results of studies on GI and body weight may in part be attributed to too few subjects to detect differences in body fat (Sloth et al. 2004) or differing macronutrient contents, particularly dietary fiber (Bouche et al. 2002). Evidence on the usefulness of low-GI diets as a preventive measure against weight gain is limited by the lack of long-term intervention studies.

Conclusion

At both the individual and population levels, strategies that improve nutrition and increase physical activity are fundamental to the control of the epidemic of overweight and obesity (Expert Panel on the Identification, Evaluation, and Treatment of Obesity in Adults 1998, WHO 1998). Whole-grain foods may be one aspect of diet that plays a role in regulation of body weight. However, current data on the potential mechanisms whereby whole-grain foods may prevent weight gain are sparse. Thus, there is a need for studies to investigate whether the low energy density of whole-grain foods helps regulate body weight by reducing the total energy intake through satiety or whether enzyme inhibitors that exist in whole grains directly affect metabolic efficiency or perhaps another mechanism exists whereby whole grains have a beneficial effect on body weight.

On the basis of current observational evidence regarding whole grains and dietary fiber in relation to weight gain, more prospective data are needed to confirm (1) whether the inverse relationship between whole grain intake and weight gain is attributed to the bran or to another component of whole grains, and (2) whether different fiber sources are related to weight gain. Although existing evidence from prospective studies suggests that individuals consuming more dietary fiber or whole grains gain less weight over time, long-term intervention studies that control dietary and other environmental factors are clearly needed.

References

Bouchard, C. and Tremblay, A. (1997). Genetic influences on the response of body fat and fat distribution to positive and negative energy balances in human identical twins. *J Nutr* 127, 943S–947S.

Bouche, C., Rizkalla, S. W., Luo, J., Vidal, H., Veronese, A., Pacher, N., Fouquet, C., Lang, V. and Slama, G. (2002). Five-week, low-glycemic index diet decreases total fat mass and improves plasma lipid profile in moderately overweight nondiabetic men. *Diabetes Care* 25, 822–8.

Brand-Miller, J. C., Thomas, M., Swan, V., Ahmad, Z. I., Petocz, P. and Colagiuri, S. (2003). Physiological validation of the concept of glycemic load in lean young adults. *J Nutr* 133, 2728–32.

Bray, G. A. and Popkin, B. M. (1998). Dietary fat intake does affect obesity! *Am J Clin Nutr* 68, 1157–73.

Brehm, B. J., Seeley, R. J., Daniels, S. R. and D'Alessio, D. A. (2003). A randomized trial comparing a very low carbohydrate diet and a calorie-restricted low fat diet on body weight and cardiovascular risk factors in healthy women. *J Clin Endocrinol Metab* 88, 1617–23.

Briefel, R. R. and Johnson, C. L. (2004). Secular trends in dietary intake in the United States. *Annu Rev Nutr* 24, 401–31.

Chan, J. M., Stampfer, M. J., Rimm, E. B., Willett, W. C. and Colditz, G. A. (1994). Obesity, fat distribution, and weight gain as risk factors for clinical diabetes in men. *Diabetes Care* 17, 961–969.

Colditz, G. A., Willett, W. C., Rotnitzky, A. and Manson, J. E. (1995). Weight gain as a risk factor for clinical diabetes mellitus in women. *Ann Intern Med* 122, 481–6.

Drapeau, V., Despres, J. P., Bouchard, C., Allard, L., Fournier, G., Leblanc, C. and Tremblay, A. (2004). Modifications in food-group consumption are related to long-term body-weight changes. *Am J Clin Nutr* 80, 29–37.

Durtshi, A. (2001). Nutritional content of whole grains versus their refined flours. Walton Feed Company. February 5, 2001. Data source: USDA Economic Research Service.

Ebbeling, C. B., Leidig, M. M., Sinclair, K. B., Seger-Shippee, L. G., Feldman, H. A. and Ludwig, D. S. (2005). Effects of an ad libitum low-glycemic load diet on cardiovascular disease risk factors in obese young adults. *Am J Clin Nutr* 81, 976–82.

Expert Panel on the Identification, Evaluation, and Treatment of Overweight in Adults. (1998). Clinical guidelines on the identification, evaluation, and treatment of overweight and obesity in adults: executive summary. *Am J Clin Nutr* 68, 899–917.

Flegal, K. M., Carroll, M. D., Ogden, C. L. and Johnson, C. L. (2002). Prevalence and trends in obesity among US adults, 1999-2000. *JAMA* 288, 1723–7.

Ford, E. S., Giles, W. H. and Mokdad, A. H. (2004). Increasing prevalence of the metabolic syndrome among U.S. Adults. *Diabetes Care* 27, 2444–9.

Foster, G. D., Wyatt, H. R., Hill, J. O., McGuckin, B. G., Brill, C., Mohammed, B. S., Szapary, P. O., Rader, D. J., Edman, J. S. and Klein, S. (2003). A randomized trial of a low-carbohydrate diet for obesity. *N Engl J Med* 348, 2082–90.

Foster-Powell, K., Holt, S. H. and Brand-Miller, J. C. (2002). International table of glycemic index and glycemic load values: 2002. *Am J Clin Nutr* 76, 5–56.

Fukagawa, N. K., Anderson, J. W., Hageman, G., Young, V. R. and Minaker, K. L. (1990). High-carbohydrate, high-fiber diets increase peripheral insulin sensitivity in healthy young and old adults. *Am J Clin Nutr* 52, 524–8.

Gross, L. S., Li, L., Ford, E. S. and Liu, S. (2004). Increased consumption of refined carbohydrates and the epidemic of type 2 diabetes in the United States: an ecologic assessment. *Am J Clin Nutr* 79, 774–9.

Hedley, A. A., Ogden, C. L., Johnson, C. L., Carroll, M. D., Curtin, L. R. and Flegal, K. M. (2004). Prevalence of overweight and obesity among US children, adolescents, and adults, 1999–2002. *JAMA* 291, 2847–50.

Helmrich, S. P., Ragland, D. R., Leung, R. W. and Paffenbarger, R. S., Jr. (1991). Physical activity and reduced occurrence of non-insulin-dependent diabetes mellitus. *N Engl J Med* 325, 147–52.

Hoffmann, K., Schulze, M. B., Schienkiewitz, A., Nothlings, U. and Boeing, H. (2004). Application of a new statistical method to derive dietary patterns in nutritional epidemiology. *Am J Epidemiol* 159, 935–44.

Howarth, N. C., Saltzman, E. and Roberts, S. B. (2001). Dietary fiber and weight regulation. *Nutr Rev* 59, 129–39.

Jacobs, D. R., Jr., Meyer, K. A., Kushi, L. H. and Folsom, A. R. (1998). Whole-grain intake may reduce the risk of ischemic heart disease death in postmenopausal women: the Iowa Women's Health Study [see comments]. *Am J Clin Nutr* 68, 248–57.

Jang, Y., Lee, J. H., Kim, O. Y., Park, H. Y. and Lee, S. Y. (2001). Consumption of whole grain and legume powder reduces insulin demand, lipid peroxidation, and plasma homocysteine concentrations in patients with coronary artery disease: randomized controlled clinical trial. *Arterioscler Thromb Vasc Biol* 21, 2065–71.

Jenkins, D. J., Wolever, T. M., Collier, G. R., Ocana, A., Rao, A. V., Buckley, G., Lam, Y., Mayer, A. and Thompson, L. U. (1987). Metabolic effects of a low-glycemic-index diet. *Am J Clin Nutr* 46, 968–75.

Jenkins, D. J., Wolever, T. M., Taylor, R. H., Barker, H., Fielden, H., Baldwin, J. M., Bowling, A. C., Newman, H. C., Jenkins, A. L. and Goff, D. V. (1981). Glycemic index of foods: a physiological basis for carbohydrate exchange. *Am J Clin Nutr* 34, 362–6.

Jensen, M. K., Koh-Banerjee, P., Hu, F. B., Franz, M., Sampson, L., Gronbaek, M. and Rimm, E. B. (2004). Intakes of whole grains, bran, and germ and the risk of coronary heart disease in men. *Am J Clin Nutr* 80, 1492–9.

Jeppesen, J., Schaaf, P., Jones, C., Zhou, M. Y., Chen, Y. D. and Reaven, G. M. (1997). Effects of low-fat, high-carbohydrate diets on risk factors for ischemic heart disease in postmenopausal women. *Am J Clin Nutr* 65, 1027–33.

Juntunen, K. S., Laaksonen, D. E., Poutanen, K. S., Niskanen, L. K. and Mykkanen, H. M. (2003). High-fiber rye bread and insulin secretion and sensitivity in healthy postmenopausal women. *Am J Clin Nutr* 77, 385–91.

Koh-Banerjee, P., Chu, N. F., Spiegelman, D., Rosner, B., Colditz, G., Willett, W. and Rimm, E. (2003). Prospective study of the association of changes in dietary intake, physical activity, alcohol consumption, and smoking with 9-y gain in waist circumference among 16 587 US men. *Am J Clin Nutr* 78, 719–27.

Koh-Banerjee, P., Franz, M., Sampson, L., Liu, S., Jacobs, D. R., Jr., Spiegelman, D., Willett, W. and Rimm, E. (2004). Changes in whole-grain, bran, and cereal fiber consumption in relation to 8-y weight gain among men. *Am J Clin Nutr* 80, 1237–45.

Kroke, A. (2004). Application of a new statistical method to derive dietary patterns in nutritional epidemiology. *Am J Epidemiol* 160, 1132; author reply 1132–3.

Kuczmarski, M. F., Kuczmarski, R. J. and Najjar, M. (2001). Effects of age on validity of self-reported height, weight, and body mass index: findings from the Third National Health and Nutrition Examination Survey, 1988-1994. *J Am Diet Assoc* 101, 28–34; quiz 35–6.

Liese, A. D., Roach, A. K., Sparks, K. C., Marquart, L., D'Agostino, R. B., Jr. and Mayer-Davis, E. J. (2003). Whole-grain intake and insulin sensitivity: the Insulin Resistance Atherosclerosis Study. *Am J Clin Nutr* 78, 965–71.

Liu, S. and Manson, J. E. (2001). What is the optimal weight for cardiovascular health? *BMJ* 322, 631–2.

Liu, S., Manson, J. E., Stampfer, M. J., Hu, F. B., Giovannucci, E., Colditz, G. A., Hennekens, C. H. and Willett, W. C. (2000a). A prospective study of whole-grain intake and risk of type 2 diabetes mellitus in US women. *Am J Public Health* 90, 1409–15.

Liu, S., Manson, J. E., Stampfer, M. J., Rexrode, K. M., Hu, F. B., Rimm, E. B. and Willett, W. C. (2000b). Whole Grain Consumption and Risk of Ischemic Stroke in Women: A Prospective Study. *JAMA* 284, 1534–1540.

Liu, S., Stampfer, M. J., Hu, F. B., Giovannucci, E., Rimm, E., Manson, J. E., Hennekens, C. H. and Willett, W. C. (1999). Whole-grain consumption and risk of coronary heart disease: results from the Nurses' Health Study [see comments]. *Am J Clin Nutr* 70, 412–9.

Liu, S., Willett, W. C., Manson, J. E., Hu, F. B., Rosner, B. and Colditz, G. (2003). Relation between changes in intakes of dietary fiber and grain products and changes in weight and development of obesity among middle-aged women. *Am J Clin Nutr* 78, 920–7.

Liu, S., Willett, W. C., Stampfer, M. J., Hu, F. B., Franz, M., Sampson, L., Hennekens, C. H. and Manson, J. E. (2000c). A prospective study of dietary glycemic load, carbohydrate intake, and risk of coronary heart disease in US women. *Am J Clin Nutr* 71, 1455–61.

Ludwig, D. S. (2002). The glycemic index: physiological mechanisms relating to obesity, diabetes, and cardiovascular disease. *JAMA* 287, 2414–23.

Ludwig, D. S., Majzoub, J. A., Al-Zahrani, A., Dallal, G. E., Blanco, I. and Roberts, S. B. (1999a). High glycemic index foods, overeating, and obesity. *Pediatrics* 103, E26.

Ludwig, D. S., Pereira, M. A., Kroenke, C. H., Hilner, J. E., Van Horn, L., Slattery, M. L. and Jacobs, D. R., Jr. (1999b). Dietary fiber, weight gain, and cardiovascular disease risk factors in young adults [see comments]. *JAMA* 282, 1539–46.

Ma, Y., Olendzki, B., Chiriboga, D., Hebert, J. R., Li, Y., Li, W., Campbell, M., Gendreau, K. and Ockene, I. S. (2005). Association between dietary carbohydrates and body weight. *Am J Epidemiol* 161, 359–67.

McKeown, N. M., Meigs, J. B., Liu, S., Saltzman, E., Wilson, P. W.F. and Jacques, P. F. (2004a). Carbohydrate nutrition, insulin resistance, and the prevalence of the metabolic syndrome in the Framingham Offspring Cohort. *Diabetes Care* 27, 538–46.

McKeown, N. M., Meigs, J. B., Liu, S., Saltzman, E., Wilson, P. W. F. and Jacques, P. F. (2004b). Dietary Glycemic Index is related to metabolic risk factors in the Framingham Offspring Cohort. In *Federation of American Societies for Experimental Biology*, vol. Abstract #582.1. Washington.

McKeown, N. M., Meigs, J. B., Liu, S., Wilson, P. W. and Jacques, P. F. (2002). Whole-grain intake is favorably associated with metabolic risk factors for type 2 diabetes and cardiovascular disease risk in the Framingham Offspring Study. *AJCN* 76, 390–8.

Meyer, K. A., Kushi, L. H., Jacobs, D. R., Jr., Slavin, J., Sellers, T. A. and Folsom, A. R. (2000). Carbohydrates, dietary fiber, and incident type 2 diabetes in older women. *Am J Clin Nutr* 71, 921–30.

Mittendorfer, B. and Sidossis, L. S. (2001). Mechanism for the increase in plasma triacylglycerol concentrations after consumption of short-term, high-carbohydrate diets. *Am J Clin Nutr* 73, 892–9.

Moreno-Aliaga, M. J., Santos, J. L., Marti, A. and Martinez, J. A. (2005). Does weight loss prognosis depend on genetic make-up? *Obes Rev* 6, 155–68.

Morrison, D. (1990). Multivariate Statistical Methods. New York: McGraw-Hill.

Must, A., Spadano, J., Coakley, E. H., Field, A. E., Colditz, G. and Dietz, W. H. (1999). The disease burden associated with overweight and obesity. *JAMA* 282, 1523–9.

NCEP (2001). Executive Summary of the Third Report of The National Cholesterol Education Program (NCEP) Expert Panel on Detection, Evaluation, And Treatment of High Blood Cholesterol In Adults (Adult Treatment Panel III). *JAMA* 285, 2486–97.

Newby, P. K., Muller, D., Hallfrisch, J., Andres, R. and Tucker, K. L. (2004). Food patterns measured by factor analysis and anthropometric changes in adults. *Am J Clin Nutr* 80, 504–13.

Newby, P. K., Muller, D., Hallfrisch, J., Qiao, N., Andres, R. and Tucker, K. L. (2003). Dietary patterns and changes in body mass index and waist circumference in adults. *Am J Clin Nutr* 77, 1417–25.

Pereira, M. A., Jacobs, D. R., Jr., Pins, J. J., Raatz, S. K., Gross, M. D., Slavin, J. L. and Seaquist, E. R. (2002). Effect of whole grains on insulin sensitivity in overweight hyperinsulinemic adults. *Am J Clin Nutr* 75, 848–55.

Pereira, M. A., Jacobs, D. R., Slattery, M. L., Ruth, K. J., Van Horn, L., Hilner, J. E. and Kushi, L. H. (1998). The association of whole grain intake and fasting insulin in a biracial cohort of young adults: The CARDIA Study. *CVD Prevention* 1, 231–242.

Pereira, M. A. and Pins, J. J. (2000). Dietary fiber and cardiovascular disease: experimental and epidemiologic advances. *Curr Atheroscler Rep* 2, 494–502.

Popkin, B. M. (2001). The nutrition transition and obesity in the developing world. *J Nutr* 131, 871S–873S.

Quatromoni, P. A., Copenhafer, D. L., D'Agostino, R. B. and Millen, B. E. (2002). Dietary patterns predict the development of overweight in women: The Framingham Nutrition Studies. *J Am Diet Assoc* 102, 1239–46.

Reaven, G. M. (1988). Banting lecture 1988. Role of insulin resistance in human disease. *Diabetes* 37, 1595–607.

Rizkalla, S. W., Taghrid, L., Laromiguiere, M., Huet, D., Boillot, J., Rigoir, A., Elgrably, F. and Slama, G. (2004). Improved plasma glucose control, whole-body glucose utilization, and lipid profile on a low-glycemic index diet in type 2 diabetic men: a randomized controlled trial. *Diabetes Care* 27, 1866–72.

Romesburg, H.C. (1984). Cluster Analysis for Researchers. Belmont, CA: Lifetime Learning Publications.

Sahyoun, N. R., Anderson, A. L., Kanaya, A. M., Koh-Banerjee, P., Kritchevsky, S. B., de Rekeneire, N., Tylavsky, F. A., Schwartz, A. V., Lee, J. S. and Harris, T. B. (2005). Dietary glycemic index and load, measures of glucose metabolism, and body fat distribution in older adults. *Am J Clin Nutr* 82, 547–52.

Saltzman, E., Das, S. K., Lichtenstein, A. H., Dallal, G. E., Corrales, A., Schaefer, E. J., Greenberg, A. S. and Roberts, S. B. (2001). An oat-containing hypocaloric diet reduces systolic blood pressure and improves lipid profile beyond effects of weight loss in men and women. *J Nutr* 131, 1465–70.

Samaha, F. F., Iqbal, N., Seshadri, P., Chicano, K. L., Daily, D. A., McGrory, J., Williams, T., Williams, M., Gracely, E. J. and Stern, L. (2003). A low-carbohydrate as compared with a low-fat diet in severe obesity. *N Engl J Med* 348, 2074–81.

Schulz, M., Kroke, A., Liese, A. D., Hoffmann, K., Bergmann, M. M. and Boeing, H. (2002). Food groups as predictors for short-term weight changes in men and women of the EPIC-Potsdam cohort. *J Nutr* 132, 1335–40.

Schulz, M., Nothlings, U., Hoffmann, K., Bergmann, M. M. and Boeing, H. (2005). Identification of a food pattern characterized by high-fiber and low-fat food choices associated with low prospective weight change in the EPIC-Potsdam cohort. *J Nutr* 135, 1183–9.

Slavin, J. L., Jacobs, D. and Marquart, L. (2000). Grain processing and nutrition. *Crit Rev Food Sci Nutr* 40, 309–26.

Slavin, J. L., Martini, M. C., Jacobs, D. R., Jr. and Marquart, L. (1999). Plausible mechanisms for the protectiveness of whole grains. *Am J Clin Nutr* 70, 459S–463S.

Sloth, B., Krog-Mikkelsen, I., Flint, A., Tetens, I., Astrup, A., Raben, A., Bjorck, I. and Elmstahl, H. (2005). Letter: Reply to J Brand-Miller. *AJCN* 81, 723–724.

Sloth, B., Krog-Mikkelsen, I., Flint, A., Tetens, I., Bjorck, I., Vinoy, S., Elmstahl, H., Astrup, A., Lang, V. and Raben, A. (2004). No difference in body weight decrease between a low-glycemic-index and a high-glycemic-index diet but reduced LDL cholesterol after 10-wk ad libitum intake of the low-glycemic-index diet. *Am J Clin Nutr* 80, 337–47.

Steffen, L. M., Jacobs, D. R., Jr., Murtaugh, M. A., Moran, A., Steinberger, J., Hong, C. P. and Sinaiko, A. R. (2003). Whole grain intake is associated with lower body mass and greater insulin sensitivity among adolescents. *Am J Epidemiol* 158, 243–50.

Stern, L., Iqbal, N., Seshadri, P., Chicano, K. L., Daily, D. A., McGrory, J., Williams, M., Gracely, E. J. and Samaha, F. F. (2004). The effects of low-carbohydrate versus conventional weight loss diets in severely obese adults: one-year follow-up of a randomized trial. *Ann Intern Med* 140, 778–85.

Storlien, L. H., James, D. E., Burleigh, K. M., Chisholm, D. J. and Kraegen, E. W. (1986). Fat feeding causes wide-spread in vivo insulin resistance, decreased energy expenditure, and obesity in rats. *Am J Physiol* 251, E576–83.

Storlien, L. H., Jenkins, A. B., Chisholm, D. J., Pascoe, W. S., Khouri, S. and Kraegen, E. W. (1991). Influence of dietary fat composition on development of insulin resistance in rats. Relationship to muscle triglyceride and omega-3 fatty acids in muscle phospholipid. *Diabetes* 40, 280–9.

Swinburn, B. A., Caterson, I., Seidell, J. C. and James, W. P. (2004). Diet, nutrition and the prevention of excess weight gain and obesity. *Public Health Nutr* 7, 123–46.

Toeller, M., Buyken, A. E., Heitkamp, G., Cathelineau, G., Ferriss, B. and Michel, G. (2001). Nutrient intakes as predictors of body weight in European people with type 1 diabetes. *Int J Obes Relat Metab Disord* 25, 1815–22.

Togo, P., Osler, M., Sorensen, T. I. and Heitmann, B. L. (2004). A longitudinal study of food intake patterns and obesity in adult Danish men and women. *Int J Obes Relat Metab Disord* 28, 583–93.

U.S. Department of Health and Human Services and the U.S. Department of Agriculture. Dietary Guidelines for Americans 2005. Internet: http://www.healthierus.gov/dietaryguidelines/ (accessed 18 December 2005).

Vega, G. L. (2004). Obesity and the metabolic syndrome. *Minerva Endocrinol* 29, 47–54.

Wang, Y., Rimm, E. B., Stampfer, M. J., Willett, W. C. and Hu, F. B. (2005). Comparison of abdominal adiposity and overall obesity in predicting risk of type 2 diabetes among men. *Am J Clin Nutr* 81, 555–63.

Westman, E. C., Mavropoulos, J., Yancy, W. S. and Volek, J. S. (2003). A review of low-carbohydrate ketogenic diets. *Curr Atheroscler Rep* 5, 476–83.

Willett, W. C. and Leibel, R. L. (2002). Dietary fat is not a major determinant of body fat. *Am J Med* 113 Suppl 9B, 47S–59S.

Wolever, T. M., Jenkins, D. J., Vuksan, V., Jenkins, A. L., Buckley, G. C., Wong, G. S. and Josse, R. G. (1992). Beneficial effect of a low glycaemic index diet in type 2 diabetes. *Diabet Med* 9, 451–8.

Wolever, T. M. and Mehling, C. (2002). High-carbohydrate-low-glycaemic index dietary advice improves glucose disposition index in subjects with impaired glucose tolerance. *Br J Nutr* 87, 477–87.

World Health Organization, (1998). Obesity: preventing and managing the global epidemic. Report of a WHO consultation on obesity. Geneva: World Health Organization.

Yancy, W. S., Jr., Olsen, M. K., Guyton, J. R., Bakst, R. P. and Westman, E. C. (2004). A low-carbohydrate, keto-genic diet versus a low-fat diet to treat obesity and hyperlipidemia: a randomized, controlled trial. *Ann Intern Med* 140, 769–77.

5   Whole Grains and Cardiovascular Disease

Joanne Slavin

Introduction

Epidemiologic studies find that whole grains protect against cardiovascular disease. Whole grains are rich in nutrients and phytochemicals with known health benefits, including dietary fiber, antioxidants such as trace minerals, and phenolic compounds. Other protective compounds in whole grains include phytate; phytoestrogens such as lignan; plant stanols and sterols; and vitamins and minerals. Feeding studies report improvements in biomarkers with whole grain consumption, such as weight loss, blood lipid improvement, and antioxidant protection. Although it is difficult to separate the protective properties of whole grains from dietary fiber and other components, the disease protection seen from whole grains in prospective epidemiologic studies exceeds the protection from isolated nutrients and phytochemicals in whole grains. Inclusion of at least three servings of whole grains per day is recommended to reduce the risk of cardiovascular disease.

Historical Background on Whole Grains

Whole grains became part of the human diet with the advent of agriculture about 10,000 years ago (Spiller et al. 2002). For the last 3,000 to 4,000 years, a majority of the world's population has relied upon whole grains as a main portion of the diet. In North America, wheat, oats, barley, and rye were harvested as staple foods as early as the American Revolution. It is only within the past one hundred years that most people have consumed refined grain products.

Health aspects of whole grains have long been known. In the fourth century B.C., Hippocrates, the father of medicine, recognized the health benefits of whole grain bread. More recently, physicians and scientists in the early 1800s to mid-1900s recommended whole grains to prevent constipation. The "fiber hypothesis," published in the early 1970s, suggested that whole foods, such as whole grains, fruits, and vegetables, provide fiber along with other constituents that have health benefits.

What Are Whole Grains?

The major cereal grains include wheat, rice, and corn, with oats, rye, barley, triticale, sorghum, and millet as minor grains. In the U.S., the most commonly consumed grains are wheat, oats, rice, corn, and rye, with wheat constituting 66% to 75% of the total. Buckwheat, wild rice, and amaranth are not botanically true grains but are typically associated with the grain family due to their similar composition (Table 5.1).

About 50% to 75% of the endosperm is starch, and it is the major energy supply for the embryo during germination of the kernel. The endosperm also contains storage proteins, typically 8% to 18%, along with cell wall polymers. Relatively few vitamins, minerals, fiber, or phytochemicals are located in the endosperm fraction. The germ is a relatively minor contributor to the dry weight of most grains (typically 4% to 5% in wheat and barley). The germ

Table 5.1. Available whole grains.

Whole wheat
Wild rice
Whole oats/oatmeal
Buckwheat
Whole-grain corn
Triticale
Popcorn
Bulgur (cracked wheat)
Brown rice
Millet
Whole rye
Quinoa
Whole-grain barley
Sorghum

Source: 2005 Dietary Guidelines for Americans

of corn contributes a much higher proportion to the total grain structure than that of wheat, barley, or oats.

Components in Whole Grains

The bran and germ fractions derived from conventional milling provide a majority of the biologically active compounds found in a grain. Specific nutrients include high concentrations of B vitamins (thiamin, niacin, riboflavin, and pantothenic acid) and minerals (calcium, magnesium, potassium, phosphorus, sodium, and iron), elevated levels of basic amino acids (e.g., arginine and lysine), and elevated tocol levels in the lipids. Numerous phytochemicals, some common in many plant foods (phytates and phenolic compounds) and some unique to grain products (avenanthramides, avenalumic acid), are responsible for the high antioxidant activity of whole grain foods (Miller et al. 2002).

Generally, grains are ground into flour and processed into grain-based foods. A nutrient comparison of whole wheat flour and enriched, white wheat flour in shown in Table 5.2. Most

Table 5.2. Comparison of 100 grams of whole grain wheat flour and enriched, white, all-purpose flour.

	Whole-grain wheat flour	White flour
Calories	339	364
Dietary fiber—g	12.2	2.7
Calcium—mg	34	15
Magnesium—mg	138	22
Potassium—mg	405	107
Folate—ug	44	291
Thiamin—mg	0.5	0.8
Riboflavin—mg	0.2	0.5
Niacin—mg	6.4	5.9
Iron—mg	3.9	4.6

Source: 2005 Dietary Guidelines for Americans

Table 5.3. Differences in dietary fiber content among whole grains (100 grams as eaten).

	Dietary fiber—grams
Brown rice	1.8
Whole grain cornmeal	7.3
Whole oats	10.3
Whole grain wheat	12.2

of the dietary fiber is lost in the milling process, with significant losses in calcium, magnesium, and potassium also particularly evident. White flour is enriched in thiamin, riboflavin, niacin, iron, and folic acid; some whole grain products are also enriched with folic acid.

Components in whole grains associated with improved health status include lignans, tocotrienols, phenolic compounds, and antinutrients including phytic acid, tannins, and enzyme inhibitors. In the grain refining process the bran is removed, resulting in loss of dietary fiber, vitamins, minerals, lignans, phytoestrogens, phenolic compounds, and phytic acid. Thus, refined grains are more concentrated in starch because most of the bran and some of the germ is removed in the refining process. Even though dietary fiber is an important component of grains, not all whole grains are high in dietary fiber (Table 5.3).

Whole Grains and Cardiovascular Disease

Cardiovascular disease (C.V.D.) is the number one cause of death and disability of both men and women in this country. There is strong epidemiological and clinical evidence linking consumption of whole grains to a reduced risk for coronary heart disease (Anderson 2002). Morris et al. (1977) followed 337 subjects for ten to twenty years and concluded that a reduction in heart disease risk was attributable to a higher intake of cereal fiber, while indicating soluble sources such as pectin and guar did not account for the lower coronary heart disease (C.H.D.). Brown et al. (1999) concluded that soluble fiber from different fiber sources was associated with small but significant decreases in total cholesterol. A pooled analysis of cohort studies on dietary fiber and the risk of coronary heart disease found that consumption of dietary fiber from cereals was inversely associated with risk of coronary heart disease (Pereira et al. 2004).

Other compounds in grains, including antioxidants, phytic acid, lectins, phenolic compounds, amylase inhibitors, and saponins have all been shown to alter risk factors for C.H.D. It is likely that the combination of compounds in grains, rather than any one component, explains its protective effects in C.H.D.

Large prospective epidemiologic studies have found a moderately strong association between whole grain intake and decreased C.H.D. risk. Post-menopausal women (34,492), age 55 to 69 years and free of C.H.D., were followed in the large prospective Iowa Women's Health Study for occurrence of C.H.D. mortality (n = 387) between baseline (1986) and 1994 (Jacobs et al. 1998). Whole grain intake was determined by seven items in a 127-item food frequency questionnaire which was used to divide participants into quintiles based on mean servings of whole-grain intake per day. The risk reduction in higher whole grain intake quintiles was controlled for more than fifteen confounding variables, and was not explained by adjustment for dietary fiber intake. This suggests that whole grain components other than dietary fiber may reduce risk for C.H.D.

In a Finnish study, 21,930 male smokers (aged 50 to 69 years) were followed for 6.1 years (Pietinen et al. 1996). Reduced risk of C.H.D. death was associated with an increased intake of rye products. Rimm et al. (1996) examined the association between cereal intake and a risk for myocardial infarction (M.I.) in 43,757 U.S. health professionals, aged 40 to 75 years. Cereal fiber was most strongly associated with reduced risk for M.I. with a 0.71 decrease in risk for each 10-gram-increase in cereal fiber intake.

The Nurses' Health Study, a large, prospective cohort study of U.S. women followed up for ten years, also was used to examine the relationship between grain intake and cardiovascular risk (Liu et al., 1999). A total of 68,782 women aged 37 to 64 years without previously diagnosed angina, myocardial infarction, stroke, cancer, hypercholesterolemia, or diabetes at baseline were studied. Dietary data were collected with a validated semiquantitative food frequency questionnaire. After controlling for age, cardiovascular risk factors, dietary factors, and multivitamin supplement use, the relative risk was 0.77 (95% C.I., 0.57 to 1.04). For a 10 gram/day increase in total fiber intake (the difference between the lowest and highest quintiles), the multivariate relative risk (R.R.) of total C.H.D. events was 0.81 (95% C.I., 0.66 to 0.99). Among different sources of dietary fiber (cereal, vegetable, fruit), only cereal fiber was strongly associated with a reduced risk of C.H.D. (multivariate RR, 0.63; 95% C.I., 0.49 to 0.81 for each 5 gram/day increase in cereal fiber). The authors conclude that higher fiber intake, particularly from cereal sources, reduces the risk of C.H.D.

Because whole grains are the predominant dietary fiber source in the United States, it is difficult to separate out the protection of dietary fiber from whole grains. Jensen et al. (2004) examined intake of whole grains, bran, and germ and risk of coronary heart disease from food frequency data in the Health Professionals Follow-up study. Added germ was not associated with C.H.D. risk and the authors conclude that the study supports the reported beneficial association of whole-grain intake with C.H.D. and suggests that the bran component of whole grain could be a key factor in this relation.

Food consumption patterns that include whole grains also appear protective for cardiovascular disease. Van Dam et al. (2003) report that intake of refined diets which do not include whole grains were associated with higher serum cholesterol levels and lower intakes of micronutrients. A prudent dietary pattern, including intake of whole grains, was associated with lower C-reactive protein levels and endothelial dysfunction, an early step in the development of atherosclerosis (Lopez-Garcia et al. 2004). Whole grain food intake was also associated with lower levels of C-reactive protein in the Nurses' Health Study (Wu et al. 2004). A prospective cohort study of post-menopausal women found that consumption of cereal fiber and whole grain intake was associated with reduced progression of coronary-artery atherosclerosis (Erkkila et al. 2005).

Feeding Studies

Whole grain feeding studies have looked at biomarkers relevant to cardiovascular disease. Katz et al. (2001) measured the effect of oat and wheat cereals on endothelial responses in human subjects. They report that month-long, daily supplementation with either whole grain oat or wheat cereal may prevent postprandial impairment of vascular reactivity in response to a high-fat meal. In a randomized controlled clinical trial, consumption of whole grain and legume powder reduced insulin demand, lipid peroxidation, and plasma homocysteine concentrations in patients with coronary artery disease (Jang et al. 2001). Finally, consumption of whole grain oat cereal was associated with improved blood pressure control and reduced the need for antihypertensive medications (Pins et al. 2002). Thus, clinical studies to date support that whole grain consumption can improve biomarkers relevant to diabetes and cardiovascular disease.

Some feeding studies have been conducted to evaluate the relationship between whole grains and glucose metabolism. Pericra et al. (2002) tested the hypothesis that whole grain consumption improves insulin sensitivity in overweight and obese adults. Eleven overweight or obese hyperinsulinemic adults aged 25 to 56 years consumed two diets, each for six weeks. Diets were identical, except that refined grain products were replaced by whole grain products. At the end of each treatment, subjects consumed 355 ml of a liquid mixed meal, and blood samples were taken over two hours. Fasting insulin was 10% lower during consumption of the whole grain diet. The authors conclude that insulin sensitivity may be an important mechanism whereby whole grain foods reduce the risk of type 2 diabetes and heart disease.

Juntunen et al. (2002) evaluated what factors in grain products affected human glucose and insulin responses. They fed the following grain products: whole-kernel rye bread, whole-meal rye bread containing oat beta-glucan concentrate, dark durum wheat pasta, and wheat bread made from white wheat flour. Glucose responses and the rate of gastric emptying after consumption of the two rye breads and pasta did not differ from those after consumption of white wheat bread. Insulin, glucose-dependent insulinotropic polypeptide, and glucagon-like peptide 1 were lower after consumption of rye breads and pasta than after consumption of white wheat bread. These results support that postprandial insulin responses to grain products are determined by the form of food and botanical structure rather than by the amount of fiber or the type of cereal in the food.

McKeown et al. (2002) reported that whole grain intake was inversely associated with body mass index and fasting insulin in the Framingham Offspring Study. Juntunen et al. (2003) fed high-fiber rye bread and white-wheat bread to postmenopausal women and measured glucose and insulin metabolism. Acute insulin response increased significantly during the rye bread periods than during the wheat bread period. They suggest that high-fiber rye bread appears to enhance insulin secretion, possibly indicating improvement of beta cell function.

McIntosh et al. (2003) fed rye and wheat foods to overweight middle-aged men and measured markers of bowel health. The men were fed low-fiber cereal grain foods providing 5 grams of dietary fiber for the refined grain diet and 18 grams of dietary fiber for the whole grain diet, either high in rye or wheat. This was in addition to a baseline diet that contained 14 grams of dietary fiber. Both the high-fiber rye and wheat foods increased fecal output by 33% to 36% and reduced fecal β-glucuronidase activity by 29%. Postprandial plasma insulin was decreased by 46% to 49% and postprandial plasma glucose by 16% to 19%. Rye foods were associated with significantly increased plasma enterolactone and fecal butyrate, relative to wheat and low-fiber diets. The authors conclude that rye appears more effective than wheat in overall improvement of biomarkers of bowel health.

Bioactive Compounds in Whole Grains That Protect Against C.V.D.

There are many theories how whole grains help lower the risk of cardiovascular disease. Whole grains are rich in compounds such as tocotrienols, a form of vitamin E, which play an important role in disease prevention, including reducing the risk of heart disease (Slavin et al. 1999). Whole grains are also a source of plant sterols, such as beta-sitosterol, which can lower cholesterol. And, whole grains are an excellent source of dietary fiber, resistant starch, and oligosaccharides, which are fermented by intestinal microflora to short chain fatty acids, such as acetate, butyrate, and propionate. Short chain fatty acids have been shown to lower serum cholesterol (Hara et al. 1999).

Whole grains are good sources of dietary magnesium, fiber, and vitamin E, which are involved in insulin metabolism. Relatively high intakes of these nutrients from whole grains may prevent hyperinsulinemia. Whole grains also may influence insulin levels through beneficial effects on satiety and body weight. However, even after adjusting for body mass index, studies have found a strong inverse relationship between whole grain intake and fasting insulin levels.

Dietary Fiber

In 2002, the Dietary Reference Intakes (D.R.I.s) included fiber as a nutrient. Dietary fiber was defined as nondigestible carbohydrates and lignin that are intrinsic and intact in plants. Foods high in dietary fiber include whole grains, legumes, vegetables, and fruits. Another class of fiber, functional fiber, was defined as nondigestible carbohydrates extracted from foods that have beneficial physiological effects in humans. Functional fiber is found in bulk laxatives, fortified foods, beverages, and dietary supplements. Total fiber was then defined as the sum of dietary fiber and functional fiber.

Previously, dietary fiber was divided into soluble and insoluble fiber in an attempt to assign physiological effects to chemical types of fiber. Oat bran and psyllium, two mostly soluble fibers, have health claims for their ability to lower serum lipids. Wheat bran and other more insoluble fibers are linked to laxation. Yet, scientific support that soluble fibers lower blood cholesterol, while insoluble fibers increase stool size, is inconsistent at best. Resistant starch and inulin, both considered soluble fibers, do not lower blood cholesterol. Thus, not all soluble fibers lower blood cholesterol, and other traits such as viscosity of fiber play roles.

The 2005 Dietary Guidelines support a fiber intake of 14 grams per 1,000 kcal to reduce the risk of cardiovascular disease and promote healthful laxation. Average fiber intakes in the United States are only about 14 grams/day, so most of us fall woefully short on fiber intake. In contrast, the vegetarians among us routinely consume 50 grams/day of fiber, and fiber intake of Paleolithic man (the fruit and nut gatherer and wild game slayer) has been estimated at 100 grams/day.

Antioxidants

Whole grain products are relatively high in antioxidant activity. Antioxidants found in whole grain foods are water-soluble and fat-soluble, and approximately half are insoluble. Soluble antioxidants include phenolic acids, flavonoids, tocopherols, and avenanthramides in oats. A large part of insoluble antioxidants are bound as cinnamic acid esters to arabinoxylan side chains of hemicellulose. Wheat bran insoluble fiber contains approximately 0.5% to 1% phenolic groups. Covalently bound phenolic acids are good free radical scavengers. About two-thirds of whole grain antioxidant activity is not soluble in water, aqueous methanol, or hexane.

In addition to natural antioxidants, antioxidant activity is created in grain-based foods by browning reactions during baking and toasting processes that increase total activity in the final product as compared to raw ingredients. For example, the crust of white bread has double the antioxidant activity of the starting flour or crust-free bread. Reductone intermediates from Maillard reactions may explain the increase in antioxidant activity. The total antioxidant activity of whole grain products is similar to that of fruits or vegetables on a per-serving basis (Miller et al. 2002).

Adom and Liu (2002) suggest that the antioxidant activity of grains reported in the literature has been underestimated because only unbound antioxidants are usually studied. They report that 90% of the antioxidants are bound in wheat. Bound phytochemicals could survive stomach and intestinal digestion, but would then be released in the large intestine and potentially play a protective role. When they compared antioxidant activity of various grains, corn had the highest total antioxidant activity, followed by wheat, oats, and rice.

Phytic acid, concentrated in grains, is a known antioxidant. Phytic acid forms chelates with various metals, which suppresses damaging iron-catalyzed redox reactions. Colonic bacteria produce oxygen radicals in appreciable amounts and dietary phytic acid may suppress oxidant damage to intestinal epithelium and neighboring cells.

Vitamin E is another antioxidant present in whole grains that is removed in the refining process. Vitamin E is an intracellular antioxidant that protects polyunsaturated fatty acids in cell membranes from oxidative damage. Another possible mechanism for vitamin E relates to its capacity to keep selenium in the reduced state. Vitamin E inhibits the formation of nitrosamines, especially at low pH. Magnesium may mediate the favorable impact of whole grains on insulin sensitivity by acting as a mild calcium antogaonist (McCarty 2005). Whole grains are a particularly rich source of magnesium.

Lignans

Hormonally active compounds in grains called lignans may protect against hormonally mediated diseases (Adlercreutz and Mazur 1997). Lignans are compounds possessing a 2,3-dibenzylbutane structure and exist as minor constituents of many plants where they form the building blocks for the formation of lignin in the plant cell wall. The plant lignans secoisolariciresinol and matairesinol are converted by human gut bacteria to the mammalian lignans enterolactone and enterodiol. Concentrated sources of lignans include whole grain wheat, whole grain oats, and rye meal. Seeds such as flaxseed seeds (the most concentrated source), pumpkin seeds, caraway seeds, and sunflower seeds are also concentrated sources of lignans.

Grains and other high-fiber foods increase urinary lignan excretion, an indirect measure of lignan content in foods (Borriello et al. 1985). Differences in metabolism of phytoestrogens among individuals have been noted. Adlercreutz et al. (1986) found total urinary lignan excretion in Finnish women to be positively correlated with total fiber intake, total fiber intake per kg body weight, and grain fiber intake per kg body weight. Similarly, the geometric mean excretion of enterolactone was positively correlated with the geometric mean intake of dietary grain products (kcal/day) of five groups of women (r = 0.996).

Serum enterolactone was measured in a cross-sectional study in Finnish adults (Kilkkinen et al. 2001). In men, serum enterolactone concentrations were positively associated with the consumption of whole grain products. Variability in serum enterolactone concentration was great, suggesting that the role of gut microflora in the metabolism of lignans may be important. Kilkkinen et al. (2003) also report that intake of lignans is associated with serum enterolactone concentration in Finnish men and women. They suggest that serum enterolactone is a feasible biomarker of lignan intake. Jacobs et al. (2002) found similar results in a U.S. study. Subjects were fed either whole grain or refined grain foods for six weeks. Most of the increase in serum enterolactone when eating the whole grain diet occurred within two weeks, though the serum enterolactone difference between whole grain and refined-grain diets continued to increase throughout the six-week study.

Serum enterolactone is associated with reduced cardiovascular disease-related and all-cause death in middle-aged Finnish men (Vanharanta et al. 2003). The authors suggest that this evidence supports the importance of whole grain foods, fruits, and vegetables in the prevention of premature death from C.V.D.

Phytosterols

Plant sterols and stanols are found in oilseeds, grains, nuts, and legumes. These compounds are known to reduce serum cholesterol (Yankah and Jones 2001). Structurally, they are very similar to cholesterol, differing in side chain methyl and ethyl groups. It is believed that phytosterols inhibit dietary and biliary cholesterol absorption from the small intestine. Phytosterols have better solubility than cholesterol in bile salt micelles in the small intestine. Phytosterols displace cholesterol from micelles, which reduces cholesterol absorption and increases its excretion (Hallikainen et al. 2000). The sterol must be consumed at the same time as cholesterol to inhibit absorption of dietary cholesterol. The amount of plant sterols and stanols required to have significant cholesterol-lowering effect is debated. Although a significant effect has been reported for less than 1 gram/day, intakes of 1 gram to 2 grams/day are usually suggested. A dose response effect is reported for phytosterols that plateaus at about 2.5 grams/day. The average Western diet contains an estimated 200 mg to 300 mg/day of plant sterols. Vegetarians may consume up to 500 mg/day. Increased whole grain consumption would increase total phytosterol intake and potentially contribute to cholesterol reduction.

Unsaturated Fatty Acids

Whole grain wheat contains about 3% lipids and whole grain oats are about 7.5% lipids. Grain lipids are about 75% unsaturated, comprised of nearly equal amounts of oleic and linoleic acid and 1% to 2% of linolenic acid. Palmitate is the main unsaturated fat. There are approximately 2 grams of unsaturated lipid/100 grams of whole wheat and about 5.5 grams for whole oat foods. Both these fatty acids are known to reduce serum cholesterol and are an important component of a heart-healthy diet. Other studies show the cholesterol-lowering effect of grain lipids or high-lipid bran products (Gerhardt and Gallo 1998).

Antinutrients

Antinutrients found in grains include digestive enzyme (protease and amylase) inhibitors, phytic acid, hemagglutinins, and phenolics/tannins. Phytic acid, lectins, phenolics, amylase inhibitors, and saponins have also been shown to lower plasma glucose, insulin, and/or plasma cholesterol and triglycerides (Slavin et al. 1999). In grains, protease inhibitors make up 5% to 10% of the water-soluble protein and are concentrated in the endosperm and embryo.

Conclusion

Whole grains are rich in many components, including dietary fiber, starch, fat, antioxidant nutrients, minerals, vitamins, lignans, and phenolic compounds that have been linked to a reduced risk of coronary heart disease and other chronic diseases. Most of the protective components are found in the bran and germ, which are reduced in the grain refining process. Unfortunately, consumers are generally not receptive to increasing whole grain intake and usual intake is only one serving per day while a minimum of three whole grains or half of grain servings per day of whole grains are recommended.

References

Adlercreutz H and Mazur W. Phyto-oestrogens and western diseases. *Annals of Medicine* 1997;29, 95–120.

Adlercreutz H, Fotsis T, Bannwart C, Hamalainen E, Bloigu A and Ollus A. Urinary estrogen profile determination in young Finnish vegetarian and omnivorous women. *J Steroid Biochem* 1986;24, 289–296.

Adom KK and Liu RH. Antioxidant activity of grains. *J Agric Food Chem* 2002;50:6182–6187.

Anderson, JW. Whole-grains intake and risk for coronary heart disease. *In Whole-Grain Foods in Health and Disease* pp 187–200 (Marquart, Slavin, and Fulcher, editors). St. Paul, Minn.: Eagan Press, 2002.

Borriello SP, Setchell KD, Axelson M and Lawson AM. Production and metabolism of lignans by the human faecal flora. *Journal of Applied Bacteriology* 1985;58, 37–43.

Brown L, Rosner B, Willett WW and Sacks FM. Cholesterol-lowering effects of dietary fiber: a meta-analysis. *Am J Clin Nutr* 1999;69:30–42.

Erkkila AT, Herrington DM, Mozaffarian D, and Lichtenstein AH. Cereal fiber and whole-grain intake are associated with reduced progression of coronary-artery atherosclerosis in postmenopausal women with coronary artery disease. *Am Heart J* 2005;150:94–101.

Gerhardt AL and Gallo NB. Full-fat rice bran and oat bran similarly reduce hypercholesterolemia in humans. *J Nutr* 1998; 128:865–869.

Hallikainen MA, Sarkkinen ES and Uusitupa MIJ. Plant stanols esters affect serum cholesterol concentrations of hypercholesterolemic men and women in a dose-dependent manner. *J Nutr* 2000;130, 767–776.

Hara H, Haga S, Aoyama Y and Kiriyama S. Short-chain fatty acids suppress cholesterol synthesis in rat liver and intestine. *J Nutr* 1999;129:942–948.

Jacobs DR, Meyer KA, Kushi LH and Folsom AR. Whole-grain intake may reduce the risk of ischemic heart disease death in postmenopausal women: The Iowa Women's Health Study. *Amer J Clini Nutr* 1998; 68:248–257.

Jacobs DR, Pereira MA, Stumpf K, Pins JJ and Adlercreutz H. Whole grain food intake elevates serum enterolactone. *Br J Nutr* 2002;88:111–116.

Jang Y, Lee JH, Kim OY, Park HY and Lee SY. Consumption of whole grain and legume powder reduces insulin demand, lipid peroxidation, and plasma homocysteine concentrations in patients with coronary artery disease: randomized controlled clinical trial. *Arterscler Thromb Vasc Biol* 2001;21, 2065–2071.

Jensen MK, Koh-Benerjee P, Hu FB, Franz M, Sampson L, Cronbak M, Rimm EB. Intakes of whole grains, bran, and germ and the risk of coronary heart disease in men. *Am J Clin Nutr* 2004; 80:1492–1499.

Juntunen KS, Niskanen LK, Liukkonen KH, Poutanen KS, Holst JJ and Hykkanen HM. Postprandial glucose, insulin, and incretin responses to grain products in healthy subjects. *Am J Clin Nutr* 2002;75, 254–262.

Juntunen KS, Laaksonen DE, Poutanen KS, Niskanen LK and Mykkanen HM. High-fiber rye bread and insulin secretion and sensitivity in healthy postmenopausal women. *Am J Clini Nutr* 2003; 77:385–391.

Katz DL, Nawaz H, Boukhalil J, Chan W, Ahmadi R, Giannamore V and Sarrel PM. Effects of oat and wheat cereals on endothelial responses. *Prevent Medicine* 2001;33, 476–484.

Kilkkinen A, Stumpf K, Pietinen P, Valsta LM, Tapanainen H and Adlercreutz H. Determinants of serum enterolactone concentration. *Am J Clin Nutr* 2001; 73, 1094–1100.

Kilkkinen A, Valsta LM, Virtamo J, Stumpf K, Adlercreutz H and Pietinen P. Intake of lignans is associated with serum enterolactone concentration in Finnish men and women. *J Nutr*; 2003;133:1830–1833.

Liu SM, Stampfer, MJ., Hu FB, Giovannucci E, Rimm E, Manson JE, Hennekens CH and Willett WC. Whole-grain consumption and risk of coronary heart disease: results from the Nurse's Health Study. *Am J Clin Nutr* 1999;70:412–429.

Lopez-Garcia E, Schulze MB, Fung TT, Meigs JB, Rifai N, Monson JE, and Hu FB. Major dietary patterns are related to plasma concentrations of markers of inflammation and endothelial dysfunction. *Am J Clin Nutr* 2004; 80:1029–1035.

McCarty MF. Magnesium may mediate the favorable impact of whole grains on insulin sensitivity by acting as a mild calcium antagonist. *Medical Hypothesis* 2005; 64:619–627.

McIntosh GH, Noakes M, Royle PJ and Foster PR. Whole-grain rye and wheat foods and markers of bowel health in overweight middle-aged men. *Am J Clin Nutr* 2003;77:967–974.

McKeown NM, Meigs JB, Liu S, Wilson PWF and Jacques PF. Whole-grain intake is favorably associated with metabolic risk factors for type 2 diabetes and cardiovascular disease in the Framingham Offspring Study. *Am J Clin Nutr* 2002; 76:390–398.

Miller G, Prakash A and Decker E. (2002) Whole-grain micronutrients. *In Whole-Grain Foods in Health and Disease* pp 243–258 (Marquart, Slavin, and Fulcher, editors). St. Paul, Minn.:Eagan Press.

Morris J, Marr J and Clayton D. Diet and heart: a postscript. *Br Med J* 1977; 2: 1307-1314.

Pereira MA, O'Reilly E, Augustsson K, Fraser GE, Goldbourt U, Heitmann BL, Hallmans G, Knekt P, Liu S, Pietinen P, Spiegelman D, Stevens J, Virtamo J, Willett WC, and Ascherio A. Dietary fiber and risk of coronary heart disease. A pooled analysis of cohort studies. *Arch Intern Med* 2004;164:370–376.

Pereira MA, Jacobs DJ, Pins JJ, Raatz SK, Gross MD, Slavin JL and Seaquist ER. Effect of whole grains on insulin sensitivity in overweight hyperinsulinemic adults. *Am J Clin Nutr* 2002;75, 848–855.

Pietinen P, Rimm EB, Korhonen P, Hartman AM, Willett WC, Albanes D, and Virtamo J. Intake of dietary fiber and risk of coronary heart disease in a cohort of Finnish men. The Alpha-Tocopherol, Beta-Carotene Cancer Prevention Study. *Circulation* 1996;94:2720–2727.

Pins JJ, Geleva D. Leemam K. Frazer C, O'Connor PJ and Cherney LM. Do whole-grain oat cereals reduce the need for antihypertensive medications and improve blood pressure control? *J Family Practice* 2002;51, 353–359.

Rimm EB, Ascherio A, Giovannucci E, Spiegelman D, Stampfer MJ and Willett WC. Vegetable, fruit and cereal fiber intake and risk of coronary heart disease among men. *J.A.M.A.* 1996;275:447–451.

Slavin JL, Martini MC, Jacobs DR and Marquart L. Plausible mechanisms for the protectiveness of whole grains. *Am J Clin Nutr* 1999;70, 459S–463S.

Spiller GA. (2002) Whole grains, whole wheat, and white flours in history. *In Whole-Grain Foods in Health and Disease* pp 1–7 (Marquart, Slavin, and Fulcher, editors). St. Paul, Minn.:Eagan Press.

Van Dam RM, Grievink L, Ocke MC and Feskens EJM. Patterns of food consumption and risk factors for cardiovascular disease in the general Dutch population. *Am J Clin Nutr* 2003;77:1156–1163.

Vanharanta M, Voutilainen S, Rissanen TH, Adlercreutz H and Salonen JT. Risk of cardiovascular disease-related and all-cause death according to serum concentrations of enterolactone. Kuopio Ischaemic Heart Disease Risk Factor Study. *Arch Internal Med* 2003;163:1099–1104.

Wu T, Giovannucci E, Pischon T, Hankinson SH, Ma J, Rifai N, and Rimm EB. Fructose, glycemic load, and quantity and quality of carbohydrate in relation to plasma C-peptide concentrations in U.S. women. *Am J Clin Nutr* 2004;80:1043–1049.

Yankah VV and Jones PJH. Phytosterols and health implications-efficacy and nutritional aspects. *Inform.*2001;12:899–903.

6 Whole Grains and Cancer Prevention

Graeme H. McIntosh

Introduction

Cancer has been a growing public health problem throughout the last century. In Australia (according to data taken from the Australian Bureau of Statistics 1995 national nutrition survey), of the 350 female and 430 male cases diagnosed per 100,000 people, breast and prostate cancers accounted for about one quarter of all cases in women and men, respectively. The next most frequently occurring in both sexes has been colorectal cancers, accounting for about 14%, with lung cancer and melanoma in men following closely behind, 12.2% and 10%, respectively. For women, lung cancer is less than melanoma, 6.9% and 9.9%, respectively.

The expression of these cancers in our society shows a pattern that reflects differing environmental hazards and lifestyles. It is generally recognized that whereas mouth, esophagus, and stomach cancers are associated with poor socioeconomic circumstances (environments lacking good hygiene, foods and/or food preservation systems), colorectal cancer is more associated with westernized cultures and generally high standards of living. To coin a phrase, "As the standard of living goes up the cancers go down (the gastrointestinal tract)." Cancers of the reproductive system are highly expressed—in males as prostate cancer and in females as breast and ovarian cancers—particularly in people 50 years of age and over.

Types of foods ingested can have an important bearing on the expression of such cancers. High intakes of red meats, fried foods, sweets, alcohol, and refined cereal foods, and poor intakes of fruits, vegetables, whole grain cereal foods, and low-fat dairy products, have been identified with increases in colorectal cancer risk. Sedentary lifestyles are also a significant part of the problem. The above factors are often associated with overweight or obesity, which correlates with increased risk of cancers. By contrast, people whose diets are rich in fruits, vegetables, nuts, and whole grain cereal foods, and who restrict meat and dairy products as low-fat options, consume moderate amounts of alcohol, and get significant amounts of physical exercise, are associated with significantly lower risks (one-half) of colorectal cancer. Breast and prostate cancers are significantly influenced by hormonal factors, and there is some evidence of dietary factors influencing their expression, e.g., fat intake versus fiber.

Whole grain cereal foods are widely used in diets, from poor third world cultures to wealthy industrialized cultures. The discussion regarding colon cancer and the importance of dietary fiber was significantly promoted by Burkitt (1970), who attributed the virtual absence of colon cancer in African nationals to high grain and dietary fiber consumption (as ground maize and sorghum). Whole grain foods are a major contributor to dietary fiber intake; they are one of the most concentrated sources of insoluble and soluble fibers in our diet. The availability of whole grain food choices with adequate labeling in our supermarket economy is somewhat limited, despite the extensive shelving space given over to breakfast cereals and breads, to name just two. Despite the make-your-own bread mix choices with good whole meal flours, they are unlikely to have significant impact, given the lack of time and convenience associated with a modern lifestyle.

Cereal and dairy foods provide interesting groups with a prominent and respected place in many food cultures, yet they have a small but vociferous chorus of opponents, coming particularly from "naturopaths and complementary medicine advocates" who attribute a number of intolerances and disturbances of the immune system (e.g., autoimmune diseases) to their consumption (Cordain 1999).

Epidemiological Evidence

There has been an extensive epidemiological analysis of food cultures with respect to diseases bringing on premature deaths, e.g. cancer and cardiovascular disease. Epidemiological evidence supporting whole grains and cancer prevention was reviewed previously (McIntosh and Jacobs 2002). There is a growing body of evidence for the role of whole grain foods providing significant protection against a number of degenerative diseases, including a number of cancers (Hill 1997). Significant protection against such degenerative diseases was reported with the "Mediterranean diet," which does need careful definition, but has been reported to diminish cardiovascular disease by 33% and cancers by 24% (Trichopoulou et al. 2003). In a number of protective diet lifestyles, whole grain foods are prominent, as compared with refined cereal foods, which can be associated with relatively increased risk that is not always well defined.

Such prudent food cultures have been reported from a variety of places: London, rural Sweden, northern India, the U.S., Greece, and southern Italy. They provide a picture of good foods in the face of a relative abundance of choice, with extensively processed and packaged foods not included. For example, significant protection against cancers has been reported with the "Mediterranean diet" (Gallus et al. 2004). Analysis in this report involved food groups as well as cancer sites. Risk of epithelial cancers was reduced with vegetables, fruits, fish, whole grains, and olive and other unsaturated fats. Cancers of the mouth, larynx, and esophagus showed a relative risk of about 0.3, while stomach and colon cancers were about 0.5 (La Vecchia et al. 2003a,b). Breast and prostate cancers showed little protective effect (RR = 0.9) of whole grain consumption (La Vecchia et al. 2003a, Gallus et al. 2004). In a U.S. study, rectal cancer relative risk reduction was 0.58 (Slattery et al. 2004). There is a coincidence of whole grain foods with dietary fiber and its protective effects in the large bowel, as reported in the European scientists consensus statement of 1998, with a RR reduction of 34% for colorectal cancers. Identification of relevant products which fit the description of high fiber cereal foods was an important qualification of this assessment. Inevitably, the recognition that refined cereal products fail to provide protection—indeed that they are associated with increased risk of diabetes, heart disease, and cancers—has increased the awareness and concern regarding their influence in western diets.

Mechanisms

Dietary Factors Responsible for Cancers

Increased sporadic colorectal cancer incidences have poor diet as a major causative factor; such diets include high saturated fat and grilled red meats (there is also concern about cooking methods because of mutagens formed in the process). High caloric/energy and low-residue diets, generally resulting from poor dietary fiber intakes, can lead to obesity, constipation, and inflammatory bowel conditions and increase cancer risk. Mutagens/carcinogens/cocarcinogens in foods include preservatives in processed meats such as nitrites and fungal agents such as aflatoxins, ochratoxins, some mushroom species such as morels containing hydrazines, or agents which were found in beers, stouts, etc. such as nitrosamines.

Flame grilled/barbequed meats, with production of meat mutagens (e.g. 2-amino-1-methyl-6-phenylimidazo[4,5-b]pyridine {PhIP} and 2-amino-3,4-dimethylimidazo[4,5-f] quinoline {MeIQ}) and high-saturated-fat processed meats (sausages, salami etc.), can increase risk. Products of some microbes in the colon may contribute to cancer risk, e.g. secondary bile acids (deoxycholic acid, a comutagenic agent formed from gut microbial changes to primary bile acids). Newmark et al. (2001) refer to western high-stress diets as low-fiber, high-sugar, low-calcium, high-phosphate, and poor in nutrient sources such as vitamin B_{12} and folate. High phosphate was equated with an increased risk of ulceration-inflammation (Bruce et al. 2000). High animal protein diets are thought to increase growth factor release, insulin growth factors, and insulinogenic responses which may increase cell proliferation in colonic epithelium and thereby increase cancer risk. Although high saturated fat diets are generally seen as the problem, high n6 polyunsaturated fats may also be of concern. Insulin resistance has been studied in rats using such high polyunsaturated fatty acid diets as corn or sunflower oil at 30% fat by weight (Belobrajdic et al. 2003).

High fructose diets are also associated with hyperinsulinemia in rats (Brusseroles et al. 2003) and are thought to be associated with significant overweight and obesity, which correlates with increased colon cancer risk.

The contribution of starch rich fiber depleted foods such as polished rice to type 2 diabetes in susceptible genotypes was first proposed by Trowell in 1973 (Trowell 1987). Insulin resistance observed in obese female Zucker rats was associated with colonic tumors and cancers, not seen in their lean relatives, when N-nitroso-N-methylurea (NMU) was systemically injected with the aim of inducing breast cancer (Lee et al. 2001). Hyperinsulinemia and insulin resistance is considered to be linked with increased colon cancer risk (Giovannucci 2001, Bruce et al., 2002).

Factors in Whole Grains Preventing Cancers

Grain foods and whole grain foods are major contributors to dietary fiber intake, accounting for 40% to 45% of the 25 grams dietary fiber per day intake in Australian diets (Australian Bureau of Statistics 1995). Whole grain and bran consumption has been shown to be inversely related to weight gain, suggesting they might contribute to metabolic conditions/alterations favoring reduced overweight and obesity (Koh-Banerjee et al. 2004). High-fiber diets have been associated with reduced serum inflammatory markers such as C-reactive protein (CRP) (Ajani et al. 2004).

Fermentation of carbohydrates in the colon is an important issue in the maintenance of health and prevention of inflammatory conditions and cancer (Cummings 1983, Hill 1995). Grains are good sources of dietary fiber components, which by definition, include nonstarch polysaccharides, resistant starches, sugar alcohols, and oligosaccharides. The latter (such as inulin and oligofructose), alone and in combination with probiotic bacteria, have been shown to significantly reduce colonic aberrant crypt foci and tumors induced with azoxymethane (AOM) (Femia et al. 2002).

Resistant starch has been shown to improve a number of bowel health markers, including increased butyrate (Noakes et al. 1996). Significant sugar use and lowered starch intake, however, promoted colon cancers (Caderni et al. 1994), while starch, and in particular, resistant starch, escapes digestion to undergo fermentation in the colon and provide a significant amount of short chain fatty acids (S.C.F.A.s) including butyrate. Starch in the diet was shown to correlate with reduced colon cancer expression across differing populations (Cassidy et al. 1994). Butyrate is effective as a differentiating/antineoplastic agent (Cummings 1997, Davie 2003). Butyrate has an antineoplastic effect by a number of possible mechanisms which include modulation of gene expression, inhibition of cell growth and increased differentiation, increased histone acetylation, and induced apoptosis. Propionate may have an additive effect with butyrate in this respect. This may well have contributed to the starch observations of Caderni, although they did not measure resistant starch in their studies.

Other factors produced in fermentation of dietary fibers could also be relevant in inhibiting cancer cells (Beyer-Sehlmeyer et al. 2003). Such fermentative activity and short-chain fatty acids may improve availability and uptake of cations such as calcium and magnesium by their opening influence on tight junctions in colonic epithelium, etc. (Mineo et al. 2003, Commane et al. 2004). This also may contribute to cancer prevention.

Lack of fermentation in the large bowel by repeated chronic usage of antibiotics could diminish butyrate and the production of the B vitamins, which otherwise may be beneficial to cancer prevention (Bruce et al. 2002). There may also be an influence of fermentation on the immune system, the colonic wall being a significant part of that system. Fiber effects such as bulking of feces, laxation, and shorter transit times have been reported for high-grain fiber diets. These effects also may help maintain large bowel health and prevent cancer. Binding of toxic/mutagenic components, diluting of the toxic metabolites, and reducing exposure time to bowel contents all offer potential mechanisms of protection, as well.

Other components in whole grains with anticancer effects include phytosterols, phenolics, dimethoxy-p-benzoquinone, phytate, and selenium. Phytate (inositol hexaphosphate) has a major influence as an antioxidant, locking up minerals and trace elements otherwise capable of initiating the production of free radical generation from fats, etc. (Shamsuddin et al. 1988).

Tannins/phenolics are present in significant quantities in the outer layers of grains. They can act as antibiotics or antioxidants, they have a protein-binding role (tanning), and they may be effective as anticancer agents (Newmark 1996). Phenolics such as hydroxycinnamic acids associated with fiber have been shown to be effective (Beyer-Sehlmeyer et al. 2003). Drankan et al. (2003) showed that the presence of orthophenolics in wheat correlated significantly with tumor inhibition in studies where fiber was kept constant. Wheat cultivars producing the highest caffeic acid levels in plasma were most effective in anticancer terms. The release of lignans (diphenolics) from grain foods and their metabolism in the colon has been correlated with a reduced risk of breast cancer (Adlercreutz 2001). Dimethyl benzaquinone (Avemar™) was shown to be effective as an anticancer agent in the rodent colon cancer model at low concentrations (Zalatnai et al. 2001). It is released from wheat germ following fermentation of wheat germ with yeast—Saccharomyces cerevisiae (18 hours incubation at 30°C).

Cereal grains may be a good source of selenium, with wheat from some locations such as South Dakota providing high concentrations. Wheats with selenium at 1 ppm to 2 ppm in the diet were shown to be effective in cancer prevention using the rodent colon cancer model (Finley and Davis 2001). Selenium is present in the protein-rich aleurone layers and germ of the grain as selenomethionine. This compound may contribute protective effects via the selenium-containing enzymes glutathione peroxidase or thioredoxin reductase.

In conclusion, there are a number of ways in which whole grains could contribute to cancer prevention, and these have been actively studied and elucidated, particularly with respect to colon cancer. Epidemiological observations have shown significant protective influences with whole grain consumption. There is a strong case for including them in a health-promoting/cancer-preventing diet.

References

Adlercreutz H, 2001. Cereal phytooestrogens and their association with human health. In *Whole Grains and Human Health. VTT Symposium*, Espoo, Finland, pp23–29.

Ajani UA, Ford ES, and Mokdad AH, 2004. Dietary fiber and C-reactive protein: findings from national health and nutrition examination survey data. *J Nutr* 134, 1181–1185.

Belobrajdic DP, McIntosh GH, and Owens JA, 2003. Whey proteins protect more than red meat against azoxymethane induced ACF in Wistar rats. *Cancer Lett* 198, 43–51.

Beyer-Sehlmeyer G, Glei M, Hartmann E, Hughes R, et al. , 2003. Butyrate is only one of several growth inhibitors produced during gut-flora-mediated fermentation of dietary fibre sources. *Brit J Nutr* 90, 1057–1070.

Bingham S, 2004. Epidemiology of dietary fibre and colorectal cancer. In *Dietary Fibre bioactive carbohydrates for food and feed*. Eds JW van der Kamp, N-G Asp, J Miller-Jones, and G Schaafsma. Wageningen Academic Publishers, The Netherlands pp179–180.

Bonithon-Copp C, Kronborg O, Giacosa A, Rath U and Faivre J, 2000. Calcium and fibre supplementation in prevention of colorectal adenoma recurrence: a randomised intervention trial. *Lancet* 356, 1300–1306.

Bruce WR, Wolever TMS, and Giacca A, 2000. Mechanisms linking diet and colorectal cancer: the possible role of insulin resistance. *Nutr Cancer* 37, 19–26.

Brusseroles J, Gueux E, Rock E, Demigne C, et al., 2003. Oligofructose protects against hypertriglyceridemic and pro-oxidative effects of a high fructose diet in rats. *J Nutr* 133,1903–1908.

Burkitt DP, 1970. Some disease characteristics of western civilisation. *Lancet* 2, 1237–40.

Caderni G, Luceri C, Spagnesi MC, Giannini A, Biggeri A, and Dolara P, 1994. Dietary carbohydrates modify azoxymethane-induced intestinal carcinogenesis in rats. *J Nutr* 124,517–523.

Cassidy A, Bingham SA, and Cummings JA, 1994. Starch intake and colorectal cancer risk: an international comparison. *Br J Cancer* 69,937–42.

Commane DM, Shortt CT, Silvi S, Cresci A, et al., 2005. Effects of fermentation products of pro- and prebiotics on trans-epithelial electrical resistance in an in vitro model of the colon. *Nutr Cancer* 51,102–109.

Cordain L, 1999. Cereal grains: humanity's double-edged sword. *World Rev Nutr Dietet*. 84, 19–73.

Cummings J, 1983. Fermentation in the human large intestine: evidence and implications for health. *Lancet* 1, 1206–1209.

Cummings JH, 1997. *The large intestine in nutrition and disease. Institut Danone*, Brussels. pp61–63.

Davie JR, 2003. Inhibition of histone deacetylase activity by butyrate. *J Nutr* 133, 2485S–2493S.

Drankan K, Carter J, Madl R, Klopfenstein C, et al., 2003. Antitumour activity of wheats with high orthophenolic content. *Nutr Cancer* 47,188–194.

Femia AP, Luceri C, Dolara P, Giannini A, et al., 2002. Antitumorigenic activity of the prebiotic inulin enriched with oligofructose in combination with the probiotics Lactobacillus rhamnosus and Bifidobacterium lactis on azoxymethane-induced colon carcinogenesis in rats. *Carcinogenesis* 2,1953–60.

Finley JW and Davis CD, 2001. Selenium (Se) from high selenium broccoli is utilised differently from selenite, selenate and selenomethionine, but is more effective in inhibiting colon carcinogenesis. *Biofactors* 14,191–196.

Gallus S, Bosetti C, and La Vecchia C, 2004. Mediterranean diet and cancer risk *European J Cancer Prevention* 13, 447–452.

Giovannucci E, 2001. Insulin, insulin like growth factors and colon cancer: a review of the evidence. *J Nutr* 131, 3109S–3120S.

Koh-Banerjee P, Franz M, Sampson L, Liu S, et al., 2004. Changes in whole-grain, bran, and cereal fibre consumption in relation to 8-year weight gain among men. *J Nutr* 80, 1237–45.

La Vecchia C, Chatenoud L, Negri E, and Franceschi S, 2003a. Wholegrain cereals and cancer in Italy. *Proc Nutr Soc* 62, 45–39

La Vecchia C, Franceschi S, and Levi F., 2003b. Epidemiological research on cancer with a focus on Europe. *Europ J Cancer Prevent*. 12,5–14.

Lee WM, Lu S, Medline A, and Archer MC, 2001. Susceptibility of lean and obese Zucker rats to tumorigenesis induced by N-methly-N-nitrosourea. *Cancer Letters*, 162,155–160

McIntosh GH, 2004. Experimental studies of dietary fibre and colon cancer—an overview. In *Dietary Fibre bioactive carbohydrates for food and feed*. Eds JW van der Kamp, N-G Asp, J Miller-Jones, and G Schaafsma. Wageningen Academic Publishers, The Netherlands pp 165–175.

McIntosh GH and Jacobs DR, 2002. Chapter 9, Cereal grain foods, fibers and cancer prevention. In *Whole grain foods in health and disease*. Eds L Marquart, JL Slavin, and G Fulcher. American Association of Cereal Chemists, St Paul, Minnesota, pp 201–232.

McIntosh GH, Le Leu RK, Royle PJ, and Young GP, 1996. A comparative study of the influence of differing barley brans on DMH-induced intestinal tumours in male Sprague Dawley rats. *J Gastroenterol Hepatol* 11, 113–119.

Mineo H, Amano M, Chiji H, Shigematsu N, et al., 2004. Indigestible disaccharides open tight junctions and enhance net calcium, magnesium and zinc absorption in isolated rat small and large intestinal epithelium. Digest. *Diseases and Sciences* 49, 122-132.

Newmark HL, 1996. Plant phenolics as potential cancer preventing agents. In *Dietary phytochemicals in cancer prevention and treatment*. Eds AICR. *Adv Exptl Med Biol* 401, 25–34.

Newmark HL, Yang M, Lipkin L, Kopelvich Y, et al., 2001. A western style diet induces benign and malignant neoplasms in the colon of normal C57B1 mice. *Carcinogenesis* 22, 1871–1875.

Noakes M, Clifton PM, Nestel PJ, Le Leu RK, and McIntosh GH, 1996. Effects of high-amylose starch and oat bran on metabolic variables and bowel function in subjects with hypertriglyceridemia. *Am J Clin Nutr* 64, 944–51.

Shamsuddin AM, Elsayed AM, and Ullah A, 1988. Suppression of large intestinal cancer in F344 rats by inositol hexaphosphate. *Carcinogenesis* 9, 577–80.

Slattery ML, Edwards SL, Buocher KM, Anderson K, and Caan BJ, 1999. Lifestyle and colon cancer: an assessment of factors associated with risk. *Am J Epidemiol* 150,869–77.

Slattery ML, Curtin KP, Edwards SL, and Schaffer DM, 2004. Plant foods, fiber and rectal cancer. *Am J Clin Nutr* 79, 274–81.

Trichopoulou A, Costacou T, Bamia C and Trichopoulos D. Adherence to a Mediterranean diet and survival in a Greek population. *N Eng J Med* 348, 2599–2608.

Trowell H, 1987. Diabetes mellitus and rice—a hypothesis. *Human Nutrition: Food Sciences and Nutrition* 41F,145–152.

Zalatnai A, Lapis K, Szende B, Rasao E, et al., 2001. Wheat germ extract inhibits experimental colon carcinogenesis in F344 rats. *Carcinogenesis* 22,1649–1652.

7 The Effects of Cereal Fibers and Barley Foods Rich in β-glucan on Cardiovascular Disease and Diabetes Risk

Joel J. Pins, Harminder Kaur, Ellen Dodds, and Joseph M. Keenan

Cardiovascular disease (C.V.D.) and diabetes are among the primary causes of death in the United States and many other nations. Uniquely enough, both of these chronic diseases can be predicted by the "metabolic syndrome," a condition that is increasing in prevalence and which now affects at least 25% of the U.S. adult population (Ford et al. 2004). The metabolic syndrome is characterized by a clustering of physical traits and metabolic dysfunctions that may include, but is not limited to, abdominal obesity[1], atherogenic dyslipidemia[2], elevated blood pressure[3], insulin resistance, and glucose intolerance[4] (National Cholesterol Education Program III 2002). If left unchecked, this condition can progress to diabetes and is an independent risk factor for coronary heart disease (C.H.D.) and other forms of C.V.D. (N.C.E.P. A.T.P.III 2002, Lorenzo et al. 2003).

Diabetes is a major independent risk factor for various forms of C.V.D., including C.H.D. Lifestyle factors, including diet, can contribute to the development of diabetes, its precursors, and its complications. Thus, these lifestyle factors also play an important role in prevention and management of these maladies. Additionally, modifying diabetes-related risk factors offers great potential for reducing C.V.D. incidence, morbidity, disability, and mortality. Diet can play a key role in modifying several major C.V.D. and diabetes-related risk factors, including high blood pressure, high cholesterol, and excessive body weight. In individuals with metabolic syndrome, dietary interventions that positively influence lipids, glucose metabolism, and body weight may help prevent or delay development of diabetes and C.V.D.

Specifically, there is mounting evidence supporting a role for dietary fiber, especially viscous soluble fiber, in prevention and management of C.V.D., diabetes, and related conditions. Fiber can have beneficial effects on several cardiovascular risk factors, including body weight, blood pressure, and blood cholesterol levels. Soluble fibers in particular, including pectin from fruits and β-glucans found in oats and barley, can reduce total cholesterol (T.C.) and L.D.L. cholesterol (L.D.L.-C.) levels (Federal Register 2003, Brown et al. 1999), improve blood glucose regulation (Kabir et al. 2002), and promote satiety (Marlett et al. 2002, Rigaud et al. 1998). Soluble fiber intake also may prevent the rise of triglycerides (T.G.) and reduction of H.D.L. cholesterol (H.D.L.-C.) that sometimes occurs with diets rich in carbohydrates (especially refined grains) (Marlett et al. 2002).

Major health organizations are increasingly recognizing the cardiovascular benefits of high-fiber diets. The American Heart Association (A.H.A.) dietary guidelines assert that a healthy diet including a variety of high-fiber foods is the foundation for achieving and maintaining cardiovascular health (Krauss et al. 2000). The National Cholesterol Education Program's (N.C.E.P.) A.T.P.III guidelines, which identify L.D.L.-C. as the primary target of cholesterol-lowering therapy, recognize the beneficial role of dietary fiber, and specifically soluble fibers, in improving blood cholesterol levels and decreasing C.H.D. risk. These evidence-based guidelines recommend a diet with 20 grams to 30 grams of dietary fiber and at least 5 grams to 10 grams of soluble fiber/day. Higher soluble fiber intakes of 10 grams to 25 grams/day are recommended for additional L.D.L.-C. lowering. This recommendation is supported by research showing that on average, an increase in soluble fiber of 5 grams to 10 grams/day is accompanied by a 5% or greater reduction in L.D.L.-C. (N.C.E.P. A.T.P.III 2002).

While the above recommendations are generally well accepted, other topics pertinent to a discussion of fiber and diabetes are more controversial. Glycemic index is one such topic. Many foods rich in dietary fiber/viscous soluble fiber produce a lower glycemic response than comparable low-fiber foods. While the American Diabetes Association doesn't stress using this measure to guide food choices (A.D.A. 2000), many recent studies, as well as guidelines from Europe, Australia, and the Food and Agriculture Organization/World Health Organization, do support an emphasis on low-glycemic index foods for individuals with diabetes and impaired glucose tolerance (Jarvi et al. 1999, Wolever and Mehling 2002).

Cereal Fiber and C.V.D./Diabetes Risk: Evidence from Epidemiological Observational Studies

Epidemiological observational studies demonstrate a strong association between higher intakes of fiber or whole grains and a lower risk of metabolic syndrome or its related risk factors. In one study researchers followed 4,999 Swedish men and women and demonstrated relationships between food patterns, independent of specific nutrients, and specific components of metabolic syndrome. Men's food patterns were associated with hyperglycemia and central obesity while women's food patterns were associated with hyperinsulinemia. Food patterns rich in high-fiber bread provided favorable effects, while patterns high in refined bread had adverse effects (Wirfalt 2001). Another study conducted in Tehran showed that whole grain consumption is inversely associated with the risk of development of the metabolic syndrome (Esmailzadeh et al. 2005).

Benefits of whole grain consumption have been observed in adults and adolescents. In a large study that followed 74,091 U.S. female nurses over twelve years, women who consumed more whole grains consistently weighed less and had a 49% lower risk of major weight gain than women who consumed fewer whole grains (odds ratio = 0.51) (Liu et al. 2003). In 285 Minnesota adolescents, higher levels of whole grain intake were associated with a lower body mass index (B.M.I.) and greater insulin sensitivity. The association between whole grain intake and insulin sensitivity was stronger among adolescents with higher B.M.I.s (Steffen et al. 2003). Data from 2,909 healthy young black and white adults over ten years of follow-up revealed a strong association between higher dietary fiber intake and lower body weight, waist-to-hip ratio, fasting insulin, and two-hour post-glucose insulin. Weaker relationships were found between higher fiber intakes and lower blood pressure, T.G., and L.D.L. cholesterol, and between higher fiber intakes and higher H.D.L. levels (Ludwig et al. 1999). Similar trends were shown in the Framingham Offspring Study cohort, where high whole grain intake was inversely associated with B.M.I., waist-to-hip ratio, T.C., L.D.L.-C., and fasting insulin. The inverse association between whole grain intake and fasting insulin was strongest among obese participants (McKeown 2002).

Higher fiber intake and/or whole grain consumption may also help prevent type 2 diabetes. Among 75,521 women, those with the highest intake of whole grain fiber had a 38% lower risk of diabetes compared to those with the lowest whole grain fiber intake (odds ratio = 0.62) (Liu et al. 2000). Data from 35,988 older Iowa women showed a 21% and 36% lower risk of diabetes for women who ate the most whole grain foods and cereal fiber, respectively, compared to those who ate the least (Meyer et al. 2000). For 42,898 men from the Health Professionals Follow-up Study, the incidence of diabetes was 30% lower (relative risk = 0.70) for those with the highest whole grain intake compared to those with the lowest whole grain intake (adjusted for B.M.I.) (Fung et al. 2002).

A fiber-rich diet also may improve glycemic control in diabetics. In a European study involving patients with type 1 diabetes, higher fiber intake was related to improved indicators of glucose control including lower glycated hemoglobin (HbA1c) levels and reduced risk of severe ketoacidosis. In multivariate analysis, only soluble fiber intake significantly predicted HbA1c levels (Buyken et al. 1998).

Given the high C.V.D. risk associated with metabolic syndrome, insulin resistance, and diabetes, it is relevant to note that there is a large body of epidemiological research that links high intakes of fiber and whole grains to C.V.D.-protective effects. In general, dietary patterns rich in whole grains and fiber are associated with decreased risk of C.V.D., coronary events, and coronary death. Soluble fibers appear to be especially beneficial (Krauss et al. 2000, Pereira et al. 2004). Data from 68,782 women in the Nurses' Health Study (N.H.S.) revealed that those with the highest total dietary fiber intake (22.9 grams/day) had a 47% lower risk for major C.V. events (R.R. = 0.53) than women with the lowest fiber intake (11.5 grams/day) (Wolk et al. 1999). Another large study looked at 39,876 female health professionals. Those who ate the most fiber (26.3 grams/day) had a 35% lower incidence of total C.V.D. and 54% fewer heart attacks than women who ate the least fiber (12.5 grams/day) (R.R. = 0.65 for total C.V.D. and 0.46 for M.I.) (Liu et al. 2002). In a study of 43,757 male health professionals, the incidence of heart attack and fatal coronary disease was 41% and 55% lower, respectively, for those with the highest intake of fiber (28.9 grams/day) compared to those with the lowest intake (12.4 grams/day). A 10-gram increase in dietary fiber corresponded to a 19% decreased risk of heart attack (Rimm et al. 1996).

Soluble fiber intake is more strongly associated with decreased C.V.D. risk than insoluble fiber. In the N.H.S., an increase in soluble fiber of 5 grams/day led to a 25% decrease in C.H.D. (R.R. = .75); the same increase in insoluble fiber led to a 12% decrease in C.H.D. (R.R. = .88) (Lorenzo et al. 2003). Of 9,776 adults who participated in the N.H.A.N.E.S. I Follow-up Study, those with the highest soluble fiber intake (5.9 grams/day) had 15% fewer C.H.D. events (R.R. = 0.85) and 10% fewer C.V.D. events (R.R. = 0.90) than those with the lowest soluble fiber intake (0.9 grams/day) (Bazzano et al. 2003).

In studies of men, women, and elderly groups, fiber from cereal sources offered more cardiovascular protection than fiber from fruits and vegetables (Wolk et al. 1999, Rimm et al. 1996, Mozaffarian et al. 2003). When intakes of cereal-fiber food sources were examined, women who ate breakfast cereal five or more times per week had a 19% lower risk of C.H.D. than those who did not eat breakfast cereal (Wolk et al. 1999).

Additional studies have provided details about the relationship of fiber and fiber-rich food sources to specific risk factors and progression of C.V.D. The intake of soluble fiber may protect against progression of atherosclerosis as measured in the carotid arteries (Wu et al. 2003). Fiber consumption has been associated with a lower risk of major weight gain in middle-aged women (Liu et al. 2003) and the reduction of C-reactive protein (C.R.P.), an inflammatory marker associated with cardiovascular risk (King et al. 2003).

While observational investigations provide promising data about fiber and C.V. health, there are well-recognized limitations to these studies. Problems include selection biases, differing composition of study populations, inaccuracies of self-reported dietary intake, limited

Table 7.1. The effect of dietary fibers and/or whole grains on C.V.D. or diabetes risk.

	# of studies reporting + findings	# of studies reporting − findings	# of studies reporting a null outcome
Diabetes	15	None	None
C.H.D. and/or C.V.D.	17	None	None

Findings from the Epidemiologic Studies reviewed in this chapter.

information about fiber sources, and difficulty identifying and controlling for confounding factors. Additionally, the impact of food synergies, or the way nutrients act together to influence metabolism and the risk of some chronic diseases, is difficult to strategically evaluate. For example, although C.V.D. risk appears to be lower with consumption of whole grains than with consumption of refined grains, it is possible that the phytochemicals located in the fiber matrix, in addition to or instead of the fiber itself, may be responsible for some or all of the reduced risk. To understand the role of soluble fiber and pathways by which food synergies work, it seems necessary to evaluate purified soluble fiber in combination with larger units, namely foods or food patterns (Jacobs and Steffen 2003). Experimental randomized animal and human trials can be used to overcome many of these limitations and to estimate the health effects of various sources of soluble fiber, including β-glucan from barley (Table 7.1).

The Effects of Barley Foods and/or Barley β-glucan on C.V.D. and Diabetes-related Risk Factors: Findings from Human Trials

Although the majority of human studies examining the effects of β-glucan have used oat sources, a number of randomized controlled clinical trials have investigated the cholesterol-lowering effects of barley foods rich in β-glucan. In 1991 a crossover clinical trial demonstrated that a four-week diet enriched with barley foods was more effective at lowering cholesterol in twenty-one men with high cholesterol than a diet with similar wheat foods. Compared to the wheat foods period (1.5 grams β-glucan/day), the barley foods period (8 grams β-glucan/day) resulted in significantly lower T.C. (6%) and L.D.L.-C. (7%) in subjects (McIntosh et al. 1991). More recent studies have reported similar findings. One study involved adding 6 grams of barley soluble fiber per 2,800 calories to the A.H.A. Step 1 diets of eighteen men with moderately high cholesterol. After five weeks there were significant reductions of total cholesterol (20%), L.D.L.-C. (24%), and T.G. (16%). Additionally, HDL-C was increased by 18% (Behall et al. 2004).

Rendell et al. (2005) conducted a breakfast study using Prowash barley meal and oatmeal on sixteen non-diabetic and eighteen diabetic patients. It was observed that a standardized Prowash barley meal produced a lower postprandial glucose response in both diabetic as well as non-diabetic subjects than an equivalent weight quantity of oatmeal.

Another recent trial was conducted with ten healthy women following a diet standardized to match the average carbohydrate, protein, and fat intakes of the Japanese. When whole grain barley was substituted into the diet (average approximately 1.8 grams/kg/day) for four weeks, lab values showed 14.5% lower T.C., 13.9% lower T.G., and 7.5% lower free fatty acid concentration compared to the standard diet control. The barley group also showed significantly lower L.D.L.-C. with no change in H.D.L. (Li et al. 2003).

One study evaluated the lipid responses in eleven men after they ate low-fat test meals with one of three pasta types: a low-fiber wheat pasta (0.3 grams β-glucan), a barley pasta naturally high in β-glucan (5.2 grams β-glucan), or a barley pasta enriched with β-glucan (5 grams β-glucan). Four hours after the barley meals, T.C. levels dropped below fasting levels; no significant change in cholesterol occurred after eating the wheat pasta meal. In the same study, insulin response, but not glucose response, was more blunted after the barley-containing meals than after meals containing the wheat pasta control (Bourdon et al. 1999).

Not all studies involving barley β-glucan have shown significant reductions in lipid parameters. In a crossover study of eighteen men with mildly high cholesterol, the addition of a β-glucan-enriched form of barley (8.1 grams to 11.9 grams β-glucan/day) to diets with 38% calories from fat did not result in significant changes in blood lipid measurements. Small, non-significant reductions in T.C. (1.3%) and L.D.L.-C. (3.8%) were reported (Keogh et al. 2003).

Some researchers have suggested that components of barley other than β-glucan may have lipid-lowering properties. Researchers treated seventy-nine mildly hypercholesterolemic subjects with cellulose, barley bran flour (primarily insoluble fiber), or barley oil added to the N.C.E.P. Step 1 diet. The barley bran flour group showed significant reductions in T.C., L.D.L.-C., and H.D.L. The barley oil group showed significant reductions in T.C. and L.D.L.-C. but showed no change in H.D.L.-C. levels. While a significant reduction in energy, dietary cholesterol, and fat consumption did occur in both flour and oil groups, changes in lipid values were greater than expected from diet changes alone (Lupton et al. 1994). However, most experts agree that most of the lipid-altering properties of barley are due to the soluble β-glucan fibers.

Moreover, benefits of barley foods may go beyond cholesterol lowering. Results of some recent studies are especially relevant due to the increase in the prevalence of the metabolic syndrome and pre-diabetes, both conditions which increase C.V.D. risk. Soluble fiber has been shown to delay glucose absorption in the gut and to decrease postprandial blood glucose in healthy individuals and diabetics. Cavallero and colleagues (2002) found that when four different barley-containing breads, each with the same amount of available carbohydrate (50 grams), were fed to healthy volunteers, a linear decrease in glycemic response was reported as β-glucan increased (β-glucan range: 0.1 grams to 6.3 grams/100grams dry weight.

A number of well-designed, randomized human clinical trials indicate that barley foods and barley β-glucan can improve glucose metabolism in people without diabetes. However, some studies have examined the acute effects of barley foods but have not quantified β-glucan content. Thorburn and colleagues (1993) examined glucose tolerance and hepatic glucose production (H.G.P.) in ten healthy subjects the morning after they had eaten either brown rice or barley for dinner (90 grams carbohydrate/portion). Subjects showed improved glucose tolerance and a 30% reduction in H.G.P. after the barley meal (3.9 grams soluble fiber) compared to the rice meal (trace amounts soluble fiber).

A more recent study indicates that eating certain high-fiber barley foods at breakfast can improve glucose tolerance at lunch (Liljeberg et al. 1999). The effects of seven different breakfasts, four of which contained barley, each with a known glycemic index (52 to 99) and dietary fiber content (2 grams to 36 grams) were evaluated in ten healthy adults. Glucose tolerance at the lunch meal was significantly improved when breakfast consisted of a lower glycemic index barley food rich in β-glucan. The highest level of satiety was also associated with this breakfast. In a study of ten women, two of whom had impaired glucose tolerance, test meals containing high-soluble-fiber barley (barley flour or barley cereal) were more effective at reducing glucose and insulin responses than test meals containing oats (oat flour or oatmeal) (Behall et al. 1999).

Other studies have examined the effects of barley foods on glucose metabolism with measured or estimated β-glucan content. In one study, barley porridge and breads were enriched with barley flour from a barley genotype with elevated levels of β-glucan (flour: 17.5 grams β-glucan/100 grams dry weight). In nine healthy subjects these enriched products induced significantly lower postprandial glucose and insulin responses than control products made only with common oat flour (4 grams β-glucan/100 grams dry weight), common barley flour (4.7 grams β-glucan/100 grams dry weight.), or white wheat flour. The most pronounced lowering of glycemic and insulinemic responses occurred with the bread that had the highest proportion of high-fiber barley flour (80% high-fiber barley flour: 20% common barley flour) (Liljeberg et al. 1996).

Processing of cereal products can affect fiber content as well as glycemic and insulinemic properties. A recent study compared glucose and insulin responses after the consumption of oats, barley, and high β-glucan oat and barley extracts. When fed to twenty healthy subjects (0.33 grams/kg body weight), the oat and barley extracts, potentially usable as fat substitutes in some products, seemed to retain the beneficial effects of the grains from which they were extracted. Glucose responses and areas under the curve for all test foods were significantly lower than responses to a control glucose solution. Insulin responses for the barley extract were lowest and were significantly lower than for the glucose solution (Hallfrisch et al. 2003).

Barley products also may improve glycemic control in diabetic populations. Barley breads improved glycemic response in fifteen patients with well-controlled type 2 diabetes. Responses to either pearled barley bread (6.7% total fiber, 2.5% soluble fiber) or whole barley bread (8.5% total fiber, 2.6% soluble fiber) compared to white bread (3.3% total fiber, 0.5% soluble fiber) were evaluated. Both test meals produced significantly lower blood glucose levels than the white bread; whole barley bread promoted the lowest postprandial rise in blood glucose (Urooj et al. 1998).

One study showed beneficial acute effects of barley foods in both healthy and diabetic subjects. Fourteen patients with diabetes and eighteen healthy volunteers consumed white bread meals and barley meals (50 grams carbohydrate/meal) on different days. In diabetic patients the incremental glycemic response to barley was significantly lower than that to white bread at 0.5 hour, 1 hour, and 1.5 hours after eating, and in healthy subjects it was significantly lower at 1 hour, 1.5 hours, and 2 hours after eating. The insulinemic response in healthy subjects was significantly lower after eating the barley meal compared to the white bread. There was no significant difference in insulinemic response in diabetic subjects, but there was a non-significant tendency for higher insulin response to barley at 0.5 hour (Shukla et al. 1991). In another trial, some type 2 diabetics were able to reduce their doses of oral hypoglycemic medications during a twelve-week period of incorporating barley bread products into their diets (Pick et al. 1998). Eleven men with diabetes completed two twelve-week diet periods: a white bread period (mean fiber intake = 28 grams/day) and a barley bread period (mean fiber intake = 39 grams/day). Glycemic response improved and postprandial insulinemic response was significantly higher during the barley bread period (average of 9.8 grams fiber, 4.1 grams soluble fiber, and 5.2 grams β-glucan via barley per day).

A recent study conducted by Biorklund et al. (2005) compared the effect of oat β-glucan and barley β-glucan on serum lipids and postprandial glucose and insulin concentrations. One hundred volunteers were divided into five different groups with four groups receiving two different doses (5 grams or 10 grams) of oat or barley β-glucan-containing beverages, each with the final group serving as the control. It was observed that compared to the control group, 5 grams of β-glucan from oats significantly lowered T.C. and postprandial glucose and insulin concentrations. But, the 10-gram oat group experienced no significant changes in blood lipids. Neither barley group experienced any significant changes in blood lipids or glucose regulation. These findings suggest a possible threshold effect and that extracted β-glucan from oats might be more effective than that extracted from barley. It is significant to note that the β-glucan from barley had a significantly lower average molecular weight, which might have affected the water-holding/viscosity capacity of these fibers and thereby reduced their lipid/glucose altering properties (Biorklund et al. 2005). See Figure 7.1 for a discussion of the mechanism of action of soluble fibers.

To further investigate the effects of barley β-glucan on C.V.D. and diabetes-related risk factors, our group recently conducted a randomized, controlled study to evaluate whether a concentrated β-glucan extract added to food products could effectively lower L.D.L.-C. in hyperlipidemic subjects with and without the metabolic syndrome. Because the molecular weight of polymers is known to influence viscosity and palatability, both high- and low-molecular-weight (H.M.W. and L.M.W., respectively) β-glucan extracts were tested at daily doses of 3 grams and 5 grams. After a four-week diet stabilization phase, subjects consumed the treatment twice per day via a ready-to-eat cereal and 5% fruit juice beverage. After six weeks of treatment, mean L.D.L.-C. levels fell by 15% in the 5-gram H.M.W. group, 13% in the 5-gram L.M.W. group, and 9% in both the 3 gram/day groups, versus baseline. Although the reduction was significant for all treatment groups, the 5 gram/day dose was more effective than the 3 gram/day dose. Molecular weight did not significantly influence the findings (Pins et al. 2005). Additionally, postprandial glucose and free fatty acids were beneficially affected by the treatment groups with the greatest effect being observed in the 5-gram H.M.W. group.

These human studies (Table 7.2) appear to confirm what was indicated by the epidemiologic data: that the soluble fiber fraction of certain grains does alter C.V.D. and diabetes

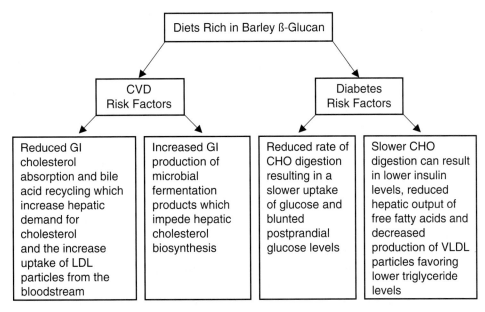

Figure 7.1. Mechanisms of action of soluble fibers from barley on C.V.D. and diabetes risk factors (Wang et al. 1992, Danielson et al. 1997).

Table 7.2.   Summary of human trials using barley foods rich in β-glucan.

	C.V.D. Risk Factors				Diabetes Risk Factors	
Author	T.C.	L.D.L.-C.	T.G.	H.D.L.-C.	Insulin Response	Glucose Response
McIntosh 1991	↓	↓	N.D.	N.D.	N.D.	N.D.
Behall 2004	↓	↓	↓	↑	N.D.	N.D.
Li 2003*	↓	↓	↓	—	N.D.	N.D.
Bourdon 1999	↓	N.D.	N.D.	N.D.	N.D.	Blunted
Keogh 2003	N.S.	N.S.	N.D.	N.D.	N.D.	N.D.
Lupton 1994	↓	↓	N.D.	—	N.D.	N.D.
Liljeberg 1999	N.D.	N.D.	N.D.	N.D.	N.D.	Improved
Behall 1999	N.D.	N.D.	N.D.	N.D.	N.D.	Improved
Liljeberg 1996	N.D.	N.D.	N.D.	N.D.	Blunted	Improved
Hallfrisch 2003	N.D.	N.D.	N.D.	N.D.	Blunted	Improved
Urooj 1998	N.D.	N.D.	N.D.	N.D.	N.D.	Improved
Shukla 1991	N.D.	N.D.	N.D.	N.D.	Blunted	N.D.
Pick 1998	N.D.	N.D.	N.D.	N.D.	Blunted	Improved
PiN.S. 2005*	↓	↓	↓	—	↓	↓
ReN.D.ell 2005	N.D.	N.D.	N.D.	N.D.	N.D.	N.D.
BiorkluN.D. 2005	N.S. ↓	N.S. ↓	N.S. ↓	N.S. ↓	N.S.	N.S.

* These two studies measured free fatty acid changes and observed that there is a significant fall in free fatty acids in blood after consming barley foods.
N.D. = not determined
N.S. = not significant

risk. However, there are inconsistencies in the human data which may be due to a variety of factors, including dose of treatment, molecular weight of treatment, dietary control, sample size, and/or variation in types of barley foods/supplements. These questions will require additional science for clarification.

Conclusion

Recent guidelines strongly recommend increased total and soluble fiber intake to achieve general and cardiovascular health and to help prevent diabetes. High soluble fiber consumption protects against C.H.D., and there is strong evidence that soluble fiber decreases total cholesterol and L.D.L.-C., while improving blood glucose regulation. Moreover, the N.C.E.P. in the A.T.P.III guidelines recommend intensive therapeutic lifestyle changes (T.L.C.) for L.D.L.-C. goal attainment before initiating drug therapy. Increased soluble fiber intake is a cornerstone to this plan and can help patients attain their L.D.L.-C. goal without the use of pharmaceuticals, or it can help reduce total medication need. Similar recommendations regarding soluble fiber intake have been established for the American Diabetes Association to help diabetic patients improve glycemic control.

Specifically, barley β-glucan fiber has demonstrated its ability to reduce total cholesterol and L.D.L.-C. and to improve glucose metabolism in different populations in several studies. Therefore, barley foods and functional foods containing extracted barley β-glucan should be considered a safe and effective option for improving lipids and glycemic control in populations with moderate dyslipidemia and/or diabetes.

Notes

1. Waist circumference $> 40''$ in males and $> 35''$ in females.
2. Elevated triglycerides $\geq$ 150 mg/dl, small L.D.L. particles, low H.D.L. cholesterol: $<$ 40mg/dl in males and $<$ 50mg/dl in females.
3. $\geq$ 130/ $\geq$ 85 mm Hg
4. $\geq$ 110 mg/dl

References

American Diabetes Association. Nutrition recommendations and principles for people with diabetes mellitus. *Diabetes Care*. 2000;23(Suppl 1):S43–S46

Bazzano, L.A.; He, J.; Ogden, L.G.; Loria, C,M,; Whelton, P.K. Dietary fiber intake and reduced risk of coronary heart disease in US men and women. *Arch Intern Med*. 2003;163(16):1897–1904.

Behall, K.M.; Scholfield, D.J.; Hallfrisch, J.G. Comparison of glucose and insulin responses to barley and oats. *Diabetes*. 1999;48(Suppl 1):Abstract 2055

Behall, K.M.; Scholfield, D.J.; Hallfrisch, J.G. Lipids significantly reduced by diets containing barley in moderately hypercholesterolemic men. *J Am Coll Nutr*. 2004;23(1):55–62

Biorklund, M.; van Rees, A.; Mensink, R.P.; Onning, G. Changes in serum lipids and postprandial glucose and insulin concentrations after consumption of beverages with beta-glucans from oats or barley: a randomized dose-controlled trial. *Euro J Clin Nutr* (2005), 1–10

Bourdon, I.; Yokoyama, W.; Davis, P., et al. Postprandial lipid, glucose, insulin, and cholecystokinin responses in men fed barley pasta enriched with beta-glucan. *Am J Clin Nutr*. 1999;69:55–63.

Brown, L.; Rosner, B.; Willett, W.W.; Sacks, F.M. Cholesterol-lowering effects of dietary fiber: a meta-analysis. *Am J Clin Nutr* 1999 January;69(1):30–42.

Buyken, A.E.; Toeller, M.; Heitkamp, G., et al. Relation of fibre intake to HbA_{1c} and the prevalence of severe ketoacidosis and severe hypoglycaemia. *Diabetologia*. 1998;41:882–90.

Cavallero, A.; Empilli, S.; Brighenti, F.; Stanca, A.M. High $(1 \to 3, 1 \to 4)$-beta-glucan barley fractions in bread making and their effects on human glycemic response. *J Cereal Sci*. 2002;36(1):59–66

Danielson, A.D.; Newman, R.K.; Newman, C.W.; Berardinelli, J.G. Lipid levels and digesta viscosity of rats fed a high-fiber barley milling fraction. *Nutr Res*. 1997;17(3):515–22.

Esmailzadeh, A.; Mirmiran, P.; Azizi, F. Whole grain consumption and the metabolic syndrome: a favorable association in Tehranian adults. *Eur J Clin Nutr* 2005; 59(3): 353–62

Food labeling: health claims; soluble dietary fiber from certain foods and coronary heart disease. Final rule. *Fed Regist* 2003 July 28;68(144):44207–9.

Ford, E.S.; Giles, W.H.; Mokdad, A.H. Increasing prevalence of the metabolic syndrome among U.S. adults. *Diabetes Care* 2004 October;27(10):2444–9.

Fung, T.T.; Hu, F.B.; Pereira, M.A., et al. Whole-grain intake and the risk of type 2 diabetes: a prospective study in men. *Am J Clin Nutr*. 2002;76(3):535–40.

Hallfrisch, J.; Scholfield, D.J.; Behall, K.M. Physiological responses of men and women to barley and oat extracts (Nu-trimX). II. Comparison of glucose and insulin responses. *Cereal Chem*. 2003;80(1):80–3.

Jacobs, D,R., Jr.; Steffen, L.M. Nutrients, foods, and dietary patterns as exposures in research: a framework for food synergy. *Am J Clin Nutr* 2003 September; 78(3 Suppl):508S–13S.

Jarvi, A.E.; Karlstrom, B.E.; Granfeldt, Y.E.; Bjorck, I.E.; Asp, N.G.; Vessby, B.O. Improved glycemic control and lipid profile and normalized fibrinolytic activity on a low-glycemic index diet in type 2 diabetic patients. *Diabetes Care*. 1999;22(1):10–8.

Kabir M, Oppert JM, Vidal H et al. Four-week low-glycemic index breakfast with a modest amount of soluble fibers in type 2 diabetic men. *Metabolism* 2002 July;51(7):819–26.

Keogh, G.F.; Cooper, G.J.; Mulvey, T.B., et al. Randomized controlled crossover study of the effect of a highly beta-glucan-enriched barley on cardiovascular disease risk factors in mildly hypercholesterolemic men. *Am J Clin Nutr*. 2003;78(4):711–8.

King, D.E.; Egan, B.M.; Geesey, M.E. Relation of dietary fat and fiber to elevation of C-reactive protein. *Am J Cardiol*. 2003;92:1335–9.

Krauss, R.M.; Eckel, R.H.; Howard, B. et al. AHA Dietary Guidelines: revision 2000: A statement for healthcare professionals from the Nutrition Committee of the American Heart Association. *Circulation* 2000 October 31;102(18):2284–99.

Li, J.; Kaneko, T.; Qin, L.Q.; Wang, J.; Wang, Y. Effects of barley intake on glucose tolerance, lipid metabolism, and bowel function in women. *Nutrition*. 2003;19(11–12):926–9.

Liljeberg, H.G.; Akerberg, A.K.; Bjorck, I.M. Effect of the glycemic index and content of indigestible carbohydrates of cereal-based breakfast meals on glucose tolerance at lunch in healthy subjects. *Am J Clin Nutr.*1999;69:647–55.

Liljeberg, H.G.; Granfeldt, Y.E.; Bjorck, I.M. Products based on a high fiber barely genotype, but not on common barley or oats, lower postprandial glucose and insulin responses in healthy humans. *J Nutr*. 1996;126:458–66.

Liu, S.; Buring, J.E.; Sesso, H.D.; Rimm, E.B.; Willett, W.C.; Manson, J.E. A prospective study of dietary fiber intake and risk of cardiovascular disease among women. *J Am Coll Cardiol*. 2002;39:49–56.

Liu, S.; Manson, J.E.; Stampfer, M.J., et al. A prospective study of whole-grain intake and risk of type 2 diabetes mellitus in US women. *Am J Public Health*. 2000;90(9):1409–15.

Liu, S.; Willett, W.C.; Manson, J.E.; Hu, F.B.; Rosner, B.; Colditz, G. Relation between changes in intakes of dietary fiber and grain products and changes in weight and development of obesity among middle-aged women. *Am J Clin Nutr*. 2003;78(5):920–7.

Lorenzo, C.; Okoloise, M.; Williams, K.; Stern, M.P.; Haffner, S.M. The metabolic syndrome as predictor of type 2 diabetes: the San Antonio heart study. *Diabetes Care* 2003 November;26(11):3153–9.

Ludwig, D.S.; Pereira, M.A.; Kroenke, C.H., et al. Dietary fiber, weight gain, and cardiovascular disease risk factors in young adults. *J.A.M.A*. 1999;282(16):1539–46.

Lupton, J.R.; Robinson, M.C.; Morin, J.L. Cholesterol-lowering effect of barley flour and oil. *J Am Diet Assoc*. 1994;94:65–70.

Marlett, J.A.; McBurney, M.I.; Slavin, J.L. Position of the American Dietetic Association: health implications of dietary fiber. *J Am Diet Assoc* 2002 July;102(7):993–1000.

McIntosh, G.H.; Whyte, J,; McArthur, R.; Nestel, P.J. Barley and wheat foods: influence on plasma cholesterol concentration in hypercholesterolemic men. *Am J Clin Nutr*. 1991;53:1205–9

McKeown, N.M.; Meigs, J.B.; Liu, S.; Wilson, P.W.; Jacques, P.F. Whole-grain intake is favorably associated with metabolic risk factors for type 2 diabetes and cardiovascular disease in the Framingham Offspring Study. *Am J Clin Nutr.*2002;76(2):390–8.

Meyer, K.A.; Kushi, L.H.; Jacobs, D.R., Jr.; Slavin, J.; Sellers, T.A.; Folsom, A.R. Carbohydrates, dietary fiber, and incident type 2 diabetes in older women. *Am J Clin Nutr*. 2000;71(4):921–30.

Mozaffarian, D.; Kumanyika, S.K.; Lemaitre, R.N.; Olson, J.L.; Burke, G.L.; Siscovick, D.S. Cereal, fruit, and vegetable fiber intake and the risk of cardiovascular disease in elderly individuals. *J.A.M.A*. 2003;289(13):1659–66.

Pereira, M.A.; O'Reilly, E.; Augustsson, K., et al. Dietary fiber and risk of coronary heart disease: a pooled analysis of cohort studies. *Arch Intern Med*. 2004;164(4):370–6.

Pick, M.E.; Hawrysh, Z.J.; Gee, M.I.; Toth, E. Barley bread products improve glycemic control of type 2 subjects. *Int J Food Sci Nutr*. 1998;49:71–8.

Pins, J.; Keenan, J.M.; Curry, L.L.; Goulson, M.J.; Kolberg, L.W. Extracted Barley Beta-Glucan Improves CVD Risk Factors and Other Biomarkers in a Population of Generally Healthy Hypercholesterolemic Men and Women. *Prevent Control* 2005; 1(1):131.

Rendell, M.; Vanderhoof, J.; Venn, M.; Shehan, M.A.; Arndt, E.; Rao, C.S.; Gill, G.; Newman, R.K.; Newman, C.W. Effect of barley breakfast cereal on blood glucose and insulin response in normal and diabetic patients. *Plant Foods Hum Nutr* 60(2): 63–7, 2005 Jun

Rigaud, D.; Paycha, F.; Meulemans, A.; Merrouche, M.; Mignon, M. Effect of psyllium on gastric emptying, hunger feeling and food intake in normal volunteers: a double blind study. *Eur J Clin Nutr* 1998 April;52(4):239–45.

Rimm, E.B.; Ascherio, A.; Giovannucci, E.; Spiegelman, D.; Stampfer, M.J.; Willett, W.C. Vegetable, fruit, and cereal fiber intake and risk of coronary heart disease among men. *J.A.M.A*. 1996;275:447–451.

Shukla, K.; Narain, J.P.; Puri, P., et al. Glycaemic response to maize, bajra and barley. *Indian J Physiol Pharmacol*. 1991;35(4):249–54.

Steffen, L.M.; Jacobs, D.R., Jr.; Murtaugh, M.A., et al. Whole grain intake is associated with lower body mass and greater insulin sensitivity among adolescents. *Am J Epidemiol*. 2003;158(3):243–50.

Third Report of the National Cholesterol Education Program (NCEP) Expert Panel on Detection, Evaluation, and Treatment of High Blood Cholesterol in Adults (Adult Treatment Panel III) final report. *Circulation* 2002 December 17;106(25):3143–421.

Thorburn, A.; Muir, J.; Proietto, J. Carbohydrate fermentation decreases hepatic glucose output in healthy subjects. *Metabolism*. 1993;42(6):780–5.

Urooj, A.; Vinutha, S.R.; Puttaraj, S.; Leelavathy, K.; Rao, P.H. Effect of barley incorporation in bread on its quality and glycemic responses in diabetics. *Int J Food Sci Nutr*. 1998;49:265–70.

Wang, L.; Newman, R.K.; Newman, C.W.; Hofer, P.J. Barley beta-glucans alter intestinal viscosity and reduce plasma cholesterol concentrations in chicks. *J Nutr.* 1992;122:2292–7.

Wirfalt, E.; Hedblad, B.; Gullberg, B. et al. Food patterns and components of the metabolic syndrome in men and women: a cross-sectional study within the Malmo Diet and Cancer Cohort. *Am J Epidemiol.* 2001;154(12):1150–9.

Wolever, T.M.; Mehling, C. High-carbohydrate-low-glycaemic index dietary advice improves glucose disposition index in subjects with impaired glucose tolerance. *Br J Nutr.* 2002;87(5):477–87.

Wolk, A.; Manson, J.E.; Stampfer, M.J., et al. Long-term intake of dietary fiber and decreased risk of coronary heart disease among women. *J.A.M.A.* 1999;281:1998–2004.

Wu, H.; Dwyer, K.M.; Fan, Z.; Shircore, A.; Fan, J.; Dwyer, J.H. Dietary fiber and progression of atherosclerosis: the Los Angeles Atherosclerosis Study. *Am J Clin Nutr.* 2003;78(6):1085–91.

Part III

Grain Technology and Health-related Outcomes

8 Biochemistry and Compartmentalization of Cereal Grain Components and Their Functional Relationship to Mammalian Health

David A. Pascoe and R. Gary Fulcher

Cereal grains provide the majority of the calories (primarily as starch) in the American diet, as they do in other cultures. Worldwide, it has been estimated that humans obtain more than 50% of their calories and protein from cereal consumption and animals obtain approximately 25% to 50%. A variety of methods have been used to prepare cereal grains and use them in foods and beverages. Wheat, rye, and barley have been used in bread and bread-like products, with wheat and rye gaining favor over time due to the protein complexes required for yeast-leavened bread. Rye, barley, sorghum, and rice also have been used in fermentative processes to produce whiskey, beer, sake, and miso.

By definition, the term "cereal" applies strictly to those genera and species of the grass family (Gramineae) that have been domesticated for food and feed production, most often as seed products (e.g. flour, bran, germ, grits, malt, rolled oats, starch, etc.). The group includes common staples such as corn (*Zea mais*); common, durum, and club wheats (*Triticum aestivum, T. durum,* and *T. compactum*); barley (*Hordeum vulgare*); rye (*Secale cereale*); oats (*Avena sativa*); rice (*Oryza sativa*); sorghum (*Sorghum bicolor*); and various millets, wild rice, and other miscellaneous grasses. All of these grains are closely related structurally and biochemically, but they are quite distinct from the other major dietary grains—such as soy, peas, lentils, canola, etc.—which are botanically distinct, storing their seed reserves primarily as proteins, lipids, and fiber, with comparatively smaller amounts of starch. There continues to be a shift toward high starch levels in the cereals, and this has been accentuated by centuries of breeding for malt, bread, and cookie flour, and starch extraction and modification. Recent developments also include production of modified starch forms, including high amylose, waxy (high amylopectin), and resistant starches for novel food applications.

The Economic Research Service of the U.S. Department of Agriculture (ERS/USDA) surveys indicate recent and dramatic increases in per capita consumption of refined grains in a relatively short time (20 to 30 years). Typical cereal grains are energy-dense, containing 50% to 80% starch, depending on the species, origin, and environmental growing conditions. Their products are thus dominated by starch, and are further characterized by having most (in some cases all) of their important biologically active components (fiber, antioxidants, minerals, vitamins) stripped from the grains during milling, malting, and other conventional fractionations.

In 2000, Americans consumed, on average, 200 pounds of refined flour and other cereal products (unadjusted data) compared to 147 pounds in the early 1980s and 135 pounds in the early 1970s (ERS/USDA 2005). During the same period, total consumption of caloric sweeteners manufactured from cereal starches have also increased dramatically, including a 4,080% increase in high fructose corn syrup (ERS/USDA).

While Americans are consuming more refined cereals and sweeteners, recent market trends show they are also choosing to supplement their food choices. The United States holds the

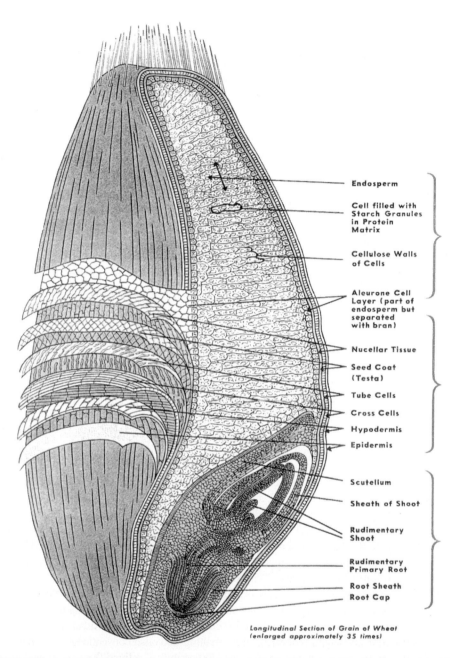

Endosperm

Cell filled with
Starch Granules
in Protein
Matrix

Cellulose Walls
of Cells

Aleurone Cell
Layer (part of
endosperm but
separated
with bran)

Nucellar Tissue

Seed Coat
(Testa)

Tube Cells

Cross Cells

Hypodermis

Epidermis

Scutellum

Sheath of Shoot

Rudimentary
Shoot

Rudimentary
Primary Root

Root Sheath

Root Cap

*Longitudinal Section of Grain of Wheat
(enlarged approximately 35 times)*

Figure 8.1. Longitudinal section of a wheat kernel showing typical tissue relationships in a cereal grain. The architecture is similar in all cereals, although the chemistry of each fraction differs considerably. (Courtesy of Hoseney 1994.)

largest portion of the world's functional food sales, with grain and beverage products comprising the top two segments of the market (Sloan 2002). Functional foods and functional food ingredients are a high priority in the food industry due to consumer demands and the market potential for specific food products that could potentially improve human health (Sloan 2002).

Since the 1980s, the availability of information to consumers about healthcare, nutrition, exercise, and food has driven a dietary supplement market and a growing trend of "hands-on healthcare." Currently, consumers choose to use fortified foods over dietary supplements (as in previous years), with fortified food sales up almost 60% since 1998, representing "health conscious" consumer selection and purchasing decisions at the grocery store (FMI 2001). An increasing number of consumers want more foods containing vitamins, minerals, antioxidants, and fiber. These "bioactive" components are all found in whole grains.

Americans have increased their use of fiber, and whole grain consumption has increased by almost 40% since the early 1990s (Kantor et al. 2001, Milner 2002). Consumers associate the consumption of fiber with increased energy, and prevention of disease, cancer, and weight gain. However, cardiovascular disease (CVD), diabetes, high blood pressure, obesity, and cholesterol are still on the rise in many developed countries, including the United States (WHO/FAO 2003).

While cereal grains contain more starch than any other single component, the mature kernel is not devoid of other important and potentially beneficial nutrients that could help prevent disease. As in all biological systems, each grain constituent is synthesized and stored in discrete locations and structures, some of which are easily digested while many others are not. More importantly, all cereal grains are organized on a common architectural template, the commercial manipulation of which allows systematic disruption, fractionation, and concentration of the major internal storage compounds. The structure of a typical unprocessed cereal (wheat) is shown in Figure 8.1.

The structure, composition, and spatial relationships of cereal tissues lend themselves to ready dissociation of the three primary industrial fractions: the germ, bran, and starchy endosperm (Kent and Evers 1994, Hoseney 1994). Whole grain products contain all three of these fractions intact, while products made from refined material (starchy endosperm, bran, or germ) contain completely different constituent profiles. Some of these fractions can be further subdivided to produce concentrates with additional differences in composition and potentially more importantly, biological activity.

The following section summarizes the biochemistry of the major bioactive components of cereal grains from their respective structural organization in the seed. The latter portion of the chapter focuses on specific differences between domesticated cereal grains, as defined in this chapter. When appropriate the reader will be directed to investigations of specific topics that will more clearly define details not covered in this chapter.

Biochemistry of Cereal Grains

Endosperm

The starchy endosperm is non-viable and serves as an energy store for the growing embryo or, after many centuries of genetic improvement, as a source of commercial raw materials for food and feed manufacture. The endosperm is the primary source of visco-elastic gluten proteins for breads, starch for syrups and malt, and soluble fibers. Regardless of the type of cereal, the endosperm is the primary ingredient of cereal product manufacturers.

The endosperm, the largest of the grain tissues, is primarily a storage tissue containing starch-filled cells with smaller and variable amounts of relatively poor-quality protein, encased in cell walls composed of various mixed linkage β-glucans, arabinoxylans (pentosans), and minor amounts of lipids, nucleic acids, and minerals. While the quality of the endosperm proteins is considered nutritionally poor, their biochemistry provides for unique developments in baking and health. The extraction of proteins from cereal grains results in the presence of four types and their ratios vary according to each cereal: albumins, globulins, glutelins, and prolamins (Table 8.1). Endosperm components in oats have been reviewed (Peterson and Brinegar 1986) and a biological review of endosperm development and function has been provided by Lopes and Larkins (1993).

Storage proteins found in the endosperm encompass the prolamins and glutelins, normally accumulating with nitrogen availability in the soil, but over-accumulating during drought, disease, and early frost. These storage proteins give rise to the gluten complex, providing the functional properties to wheat dough (Shewry et al. 1985, Shewry and Tatham 1990, Tilley et al. 2001), and consist of low molecular weight gliadins (approximately 40 Kd) and high molecular weight (approximately 100 Kd) glutenins (Lasztity 1996). A complex interaction between appropriate amino acids, disulfide bonding, ratio of gliadin/glutenins, and an interaction with water allows these gluten proteins to yield a dough mixture with cohesive and elastic properties for making bread with a satisfactory loaf volume (Eliasson and Larrson 1993).

Amino acid analysis of corn and oat endosperm demonstrates the quality and general amino acid composition of storage proteins (Table 8.2). While the nutritional quality of protein in the bran is of higher grade, the reduced quality of storage proteins generally reflects a reduced level of lysine, methionine, cysteine, and trytophan and a higher proportion of glutamic acid and proline, two important amino acids in gluten formation.

Glutamic acid and proline-rich specific sequences of storage proteins also cause unwanted immunological activity in an increasing number of consumers (Robins and Howdle 2005). Cereal-related allergy has become a prevalent problem in our society because cereals play a central role in our diet. An estimated one in 150 Americans must avoid them due to celiac sprue disease, and many other people can be affected through ulcerative colitis or irritable bowel disease (Shan et al. 2002).

Celiac disease is a multifactorial condition which restricts an individual from eating food products that contain gluten, including wheat, spelt, barley, and rye. This is significant because gluten is the second most prevalent food ingredient next to sugar and starch in the American

Table 8.1. Compositional distribution of proteins found in major cereal grains. (Values based upon Osborne [1907] solubility fractions.)

Cereal Grain	Albumins	Prolamins	Globulins	Glutelins
Wheat	9–15	33–45	6–7	40–46
Corn	4–8	47–55	3–4	38–45
Rice	5–11	2–7	~10	77–78
Barley	~12	25–52	8–12	52–55
Oats	10–20	12–14	12–55	23–54
Rye	10–44	21–42	10–19	25–40
Sorghum	~4	~48	~9	~37

Data from Lasztity (1996) and Eliasson and Larsson (1993).

Table 8.2. Amino acid composition of wheat grain and wheat flour (% of protein).

Amino Acid	Corn Endosperm	Oat Endosperm
Alanine	8.1	4.5
Arginine	3.8	6.6
Cysteine	1.8	2.2
Glutamic Acid	21.3	23.6
Glycine	3.2	4.7
Histidine	2.8	2.2
Leucine	14.3	7.8
Lysine	2.0	3.7
Methionine	2.8	2.4
Phenylalanine	5.3	5.6
Proline	9.7	4.6
Serine	5.2	4.6
Valine	4.7	5.5

Data from Hoseney (1994).

diet (Harder 2003). Wheat proteins, specifically the prolamins, gliadin and glutenins, appear to cause the majority of inflammatory problems for celiac patients, but the globular proteins, albumin and globulin, have also demonstrated reactions *in vitro* (Battais 2003).

Wheat proteins belong to a family of plant proteins with similar characteristics that cause allergy and intolerance in affected individuals (Breiteneder and Mills 2005). Common characteristics include thermal stability and resistance to enzymatic proteolysis, with improved stabilization through binding of metals, lipids, and some hydrophobic signaling molecules (Platt and Mensink 2005). These interactions can happen in the gastrointestinal tract, but they may also happen during processing of salad dressings, sauces, and mayonnaises with casein, whey, or soy proteins present. Many proteins unfold during interaction with lipid bilayers to reveal hydrophobic areas. These types of protein interactions can pose problems for the immune system in identifying self and non-self food epitopes in the gastrointestinal tract during absorption.

In addition to these interactions, most investigators agree that the one mechanism causing most problems comes from transglutaminase in the gastrointestinal tract, transforming glutamine to glutamic acid on proline-rich gluten peptides (Robins and Howdle 2005). This change (deamination) of an amino acid affects protein structure, stimulating the host immune system. However, help for the approximately 3 million celiac patients may not be so far off with the counter use of enzymatic therapy. Bacterial prolyl endopeptidases specifically break up the proline-rich gliadin peptides and have shown significantly reduced reactions in animal models (Shan et al. 2004). This may pose a challenge for food scientists to build a better bread with significant loaf volume, without the all-important proline/glutamine sequences in gliadins. Celiac sprue disease has recently been reviewed by Sollid (2002) and Breiteneder and Mills 2005.

Endosperm cell walls consist of dietary fiber sources, non-starchy carbohydrates that act as scaffolding during development, and aid movement of water and materials during germination (Carpita 1996, Carpita et al. 2001). Non-starchy carbohydrates (i.e. β-glucans, arabinoxylans) demonstrate unique biological activity in the gastrointestinal tract in the purified and food matrix forms. Dietary fiber in general confers many health benefits to mammals, reducing risk factors for heart and gastrointestinal disease and diabetes. While Americans are reminded to consume 20 grams to 35 grams of total fiber a day, the average consumer takes in less than half this amount (Marlett and Slavin 1997). Soluble fiber from oat and barley has received the attention of many investigators due to its ability to lower total and LDL cholesterol, reduce postprandial glucose and insulin, and slow gastric emptying (Cumming et al. 1979, 1992; Pietinen et al. 1996; Rimm et al. 1996; Brown et al. 1999). While not as well known, some soluble fibers from oat and barley stimulate the immune system (Platt and Mensink 2005).

Recent evidence demonstrates that soluble dietary fiber fermentation in the colon affects the highly integrated immune system along the gastrointestinal tract (Lim et al. 1997), increasing CD4+ T-cells in lymph (a review of dietary fiber and the immune system by Schley and Fields 2002) while others (Field et al. 1999) show consuming high fermentable fiber diets produces higher CD8+ T-cells. This mechanism may work through production of short-chained fatty acids that traverse the intestinal wall to stimulate several components of the immune system (Watzl et al. 2005, Galvez et al. 2005). β-glucans from fungi have been used to control bacterial infections including pneumocystis, anthrax, and sepsis in infected animals (Kournikakis et al. 2003, Evans et al. 2005, Sener et al. 2005).

Cereal β-glucans are linear polymers of repeating glucopyranosyl units, connected by β-(1,3) and β-(1,4) linkages, commonly referred to as mixed-linkage β-glucans. Soluble mixed-linkage cereal β-glucans from rye and oats have stimulated monocytes to produce cytokines tumor necrosis factor (TNFα) and interleukin 1 (IL-1) (Estrada et al. 1997, Roubroeks et al. 2000). TNFα is a key chemical messenger secreted by macrophages and monocytes in response to invading microorganisms, stimulating T-cells and mediating inflammation in the host (Gonçalves et al. 2001, Kollias et al 1999). Controlling TNFα may potentially control infectious agents, insulin sensitivity, and inflammation related to cardiovascular disease and obesity (Dullemen et al. 1995, Ofei et al. 1996, Mendall et al. 1997). Here, we show that a highly purified (> 97%) mixed linkage (1,3),(1,4)- β-D-glucan preparation from oats stimulates murine macrophages (RAW 267.4) *in vitro* (Figure. 8.2). Treatment of the same oat β-glucan samples with lichenase produced significantly (p < 0.05) more TNFα (approximately 3 times) from macrophages. Mixed linkage (1,3),(1,4)- β-D-glucans from barley (± lichenase treatment) were also used to treat the same macrophages, but no increase in TNFα production was observed with enzyme treatment (data not shown).

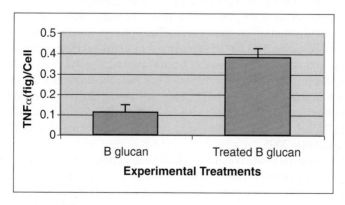

Figure 8.2. Production of TNFα from macrophages simulated by enzyme-treated (lichenase1u/ml; 40 C, 1 h) and -untreated oat β-glucan (>97% pure)(n = 3).

Increased TNFα production due to lichenase treatment may be due to increased β-(1-3) linkage exposure contacting macrophage receptors (Brown and Gordon 2001). In the last five years an increasing number of studies have revealed the complex interaction of β-(1-3) glucans and multiple immune system receptors (Brown et al. 2002, Willment et al. 2005). But of fundamental importance, it should not be forgotten that extraction methods often determine the functional characteristics of the glucans; in our experiments, oat β-glucan was extracted by an alkaline process and barley β-glucans by hot water, and this may explain TNFα production differences.

Germ

The germ is simply the embryonic plant destined for germination in favorable growth conditions, but because of these characteristics contains a small quantity of enzymes (e.g. phytase), proteins (albumins, globulins), lipid (approximately 10%), and nucleic acid (approximately 4%) (Pomeranz 1988). Protein content in cereal germs ranges from approximately 20% to 25%. They tend to have higher leucine, lysine, and threonine amino acids and low tryptophan and methionine. Lipids present in the germ include linolenic, linoleic, oleic, and palmitic acids (Ashworth et al. 1981, Barnes 1982). The germ is more complex than the endosperm, comprising a large number of tissues and storage compounds, many of which are also significantly different from those encountered in the bran. Although the bran and germ appear to be similar, both contain proteins, lipids, and phenolics, such as ferulic acid, but the extraordinary niacin reserves of the bran, for example, are totally absent from the germ, belying a number of distinctions that differentiate these tissues, both chemically and nutritionally. A large number of antioxidant and antimicrobial compounds have been identified in these tissues, but many remain unidentified (Collins 1986; McKeehen et al. 1998, 1999).

Bran

The bran, comprised of the most complex tissues in the grain, also contains the highest concentration of bioactive compounds. The bran is a diverse array of at least seven different tissues, each with different compositions and biological activities. The dry weight of the bran, including all of its several botanically distinct tissues, approaches 20% of the mature wheat kernel, but may be more or less in other cereal grains. It is relatively indigestible without further processing, and the elevated levels of antioxidants often impart bitter flavors and dark colors to finished products. Bran also contains a significant amount of both insoluble and soluble fiber in the form of pentosans, cellulose, and mixed-linkage β-glucans (Bacic and Stone 1981a,b; Fulcher and Wong 1980; Dervilly-Pinel et al. 2004). Sterols and phytoestrogens (see below) are also stored in these tissues (Bach Knudsen et al. 2000, Mazur and Adlerkreutz 1998, Piironen et al. 2002).

One of the bran tissues, the aleurone layer, constitutes approximately 50% to 70% of the bran weight and is, for example, the richest natural known source of niacin and contains many additional B-vitamins, minerals, arginine- and lysine-enriched proteins, and unique unsaturated lipids (Fulcher 1972; Fulcher et al. 1972a, b; Hargin et al. 1980; Fulcher et al. 1981). It is a substantial source of hydrolytic enzymes during germination (in some products) and it contains major groups of antioxidants, including several cinnamic acids, flavonoids, tocopherols, tocotrienols, lignin, and pigments such as anthocyanins and proanthocyanidins. The nutritional properties of isolated aleurone layers are usually higher than those exerted by the intact, commercial bran fractions that contain them. The aleurone layer of all cereals is the primary source of bioactive compounds in the bran and in general, all whole grain products.

Antioxidants/Pigments

The elevated phenolic acid antioxidant complement of aleurone layers has been recognized for many years and the compounds have received renewed interest as the primary sources of antioxidants in characterized bran (Kikuzaki et al. 2002, Adom 2003). First recognized as a primary phenolic compound, ferulic acid is by far the dominant phenolic acid in bran, and it occurs in particularly high concentrations in the aleurone cell walls (Fulcher et al. 1972b). It is accompanied by several companion compounds, notably p-coumaric, syringic, and p-hydroxybenzoic acids, among other low-molecular-weight phenolic esters (Collins 1986 McKeehen et al. 1999), and their combined effect is to contribute the majority of the antioxidant activity of wheat bran, as measured by the oxygen radical absorbance capacity (ORAC) procedure and free radical 2,2-diphenyl-1-picrylhydrazyl (DPPH) scavenging activity (see Miller et al. 2000a,b and Gavin et al. 2003 for discussion). Moreover, these elevated antioxidant profiles are expressed in processed grain products containing significant bran concentrations (Miller et al. 2000a,b).

While some of these same hydroxycinnamic acids have demonstrated chemopreventive effects *in vivo*, the direct absorption of these phenolic acids into the human circulatory system after cereal bran consumption has been demonstrated (Kawabata et al. 2000, Kern et al. 2003). Interestingly, the consumption of cereal bran, where most phenolic acids are bound in cell wall components, greatly improved the plasma half-life of phenolic acids and their antioxidant

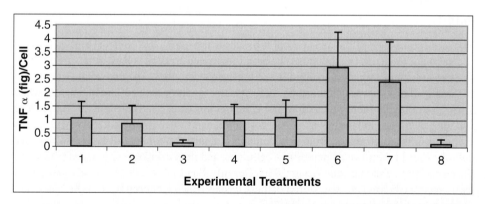

Figure 8.3. TNFα production from macrophages stimulated by oat β-glucan and curdlan, but inhibited by wheat and barley bran ethanolic extracts. (1) Oat β-glucan (300ug/ml). (2) Pretreated macrophages (2h) with wheat bran extract (2.4ug/ul) then addition of oat β-glucan (300ug/ml). (3) Pretreated macrophages (2h) with barley bran extract (2.9ug/ul) then addition of oat β-glucan (300ug/ml). (4) Pretreated macrophages (2h) with oat bran extract (1.4ug/ul) then addition of oat β-glucan (300ug/ml). (5) Pretreated macrophages (2h) with buckwheat bran extract (1.8ug/ul) then addition of oat β-glucan (300ug/ml). (6) Curdlan a strict β(1–3) glucan (50ug/ml). (7) Pretreated macrophages (2h) with wheat bran extract (2.4ug/ul) then addition of curdlan (50ug/ml). (8) Pretreated macrophages (2h) with barley bran extract (2.9ug/ul) then addition of curdlan (50ug/ml). Statistical significance (p < 0.05) only between treatments 1 and 3, 6, and 8 (n = 3).

capacity in animals over a 24-hour period, when compared to free isolated phenolic acid consumption (Rondini et al. 2004). Recent results in our lab suggest that cereal bran components also have the capacity to inhibit inflammatory cytokines. Macrophages stimulated to produce TNFα with oat β-glucan and curdlan (bacterial β-3 glucan) can be significantly ($p < 0.05$) inhibited by pretreatment with extracts from barley bran (Figure 8.3). Macrophages pretreated with wheat bran extracts also inhibited TNFα production, but to a lesser degree ($p > 0.05$). Oat bran and buckwheat bran extracts did not inhibit the production of TNFα from macrophages stimulated by oat β-glucan. Low-molecular-weight phenolic acids or other unidentified compounds may participate in this form of cytokine inhibition.

Proteins

The nutritional characteristics of wheat proteins have been of somewhat limited interest historically, except for the recent interest in food allergens. While the storage proteins of the endosperm are composed for the most part of glutamic acid-rich, insoluble, lysine-deficient polymers that are prized primarily for their gluten-forming and related rheological properties, many proteins of the bran are considered metabolically active. Metabolically active proteins include enzymes found in the active bran layers during respiration, germination, and post-harvest reactions (reviewed by Anderson et al. 1982, see below in the section on Enzymes). Like other grain components, however, there is abundant compartmentalization of protein types within the grain, and both the germ and bran are compositionally quite different from the starchy endosperm that constitutes the majority of white flour.

Wheat germ is a relatively small part of the grain, so the bran, and particularly the aleurone layer, is the primary contributor of non-endosperm proteins. Bran is well known as a negative modifier of gluten strength—the more bran present in flour, the less acceptable are the rheological properties. Some of the rheological deficiencies of bran-rich (or whole grain) flours lie in the dilution effect expressed by the non-gluten bran components (e.g. fiber). There are suggestions however, that bran proteins may actively interfere with dough formation, but the evidence is inconsistent.

Nutritionally, however, bran is another matter—it is typically higher in total protein (15% to 20%) than the adjacent endosperm (typically 10% to 15%), and usually contains elevated levels of those amino acids commonly considered to be nutritionally limiting in wheat products, especially lysine and other basic amino acids such as arginine and histidine (Fulcher et al. 1972a, Lasztity 1996). Lysine levels in isolated aleurone cell contents can be more than double the levels found in the starchy endosperm (Fulcher et al. 1972a). Germ is similar in having elevated lysine levels (as much as 30% to 50% in some cereals; Fulcher 1986) and both fractions (bran and germ) should be viewed as preferred sources of these basic amino acids. Once again, the aleurone layer contains the majority of the bran proteins, and recent assays of isolated aleurone layers confirm this notion, indicating 16.9% to 20.8% (Buri et al. 2003).

Enzymes

The primary role of the aleurone layer in the mature grain is similar for all cereals: it is the target of germ-produced hormones that stimulate the synthesis of a vast array of hydrolytic enzymes that are needed for mobilizing seed reserves, including starch and other carbohydrates, protein, lipids, and nucleic acids. Enzymes analyzed and characterized in cereal grains, like other systems, usually have been those that are detectable and at higher concentrations than others (Hoseney 1994). These include, but are not restricted to, proteases, lipases, α, β-amylases, phytases, lipoxygenase, and acid phosphatases (Hoseney 1994, Fox and Mulvihill 1982). As such, aleurone cells are capable of synthesizing significant quantities of many different enzymes, some of which may be capable of both positive (e.g. nutrient release) and negative (e.g. enzymatic rancidity) effects in aleurone-enriched products. This capacity, however, should not be viewed as a significant deterrent to consumption in most cases—appropriate processing will either stimulate or inactivate aleurone enzymes and control should not be an issue. The process of hormone-aleurone interaction has been reviewed many times (Jacobsen 1984).

Sterols and Lignans

Sterols

Although traditionally associated with soy and corn oils, recent evidence suggests that wheat and other cereals also may be sources of significant amounts of plant sterols (Zangenberg et al. 2004, Awika and Rooney 2004). Sterols, stanols, and their esters, including campesterol, campestanol, sitosterol and sitostanol, among others, have been associated with reduced serum cholesterol (Normen et al. 2000) and lower risks of colon cancer (Awad and Fink 2000, Buri et al. 2003, Normen et al. 2001). Pearling fines of hulless barley and rye contain more than 2 mg/gram of sterol compounds (Lampi et al. 2004). More importantly, the level of total sterols in commercial concentrates of wheat aleurone layers is significantly higher than that of either bran (by 25%) or whole wheat (approximately 250%). This argues strongly in favor of the bran and aleurone layers being the primary sources of cereal sterols and some are substantially enriched in aleurone preparations (e.g. sitostanol occurs in isolated aleurone layers at twice the concentrations found in whole wheat grains; see Buri et al. 2003) and total sterol content in aleurone layers approaches that of presumed therapeutic concentrations that occur in many other plants.

Both sterol and stanol esters are deemed effective at 1.3 grams/day and 3.4 grams/day in lowering cholesterol and at these levels may meet the allowable Food and Drug Administration health claims for cholesterol reduction and heart disease reduction. Most cereal grains contain significant levels of sterols and their esters (approximately 50 mg/100 grams to 100 mg/100 grams; Piironen et al. 2002) and isolated wheat aleurone layers appear to contain more than 200 mg/100 grams total plant sterols (Buri et al. 2003).

Lignans (Phytoestrogens)

Lignans and neolignans are a large group of natural products characterized by the coupling of two C_6C_3 units. As such, they are closely related to the ferulic, coumaric, syringic, and sinapic acids that are commonly found in cereal bran, being simple dimers of these and other cinnamic acids (Mazur 1998). They are presumed precursors of lignin biosynthesis and as such are found in a wide range of plant species, including cereals and other commercial plant products.

Lignans are a significant dietary component, primarily as physiological effectors of estrogen-like activity (Hallsman et al. 2003). Although they are most commonly associated with soy and other legumes, they are abundant in many cereals, particularly rye, but including wheat (Nilsson et al. 1997).

Lignans are capable of binding to estrogenic receptors in mammalian cells, thereby modifying hormonal balance. High concentrations of laricinesinol, isolariciresinol, pinoresinol, and syringaresinol have recently been discovered in rye bran. All of these compounds, except isolariciresinol, are converted to enterolactone and enterodiol by intestinal bacterial enzymes (Heinonen et al. 2001). As phenolic compounds they are also effective antioxidants (Adlercreutz 1997).

Several laboratories have developed evidence that dietary intake of lignans assists in lowering breast and prostate cancer risk, and may also reduce the risk of coronary heart disease (Bach and Knudsen et al. 2003). Once again, however, it is essential to note that the majority of the lignans that occur in wheat are concentrated primarily in the aleurone layer. Using secoisolariciresinol (SECO) and matiaresinol (MAT) as primary markers of lignan content, Mazur and Adlerkreutz (1998) report that in some aleurone concentrates, these compounds exceed the total SECO+MAT content of whole wheat by more than ten times (381 μg/100 grams vs 36 μg/100 grams) and endosperm flour by forty-fold (381 μg/100 grams vs. 8 μg/100 grams)! Both compounds are present in significantly higher levels in aleurone preparations as compared to wheat bran. More importantly, SECO and MAT contribute only about 5% of the total lignan content to wheat bran; others such as syringaresinol are much more abundant (more than 6 mg/100 grams). Quite obviously, wheat bran, and especially aleurone layers, are the primary source of lignans in the wheat kernel.

Vitamins

Cereal brans represent perhaps the richest natural source of niacin in our food supply (Hinton 1947, Hinton et al. 1953, Fulcher et al. 1981). Moreover, the niacin is contained entirely within the aleurone layer, and is accompanied by many other water-soluble vitamins such as thiamine, riboflavin, folic acid, pantothenic acid, and fat-soluble tocopherols. Isolated aleurone cell contents, for example, may contain as much as 1,500 μg of niacin (Fulcher 1972). While there is considerable influence of both genetics and environment on its synthesis, aleurone cells remain a spectacular dietary source of all members of the B-vitamin group. In an effort to maximize white flour color, as well as flavor and bake volumes, the traditional milling process removes the bran, including the aleurone layer, but this loss results directly in severe reduction of several vitamins.

Historically, widespread removal of bran from many cereals, including rice, corn, and wheat, has led directly to several well-known dietary deficiency syndromes, including beriberi and pellagra (Roe 1973). It must be emphasized, however, that while the retention of aleurone layers in processed cereal foods will no doubt increase the dietary availability of these vitamins, the manner in which the vitamins are sequestered, and the processes employed in processing, will affect both the availability of vitamins as well as the degree to which they are retained (undamaged) in products.

It has been known for some time (Mason and Kodicek 1973a,b) that at least some of the wheat aleurone niacin is sequestered as an ester, which is both poorly characterized and difficult to digest (Roe 1973) and caution is required in interpreting the results of "total" niacin assays. Nonetheless, niacin is the exclusive domain of the aleurone layer, at least in wheat (Fulcher et al. 1981), and it is easily digested after relatively mild pre-treatments that are designed to cleave the ester linkages. Perhaps more interestingly, the niacin in wheat is associated with one or more antioxidants, and the complex also exerts some antibiotic effects (Mason and Kodicek 1973a,b). Niacin deposits do not exist in wheat germ, although other members of the B-vitamin group show some partitioning into both bran and germ.

Regardless of the absolute vitamin content of any particular B-vitamin in bran, the case can certainly be made that the majority of the B-vitamins are stored primarily in the aleurone layer, and in some cases (e.g. niacin), exclusively. The layer is a remarkable source of bioactive compounds, such as vitamins, combined with antioxidants such as phenyl propanoids (primarily cinnamic acid derivatives and some lignin), tocopherols, lignans, sterols, and sterol esters. There is substantial genetic variation (McKeehen et al. 1999, Pussayaw-nawin et al. 1998, Zupfer et al. 1998) across the *Triticum* and other cereal genomes in total content of all of these materials, but the simple conclusion is that aleurone layers are perhaps the most compelling source of these compounds in the food system.

Minerals

The majority of the mineral complement in any cereal grain is sequestered primarily in the form of crystalline phytate complexes. Typically, the total mineral content is measured as "ash" after incineration at more than 550°C, but this technique belies a wealth of variation in composition, as well as distribution. First, while most of the minerals in wheat are concentrated as phytate salts in both the germ and bran, the overwhelming dominance of the latter as a proportion of the grain (approximately 20% vs approximately 5%) dictates that grain minerals are, like most other biologically active constituents, a characteristic feature of bran (thus its decades-long role as a diagnostic tool for measuring bran content in flour).

Like many other components, however, it is the aleurone layer that is the primary domain of wheat minerals. Phytin crystals are not found in any other bran structures but the aleurone cells, and it has been shown that the crystals that are synthesized and stored within each protein body in the aleurone cells are in fact the phytin reserves, despite the rather random and often clouded history of research on these structures over the last century and a half (Fulcher and Rooney Duke 2002).

Typical phytin crystals consist of a phosphate-rich myo-inositol skeleton to which are chelated an array of cations, including K, Mg, Ca, Fe, Zn, and Na. The ratios of these cations may vary and the total amount of phytin may vary, and the availability of the minerals to the digestive process has been debated for decades (Lopez et al. 2002). The fact remains, however, that the aleurone layer once again is the primary mineral reserve in the grain. Typical "ash" values for wheat bran are in the range of approximately 10 grams/100 grams (dry matter, DM) and individual cations range from 10 mg/kg to more than 900 mg/kg (DM) bran. The latter is not unusual for Ca values, indicating that Ca is stored in abundance in wheat aleurone layers (Fulcher 1972). Its nutritional availability obviously depends upon the chelating capacity of the inositol and of the processing conditions. The fact remains, however, that the aleurone layer is the primary source of minerals in wheat mill fractions.

Lipids

Wheat lipids are unique in foods, and their chemistry (and variability) has been described in some detail (Morrison 1984, Hargin et al. 1980). They are important ingredients and natural constituents of wheat products: they modify structure, lubricate and separate dough sheets, and produce some of the desired (and some undesired) sensory properties (flavor and texture). As with other constituents, however, it is important to recognize that lipids vary from tissue to tissue in the grain, and their nutritional characteristics have tended to be viewed as of minor interest, at least with respect to wheat. However, aleurone layers store a substantial percentage of the total lipid in the grain. Depending on the grain, the rest is distributed mainly to the germ or endosperm. Polyunsaturated fatty acids represent perhaps two-thirds of the total crude fat. Monounsaturated saturated fatty acids each contribute about 15% to 20% of the total (Buri et al. 2003).

Aleurone lipids also differ substantially from other grain lipids, as shown by very detailed analyses by Hargin et al. (1980). Hargin's work showed that 60% to more than 75% of the aleurone lipid is triglyceride, while the remaining aleurone lipids included non-polar lipids (7% to 12%, including sterylester, diglyceride, free fatty acids, monoglyceride, and 6-O-acylsterylglycoside), glycolipids (2.2% to 9.8%), and phospholipids (13.8% to 17.9%). In contrast, endosperm non-starch lipids contained only 16.7% to 26.2% triglyceride, with proportionally higher levels of non-polar lipids (13.3% to 19.5%), glycolipids (20.4% to 38.3%), and phospholipids (23.6 to 35.3%).

These figures are included to emphasize the variation in lipid content—even within a single tissue such as the aleurone layer—and in lipid composition between tissues or grain "compartments." Once again, the aleurone layer is unique, with elevated levels of triglycerides, and its uniqueness offers potential opportunities, both nutritionally and in processing.

Soluble and Insoluble Fiber(s)

Oat bran has received considerable attention as a source of mixed linkage β-glucans, the purported cholesterol-lowering soluble fiber that is concentrated in oat and barley bran. Although the mechanism(s) by which serum lipids are modified by these polymers is poorly under-·stood, bran-rich oat products may qualify for heart health claims, along with barley products, which were recently welcomed into the FDA health claims arena.

Wheat flour contains measurable amounts of both mixed linkage β-glucans and arabinoxylans (Wang et al. 1998), although the former are not as abundant as in oats or barley. In bran, however, there are substantial amounts of both polymer groups, contributing as much as 9% or more of the total soluble fiber that can be extracted from wheat bran after preliminary abrasion processing (Cui et al. 1999). How much of these materials reside in clean aleurone cells and how much is a product of other adhering bran layers is difficult to determine. It is apparent, however, that approximately 50% of wheat aleurone layers are comprised of "total dietary fiber" (Association of Analytical Chemists 991.43), mostly as insoluble fiber, with a relatively small amount (approximately 4%) contributing to the soluble fiber values. At the very least, the exceptionally high dietary fiber value of wheat bran has been recognized for decades, and it is likely that a substantial portion of these properties are due to the 75% of the bran that is aleurone tissue. A thorough compilation of different wheat classes/varieties, and their glucan, arabinoxylan, and related polymer contents, has been assembled by Hartunian Sowa (1997).

While not many studies are available, it is clear that the fiber in whole grains may provide a functional benefit in reducing weight gain when used in high fiber diets. Liu et al. (2003) analyzed data from the Harvard Nurses Study and found an inverse relationship with weight gain and the consumption of whole grains. While this relationship was significant, perhaps more important was the observed direct relationship between increased consumption of refined grains and increased weight gain.

Jenkins et al. (1987, 1988) and others have suggested that high fiber diets increase satiety through the reduction of postprandial insulin and glucose, resulting in a reduction in weight gain. A reduction in insulin and glucose from fiber may reduce hunger between meals and overall caloric intake of secondary meals. This may be due to the effects of increasing viscosity that some soluble fibers have in the stomach and gastrointestinal tract (Hoad et al. 2004), or it may be due to the ability of some dietary fiber sources to modulate the endocrine system through gastrointestinal hormones (Massimino et al. 1998).

Specific food components regulate food intake by stimulating appropriate receptors in the gastrointestinal tract, releasing gut hormones such as cholecystokinin (CCK), gastrin, or GLP-1. CCK has been suggested to be a short-term controlling agent on appetite and has been shown to be stimulated by the short peptide leptin, fatty acids, tyrosine and phenylalanine (Furuse et al. 1991, Barrachina et al. 1997). CCK is an endocrine hormone that is released into circulation when certain foods enter the stomach, resulting in hormonal or neuronal stimulation (Lewis and Williams 1990). While many functional food components have been studied, Holt et al. (1995) found that meals containing high-fiber cereals stimulated CCK to a greater extent than low-fiber meals. Bourden et al. (1999) and others have demonstrated that elevated and sustained CCK plasma levels can occur after consuming low- or high-fat meals containing significant amounts of fiber (Bourton-Freeman 2000). While animal and human feeding studies have demonstrated the connection between some dietary fiber consumption from cereals and CCK secretion, the literature is rather short of *in vitro* and *in vivo* evidence demonstrating CCK stimulation by different carbohydrate polymers or their different stereo-chemistry. Potential mechanisms of how dietary fiber controls body weight have been reviewed recently by Slavin (2005) and gastrointestinal satiety signals have been reviewed by Woods (2004).

The biologically active components of bran and germ are typically discarded residues from conventional wheat milling, barley malting, and other commercial processing operations, and are used primarily in animal feed formulations. A typical yield of flour (starchy endosperm) from wheat ranges from 72% to 80% of the starting dry weight of the kernel, and the remaining 20% to 28% of the grain is almost entirely destined for animal feed. Thus, refined grain is devoid of almost all of the biologically important molecules normally associated with viability and sustained metabolism of the grain during germination. An exception is corn, which is processed to provide starch from the endosperm and oil from the exceptionally large germ (Kent and Evers 1994, Hoseney 1994). However, the majority of corn's fiber, vitamins, minerals, and as yet poorly characterized antioxidants are put aside as feed, just as they are with other grains (Kent and Evers 1994, Hoseney 1994).

Although wheat, barley, and corn have received much of the attention in terms of chemical analyses, there is an enormous array of compounds in all cereals whose structures and activities are not well established. Most, however, exhibit some level of biological activity (McKeehen 1998, 1999), and the removal of the bran and germ in the refining process represents a substantial alteration in human dietary intakes in little more than a century (see *per capita* consumption data, ERS/USDA). More importantly, the non-endosperm portions of the grain represent an important source of bioactive materials that may impact mammalian systems in beneficial ways, including reduction of diabetic and cardiovascular risks through increased use of whole grain foods (Poutanen et al. 2002, Behall and Hallfrisch 2002, Slavin 2002).

It must be emphasized, however, that while the grain may contain a substantial array of bioactive compounds, the impact of recent processing innovations also remains to be evaluated. A cursory examination of the ERS/USDA data, for example, indicates that there has been a change in proportion of cereal types in the American diet, evolving from largely wheat-based intakes, with measurable oat, rye, and even barley elements, to a more limited base of wheat, corn and rice (ERS/USDA 2005). Concomitantly, there has been a substantial alteration of processing conditions, in which high fructose corn syrup has replaced a major portion of the traditional beet and cane sugar sweeteners, and in which many more products are extruded snack foods. Neither extrusion nor corn sweetener production was a significant feature of the cereal industry as recently as thirty years ago.

The continued refinement of cereal grains by removal of bran and germ (and their extensive array of bioactive materials), combined with dramatic changes in processing (extrusion and sweeteners), may provide a partial explanation for the substantial increases in non-insulin dependent diabetes mellitus (NIDDM). It also may provide an opportunity to identify the components in whole grains that may confer protective effects or reduce the negative effects of excessive whole grain consumption. At the very least, one might expect attenuation based on the simple effects of dilution and fiber addition.

Whole Grain Cereals

For purposes of further discussion, whole grains shall be viewed as consisting of the entire cereal grain kernel. The American Association of Cereal Chemists (AACC) continues to refine its definitions to encourage increased consumption of whole grains. The formal definition adopted by the AACC follows:

> "Whole grains shall consist of the intact, ground, cracked or flaked caryopsis, whose principal anatomical components: the starchy endosperm, germ and bran, are present in the same relative proportions as they exist in the intact caryopsis."

The previous sections of this chapter have outlined generic properties of the cereal grain— structure, chemical compartmentalization, and function. Each tissue is distinctly different from the others. It is also important to emphasize that each species of cereal exhibits distinctive characteristics not found in other cereals, and each is a package of significantly different bioactive compounds that are further modified in distinctly different classes or types within each species. The following section indicates some of the major differences between cereal species, and notes some of the advantages and opportunities for their use in food systems. Comments are restricted to the major cereals: wheat, corn, rice (wild and domestic), barley, rye, oats, and sorghum. Gross compositional differences between these cereals are demonstrated in Table 8.3.

Table 8.3.   Gross compositional fractions of different cereal grains. (Values are based on % dry weight.)

Cereal Grain	Protein	Lipid	Starch	Fiber	Ash
Wheat	12.2	1.9	71.9	1.9	1.7
Corn	10.2	4.6	79.5	2.3	1.3
Rice	8.1	1.2	75.8	0.5	1.4
Barley	10.9	2.3	73.5	4.3	2.4
Rye	11.6	1.7	71.9	1.9	2.0
Oats	11.3	5.8	55.5	10.9	3.2
Sorghum	11.0	3.5	65.0	4.9	2.6

Data from Lasztity (1996).

Barley

Barley has been used as a food product only sparingly in recent years (primarily as pearled barley for specialty applications). Its primary application is for animal feed and as a fermentation/distillation base for beer and ethanol. However, it presents major genetic opportunities, including exceptionally elevated levels of highly variable viscous polymers with wide-ranging solubilities, including (but not limited to) glucans and pentosans (Rooney Duke 1996, Fulcher and Rooney Duke 2002), a very large and softer kernel exhibiting hulless and waxy starch characteristics, exceptionally high antioxidant levels (two to three times those of wheat; see Zupfer et al. 1998, Pussayanawin et al. 1988, Wetzel et al. 1988, Andereasen et al. 2000a, b, 2001), antimicrobial and antifungal activity, and insect antifeedant activity (McKeehen et al. 1998, 1999; Fulcher et al. 1972a; Serratos et al. 1987; Sen et al. 1994; Bergvinsen et al. 1997).

In wheat, barley, and rye kernels, starch is synthesized in two granule types, the large "A" granules (approximately 20 μ/gram to 30 μ/gram diameter) and small "B" granules (approximately 2 μ/gram to 10 μ/gram diameter). Although their primary effects are usually related to processing properties (Haberer 1994, Rasper and DemMan 1980), each is quite different regarding digestibility, a feature of cereal starches that has been well documented in animal nutrition, brewing, and a range of other industrial contexts (Feng et al. 1997, McGregor and Bhatty 1993, Lu et al. 1999). However, granule size alone is not sufficient to define the level of digestibility, and other characteristics of the granule are also involved in starch digestibility (see Bird et al. 2000, Topping and Clifton 2001 for discussion). Some of the starch is stored as "resistant starch," a feature of cereal starches that is receiving increased attention (Slavin 2002).

Oats

Oats contain some of the largest quantities of lipids; approximately one-third are polar phospholipids and glycolipids complexes. Depending on variety, oats contain some of the highest contents of globulin proteins (15% to 55%) and some of the lowest glutelins (23% to 50%). Oats offer an unusual example of difficulties when fractionating cereals. Although products such as "oat bran" are common items of commerce, receiving almost excessive attention for their presumed ability to modify serum chemistry, the products are neither bran nor endosperm, but rather a somewhat diluted version of the latter. Because of the soft texture of the oat kernel, one cannot manufacture true bran with little or no starch as one can the other, harder textured cereals (Fulcher 1986).

Rice

Rice is a major component of the American diet, and its increased use is based in part on its low price, ready availability, blandness, and ease of processing. According to recent figures (ERS/USDA 2005), American rice consumption has increased 174% in the past thirty years, rivaling increases exhibited by corn (178%), while wheat has increased only 48% in the same period. Oat consumption has declined by 9% in the same period and does not represent a major cereal component of the U.S. diet. Furthermore, rice is consumed primarily in milled form (ERS/USDA 2005), in which the bran and germ have been removed (see also Kent and Evers 1994, Hoseney 1994).

A distinctive feature, however, relates to the fact that rice starch is similar to that of oats—they have compound granules that are compositionally and structurally similar. Oat and rice starch are known to digest more readily than that of other cereals; the basis for the difference is not obvious (Guraya et al. 1997). Although rice bran is typically rich in many vitamins and lipid-soluble antioxidants such as tocopherols/tocotrienols (Barnes 1983, Peterson and Qureshi 1993, Cahoon et al. 2003), like many cereals it also contains a number of anti-nutrition factors in the bran (embryo and germ). They include phytin (phytate), trypsin inhibitor, oryzacystatin, and haemagglutinin-lectin (Juliano 1993).

Rye

Although more closely related to wheat than many other cereals, rye is quite different compositionally. It contains starches similar to those of wheat, but the endosperm includes substantially elevated levels of phenolic acids and alk(en)ylresorcinols, as well as sterols, tocols, and lignans that are largely responsible for the strong flavor and dark color of rye and rye products (Andreasen et al. 2000a,b, 2001). These diverse compounds are readily partitioned during fractionation and the bioactive concentrations are substantially different in different mill streams. Bran and flour are very different compositionally, and the latter also contains high levels of viscous soluble polymers, including both arabinoxylans and β-glucans (Bacic and Stone 1982a,b).

Studies over several years continue to confirm the rather large variation in total and specific phenolic acid contents in different cereals grown in different locations (Pussayanawin et al. 1988, Zupfer et al. 1998, McKeehen 1998, Miller et al. 1995, Miller and Fulcher 1995, Rooney Duke 1996, Hartunian Sowa 1997). In all cases, however, the compartmentalization of these bioactive compounds is highly organized within the grains, and fractionation and/or further processing (extraction, baking, extrusion) leads directly to concentration, removal, or damage to the molecules. Cereal bran, for example may contain as much as 800 μ/gram to 1,000 μg/gram of the most common phenolic acid, 3-methoxy-4-hydroxycinnamic acid, while the adjacent starchy endosperm may have less than 100 μg/gram, much of which is derived from fractionation procedures rather than essential biological compartmentalization. Moreover, 3-methoxy-4-hydroxycinnamic acid is only one of many related compounds in the grains. There is considerable genetic diversity among the cereals, to the point of allowing phenolic biosynthetic patterns to be detected in common food grains among different genera. Effects on mammalian systems would also be expected to vary considerably in antioxidant profiles, flavor, reactivity, and antimicrobial activity.

Corn and Sorghum

Corn and sorghum share a number of common genetic traits, including strong tolerance of stress during production and compartmentalization of similar compounds in the bran and germ. Although U.S. consumption of dry-milled corn products is considerably less than that of wheat, total consumption of more highly refined corn products (such as dextrose, high fructose corn syrups, and other modified starches) moves the total corn consumption levels to those of wheat. Like rice, corn product consumption has exceeded that of wheat by a large margin. Moreover, most of the increased corn consumption has been based on materials (starch, syrups) that are much more refined than those derived from wheat flour. In addition, many snack foods are more commonly based on corn and rice starch extrusion than on wheat, rye, or oat extrusion, all of which often lead to development of undesirably strong flavors and colors. We do not yet understand the effects of high temperature and high pressure extrusion on bioactivity of the many compounds mentioned above. It is likely that they will be modified in any food processing system, be it baking, extrusion, or extraction.

Sorghum is not a common item in the U.S. human diet, but is used largely as an animal feed in areas of the country characterized by low rainfall or other environmentally stressful conditions. It is, however, a staple in many other parts of the world, and its chemistries are also of more than passing interest. Africa and the Indian subcontinent are both regions of considerable sorghum production and its use in the human diet is traditional in both baked goods and in alcoholic beverages. It appears in both red and white forms and its flavors are very strong.

Small amounts of mixed-linkage β-glucans are in both the bran and germ (Earp et al. 1983), and the phenolic content of the bran is very high (Waniska 2000). The grain is genetically highly variable, and may contain extensive pigmentation due to carotenoids, tannins (a unique trait among the major cereals), phenolic acids, flavonoids, and anthocyanins, among others. It is well known for its antimicrobial activities in the bran fractions (Ramputh et al. 1999). Phenolic compounds can occur in free or bound form and many have been identified by high-performance lipid chromatography (Waniska et al. 1989). Tannins are of particular interest because they have been implicated as anti-nutritional compounds in a number of animal systems (Mole et al. 1993). There are, however, a number of strong fungal growth inhibitors in sorghum that speak further to the strong biological activities therein (Waniska 2000). Most of these reside in the outer coverings and are removed during traditional and commercial processing.

The most rapidly increasing cereal in the American diet (ERS/USDA 2005), corn also is unique in its composition, structure, and end-use applications. The grain is much larger than other major cereals, with a proportionately larger oil-rich embryo and a significantly thinner bran layer than that of other grains. The crude protein content of corn sits between oats and wheat with some of the lowest albumin and globulin concentrations of the cereal grains. However, its large endosperm can contain some of the highest prolamin concentrations (55%).

Corn occurs in several forms in North America, including the most common dent (yellow or white) corn, flint (popcorn), and several minor specialty products, some of which are highly colored. The primary endosperm products are grits, flour, and starch; the latter is the major ingredient in a large array of cereal products. It is used to provide relatively modest amounts of clean starch, but much larger amounts of physically or chemically modified products for the human diet. Products of corn starch processing include acid-thinned starches, numerous cross-linked and/or substituted starches, enzyme-modified starches, and the majority of caloric sweeteners in the food industry. Corn sweeteners (e.g high fructose corn syrups) surpassed those from more traditional cane and beet sources many years ago (see ERS/USDA data).

Like other cereals, the unfractionated corn kernel contains a significant number of bioactive compounds that are concentrated primarily in the bran and germ. Insect antifeedant compounds are well known constituents of the bran (Sen et al. 1994, Serratos et al. 1987, Bergvinson et al. 1997), and both fungal and bacterial inhibitors are also common in both bran and germ tissues (Arnsaon et al. 1997, Serratos et al. 1997). With their removal during grit and starch isolation, the products contain few if any of these original active antioxidants, sterols, and pigments, and current breeding efforts continue to optimize starch, ethanol, and grit production while minimizing non-starch structures. An exception: corn germ continues to be used almost exclusively as an oil source and the extracted tissues, including antioxidants, minerals, and fiber, are relegated to feed markets.

In North American food markets, corn flour and starch are now the primary starting materials for an increasing array of extruded, easily digested, low density, ready-to-eat breakfast and snack food products. Rice flour and starch are also used, but at lower levels, and extruded wheat and barley products are relatively uncommon. There appears to be only minimal information regarding the effects of high energy processing on digestibility, glycemic response, and bioactivity of such compounds as low molecular weight phenolics and other antioxidants. It might be expected, however, that any residues in grit, flour, and starch fractions that remain after initial processing might well be vulnerable to rapid destruction in the extreme conditions of extrusion and steam processing (Fulcher and Rooney Duke 2002).

While the case can be made that cereal architectures are very similar, it is also apparent that different genera are each distinctive both structurally (e.g. starch granule organization, barely aleurone structure), and biochemically (e.g. the elevated phenolic content of rye and sorghum, and genetically more refined wheat and corn products). Each, however, offers a distinct opportunity to use carefully selected fractionation strategies that allow us to assess the influence of the bioactives in bran and germ in attenuating the propensity of cereal products to stimulate development of diabetic responses in test animals. Each grain can be fractionated to produce highly purified bran, germ, and endosperm, and some can be further processed to separate sub-layers that are also chemically distinct (e.g. whole bran, pericarp, and aleurone layers).

Wild Rice

Wild rice is similar to other cereals in that it has an abundance of phenolic constituents in the outer layers of the grain. The crop has received much less effort devoted to its biochemical modification or "improvement," and its content of cinnamic acid derivatives, notably ferulic acid (3-methoxy-4-hydroxycinnamic acid), is much higher than that of common grains. Where wheat and barley grains contain an average of 400 μg/gram to 700 μg/gram of this compound (Zupfer et al. 1998) in the entire grain, and perhaps 1,000 μg/gram in bran, wild rice has released almost 4,000 μg/gram on analysis (Bunzell et al. 2002). In the latter case, assuming typical compartmentalization within the grain, we might expect two to three times that amount in wild rice bran concentrates, and probably in germ as well.

It bears emphasizing that wild rice also contains substantial quantities of associated phenolics, many of which have not been completely identified, but which include p-coumaric acid, sinapic acids, as well as various of their glycosides such as FAXXO-(5-O-[trans-feruloyl]-α-L-arabinofuranosyl)-(1→3)-O-β-D-xylopyranosyl-(1→4)-D-xylopyranose. The phenolic acid patterns are not unlike those of barley aleurone (Gubler et al. 1985), wheat bran (McCallum and Walker 1991), and corn bran (Ohta et al. 1994, Wender and Fry 1997a,b), but even the most cursory analysis indicates a large number of unidentified constituents.

Conclusion

The foregoing discussion emphasizes a simple fact: all cereal grains are structurally similar, but each contains a unique combination of starches, viscous soluble polymers, and bioactives of enormous diversity and composition, with fiber, lipid, mineral, and vitamin packages that are also unique to each type of grain. In seeking to understand the impact of refined grains, whole grains, and specific fractions of whole grains, these various cereals offer opportunities to test specific fractions (inferring specific chemistry) for biological activity, particularly as it pertains to alleviating the underlying health effects of diabetes, obesity, cardiovascular disease, and cancer in mammals.

References

Adom, K.K., Sorrells, M.E., Liu, R.H. 2003. Phytochemical Profiles and Antioxidant Activity of Wheat Varieties. *J Agric Food Chem* 51:7825–34.

Adlercruetz, H., Mazur, W. 1997. Phyto-oestrogens and Western Diseases. *Ann Med* 29:95–120.

American Association of Cereal Chemists. 1991. St. Paul, Minn. Approved Methods.

Andreasen, M. F., Christensen, L. P., Meyer, A .S. and Hansen Å. 2000a. Ferulic Acid Dehydrodimers in Rye (*Secale cereale L.*). *Journal of Cereal Science*, 31, 303–307.

Andreasen, M.F., Christensen, L.P., Meyer, A.S., and Hansen, Å. 2000b. Content of Phenolic Acids and Ferulic Acids Dehydrodimers in 17 Rye (*Secale cereale L.*) Varieties. *Journal of Agricultural and Food Chemistry* 48: 2837–2842.

Andreasen, M.F., Landbo, K., Christensen, L.P., Hansen, Å. and Meyer, A.S. 2001. Antioxidant effects of phenolic rye (*Secale cereale, L.*) extracts, monomeric hydroxycinnamates and ferulic acid dimers on human low-density lipoproteins. *Journal of Agricultural and Food Chemistry*, 49, 4090–4096.

Arnason, J.T., Conilh-de-Beyssac, B., Philogene, B.J.R., Bergvinson, D.J., Serratos, J.A., Mihm, J.A. 1997. In: Mechanisms of resistance in maize grain to the maize weevil and the larger grain borer. Mihm, J.A. (ed.). *Insect Resistant Maize: Recent Advances and Utilization*. Mexico, DF (Mexico). Centro International de Mejoramiento de Maiz y Trigo.

Ashworth, E.N., Christiansen, M.N., St. John, J.B., Patterson, G.W. 1981. Effect of temperature and BASF 13 338 on the lipid composition and respiration of wheat roots. *Plant Physiol* 67(4): 711–15.

Awad, A.B. and Fink C.S. 2000. Phytosterols as Anticancer Dietary Components: Evidence and Mechanism of Action. *J. Nutr.* 130: 2127–2130.

Awika, J.M. and Rooney, L.W. 2004. Sorghum phytochemicals and their potential impact on human health. *Phytochemistry* 65(9):1199–221.

Bach Knudsen, K.E., Bjørnbak Kjær, A.S.A.K, Tetens, I., Heinonen, A.-M., Nurmi, T., and Adlercreutz, H. 2003. Rye Bread in the Diet of Pigs Enhances the Formation of Enterolactone and Increases its Levels in Plasma, Urine and Feces. *J. Nutr.* 133:1368–1375

Bacic, A., Stone, B.A. 1981a. Isolation and ultrastructure of aleurone cell walls from wheat and barley. *Aust J Plant Physiol.* 8(4/5): 453–474.

Bacic, A., Stone, B.A. 1981b. Chemistry and organization of aleurone cell wall components from wheat and barley. *Aust J Plant Physiol.* 8(4/5): 475–495.

Barrachina, M.D., Martinez, V., Wang, L., Wei, J.Y., and Tache, Y. 1997. Synergistic interaction between leptin and cholecystokinin to reduce short-term food intake in lean mice. *Proc Natl Acad Sci* 94:10455–60.

Barnes, P.J. 1982. Composition of cereal germ preparations. *Z Lebensm Unters Forsch* 174(6):467–71.

Barnes, P.J. 1983. Cereal tocopherols. *Dev. Food Sci.* 5B, 1095–1100.

Battais, F., Pineau, F. Popineau, Y., Aparicio, C., Kanny, G., Guerin, L., Moneret-Vautrin, D.A., and Dener-Papini, S. 2003. Food allergy to wheat: identification of immunoglobulin E and immunoglobulin G-binding proteins with sequential extracts and purified proteins from wheat flour. *Clin Exp Allergy* 33(7):962–70.

Behall, K.M., and Hallfrisch, J. 2002. Effects of grains on glucose and insulin responses. In: *Whole Grain Foods in Health and Disease*. L. Marquart, R.G. Fulcher, and J.L. Slavin (Eds). American Association of Cereal Chemists, St. Paul, Minn. p. 269–282.

Bergvinson, D.J., Arnason, J.T., and Hamilton, R.I. 1997. Phytochemical changes during recurrent selection for resistance to the European corn borer. *Crop Sci.* 37(5):1567–1572.

Bird, A.R., Brown, I.L., and Topping, D.L. 2000. Starches, resistant starches, the gut microflora and human health. *Curr Issues Intest Microbiol.* 2000 Mar;1(1):25–37.

Bourden, I., Yokoyama, W., Davis, P., Hudson, C., Backus, R., Richter, D., Knuckles, B., and Schneeman, B. O. 1999. Postprandial lipid, glucose, insulin, and cholecystokinin responses in men fed barley pasta enriched with β-glucan. *Am J Clin Nutr* 69(1):55–63.

Bourton-Freeman, B. 2000. Dietary Fiber and Energy Regulation. *J Nutr* 130;272S–275S.

Breiteneder, H., and Clare Mills, E.N. 2005. Molecular properties of food allergens. *J Allergy Clin Immunol* 115(1):14-23.

Brown, L., Rosner, B., Willett, W.W., and Sacks, F.M. 1999. Cholesterol-lowering effects of dietary fiber: A meta-analysis. *Am J Clin Nutr* 69:30–42.

Brown, G.D., and Gordon, S. 2001. Immune Recognition: A new receptor for β-glucans. *Nature* 413:36–37.

Brown, G.D., Taylor, P.R., Reid, D.M., Willment, J.A., Williams, D.L., Martinez-Pomares, L., Wong, S.Y., and Gordon, S. 2002. Dectin-1 is a major beta-glucan receptor on macrophages. *J Exp Med* 196(3):407–12.

Bunzell, M., Allerding, E., Sinwell, V., Ralph, J., and Steinhart, H. 2002. Cell wall hydroxycinnamates in wild rice (*Zizania aquatica L.*) insoluble fiber. *Eur Food Res Technol.* 214:482–488

Buri, R.C., von Reding, W., and Gavin, M.M. 2003. Isolation and characterization of aleurone from wheat bran. Corporate Development Report, Buhler AG, Uzwil, Switzerland.

Cahoon, E.B., Hall, S.E., Ripp, K.G., Ganzke, T.S., Hitz, W.D. and Coughlan, S.J. 2003. Metabolic redesign of vitamin E biosynthesis in plants for tocotrienol production and increased antioxidant content. *Nature Online*: Volume 21(9):1082–1087.

Carpita, N.C. 1996. Structure and biogenesis of the cell walls of grasses. *Annu Rev Plant Physiol Plant Mol Biol* 47:445–76.

Carpita, N.C., Defernez, M., Findlay, K., Wells, B., Shoue, D.A., Catchpole, G., Wilson, R.H., and McCann, M.C. 2001. Cell Wall Architecture of the Elongating Maize Coleoptile. *Plant Physiol* 127:551–65.

Collins, F.W. 1986. Oat phenolics: structure, occurrence and function. In: Oats: Chemistry And Technology, Webster, F. H. (Ed.).. American Association Of Cereal Chemists: St. Paul, Minn., Illus. p. 227–296.

Cummings, J.H., Southgate, D.A.T., Branch, W.J., Wiggins, H.S., Houston, H., Jenkins, D.J., Jivraj, T., and Hill, M.J. 1979. The digestion of pectin in the human gut and its effects on calcium absorption and large bowel function. *Br J Nutr* 41:495–503.

Cummings, J.H., Bingham, S.A., Heaton, K.W., Eastwood, M.A. 1992. Fecal weight, colon cancer risk and dietary intake of nonstarch polysaccharides (dietary fiber). *Gastroenterology* 103:1783–89.

Dervilly-Pinel, G., Tran, V., and Saulnier, L. 2004. Investigation of the distribution of arabinose residues on the xylan backbone of water-soluble arabinoxylans from wheat flour. *Carbohydrate Polymers* 55(2) :171–177

van Dullemen, H.M., van Deventer, S.J.H., Hommes, D.W., Bijl, H.A., Jansen, J., Tytgat, G.N.J., and Woody, J. 1995. Treatment of Crohn's disease with anti-tumor necrosis factor chimeric monoclonal antibody (cA2). *Gastroent* 109:129–135.

Economic Research Service, U.S.D.A., Food Consumption (Per Capita) Data System http://www.ers.usda .gov/data/foodconsumption/2005

Earp, C.F., Doherty, C.A., Fulcher, R.G., and Rooney, L. W. 1983. Beta glucans in the caryopsis of Sorghum bicolor. *Food Microstructure.* 2(2):183–188.

Eliasson, A.C., and Larsson, K. 1993. *Cereals in Breadmaking: A Molecular Colloidal Approach.* Marcel Dekker Inc., New York, NY, pp 376.

Estrada, A., Yun, C.H., Van Kessel, A., Li, B., Hauta, S., Laarveld, B. 1997. Immunomodulatory activities of oat beta-glucan in vitro and in vivo. *Microbiol Immunol* 41(12):991–8.

Evans, S.E., Hahn, P.Y., McCann, F., Kottom, T.J., Pavlovic, Z.V., and Limper, A.H. 2005. Pneumocystis cell wall beta-glucans stimulate alveolar epithelial cell chemokine generation through nuclear factor-kappaB-dependent mechanisms. *Am J Respir Cell Mol Biol* 32(6):490–7.

Feng, P., Hunt, C.W., Pritchard, G.T., and Parish, S.M. 1995. Effect of barley variety and dietary barley content on digestive function in beef steers fed grass hay-based diets. *Journal of Animal Science* 73(11):3476–3484

Field, C.J., McBurney, M.I., Massimino, S., Hayek, M.G., and Sunvold, G.D. 1999. The fermentable fiber content of the diet alters the function and composition of canine gut associated lymphoid tissue. *Vet Immunol Immunopahtol* 72(3–4):325–41.

Fox, P.F., and Mulvihill, D.M. 1982. Enzymes in wheat, flour and bread, in *Advances in Cereal Science and Technology, Vol. 5,* Pomeranz, Y., Ed. pp107–156. American Association of Cereal Chemists, St. Paul, Minn.

Fulcher, R.G. 1972. Observations on the Aleurone Layer. PhD Dissertation. Monash University, (Australia).

1972. Fulcher R. G. 1986. Morphological and chemical organization of the oat kernel. *Oats: Chemistry And Technology.* Webster, F.H. (Ed.). American Association Of Cereal Chemists: St. Paul, Minn., Illus. p. 47–74.

Fulcher, R. G. O'Brien, T.P., and Lee, J. W. 1972a. Studies on the aleurone layer. Part 1: Conventional and fluorescence microscopy of the cell wall with emphasis on phenol carbohydrate complexes in wheat. *Australian Journal of Biological Sciences.* 25(1):23–34.

Fulcher, R.G., O'Brien, T.P., and Simmonds, D.H. 1972b. Localization of arginine-rich proteins in mature seeds of some members of the gramineae. *Australian Journal of Biological Sciences.* 25(3): 487

Fulcher, R.G., O'Brien, T.P., and Wong, S. I. 1981. Microchemical detection of niacin aromatic amine and phytin reserves in cereal bran. *Cereal Chemistry.* 58(2):130–135.

Fulcher, R.G., and Rooney Duke, T.K. 2002. Whole grain structure and organization: implications for nutritionists and processors. In: *Whole Grain Foods in Health and Disease*. L. Marquart, R.G. Fulcher, and J.L. Slavin (Eds). American Association of Cereal Chemists, St. Paul, Minn. p. 9–45.

Furuse, M., Chol, Y.H., Yang, S.I., Kita, K., and Okumura, J. 1991. Enhanced release of cholecystokinin in chickens fed diets high in phenylalanine or tyrosine. *Comp Biochem Physiol A* 99(3):449–51.

Galvez, J., Rodriguesz-Cabezas, M.E., and Zarzuelo, A. 2005. Effects of dietary fiber on inflammatory bowel disease. *Mol Nutr Food Res* 49(6):601–8.

Gavin, M., Yu, L., and von Reding, W. 2003. Isolation and characterization of aleurone from Swiss wheat and their antioxidant activity. Summary report: Buhler AG, Uzwil, Switzerland, and Dept of Nutrition and Food Science, University of Maryland.

Goncalves, N.S., Maghami, M.G., Monteleone, G., Frankel, G., Dougan, G., Lewis, D.J.M., Simmons, C.P., and MacDonald T.T. 2001. Critical Role for Tumor Necrosis Factor Alpha in Controlling the Number of Lumenal Pathogenic Bacteria and Immunopathology in Infectious Colitis. *Infect Immun* 69(11)L:6651–59.

Gubler, F., Ashford, A.E., Bacic, A., Blakeney, A.B., and Stone, B.A. 1985. Release of ferulic-acid esters from barley aleurone 2. Characterization of the feruloyl compounds released in response to gibberellic-acid *Australian Journal of Plant Physiology* 12(3):307–317

Guraya, H.S., Kadan, R.S., and Champagne, E.T. 1997. Effect of Rice Starch-Lipid Complexes on In Vitro Digestibility, Complexing Index, and Viscosity. *Cereal Chem.* 74(5):561–565.

Haberer, K.M. 1994. Evaluation of Starch Quality in Relation to Mixing Characteristics of Minnesota Grown Wheat Varieties. Master's thesis, University of Minnesota, 1994, 161 pages.

Hallsman, G., Zhang, J.-X., Lundin, E., Stattin, P., Johansson, A., Johansson, I., Hulten, K., Winkvist, A., Lenner, P., Åman, P., and Adlercreutz, H. 2003 Rye, lignans and human health. *Proc Nutr Soc* 62:193–99.

Harder, B. 2003. Target: Celiac Disease, Therapies aimed to complement or replace the gluten-free diet. *Science News* 163(25):392–401.

Hargin, K.D., Morrison, W.R., and Fulcher, R.G. 1980. Triglyceride deposits in the starchy endosperm of wheat. *Cereal Chemistry.* 57(5):320–325.

Hartunian Sowa, S.M.1997. Nonstarch polysaccharides in wheat: Variation in structure and distribution. PhD Dissertation.

Heinonen, S., Nurmi, T., Liukkonen, K., Poutanen, K., Wahala, K., Deyama, T., Nishibe, S., and Adlercruetz, H. 2001. *In vitro* metabolism of plant lignans: new precursors of mamanlian lignans enterolactone and enterodiol. *J Agric Food Chem.* 49(7):3178–86.

Hinton, J.J.C. 1947. The distribution of vitamin B$_1$ and nitrogen in the wheat grain. *Proc. Roy Soc. London.* B134: 418–429.

Hinton, J.J.C., Peers, F.G., and Shaw, B. 1953. The B-vitamins in wheat: the unique aleurone layer. *Nature.* 172: 993–995.

Hoad, C.L., Rayment, P., and Spiller, R.C. 2004. In vivo imaging of intragastric gelation and its effect on satiety in humans. *J Nutr* 134:2293–300.

Holt, S., Brand, J., Soveny, C., and Hansky, J. 1992. Relationship of satiety to postprandial glycaemic, insulin and cholecystokinin responses. *Appetite* 18:129–41.

Hoseney, RC. 1994. Principles of Cereal Science and Technology. (2nd Edition). American Association of Cereal Chemists, St. Paul, Minn.

Izydorczyk, M.S., Symons, S.J., and Dexter, J.E. 2002. Fractionation of wheat and barley. Ch. 3, pp 47–82. In *Whole-Grain Foods in Health and Disease*. L. Marquart, J.L., Slavin, and R.G. Fulcher, (Eds.) American Association of Cereal Chemists, St. Paul, Minn.

Jenkins D.J., Jenkins A.L., Wolever T.M., et al. 1987. Starchy foods and fiber: Reduced rate of digestion and improved carbohydrate metabolism. *Scand J Gastroenterol.* 129(suppl):132–41.

Jenkins, D.J., Wesson, V., Wolever, T.M., et al. 1988. Wholemeal versus wholegrain breads: Proportion of whole or cracked grain and the glycemic response. *Br Med J.* 297(6654):958–60.

Juliano, B.O. 1993. Rice in human nutrition. International Rice Research Institute and Food and Agriculture Organization of The United Nations, Rome (Publishers)

Kantor, L.S., Variyam, J.N., Allshouse, J.E., Putnam, J.J., and Lin, B.H. 2001. Choose a Variety of Grains Daily, Especially Whole Grains: A Challenge for Consumers in The Dietary Guidelines: Surveillance Issues and Research Needs. *J Nutr Suppl* 131:473S–86S.

Kawataba, K., Yamamoto, T., Hara, A., Shimizu, M., Yamada, Y., Matsunaga, K., Tanaka, T., and Mori, H. 2000. Modifying effects of ferulic acid on azoxymethane induced colon carcinogenesis in F344 rats. *Cancer Lett* 157:15–21.

Kent, N.L., and Evers, A.D. 1994. *Technology of Cereals*. (4th Edition). Pergamon Press, U.K.

Kern, S.M., Bennet, R.N., Mellon, F.A., Kroon, P.A., and Garcia-Conesa, M.T. 2003. Absorption of Hydroxycinnamates in Humans after High-Bran Cereal Consumption. *J Agric Food Chem* 51:6050–55.

Kikuzaki, H., Hisamoto, M., Hirose, K., Akiyama, K., and Taniguchi, H. 2002. Antioxidant properties of ferulic acid and its related compounds. *J Agric Food Chem* 50:2161–68.

Kollias, G., Douni, E., Kassiotis, G., and Kontoyiannis. D. 1999. The function of tumour necrosis factor in models of multi-organ inflammation, rheumatoid arthritis, multiple sclerosis and inflammatory bowel disease. *Ann. Rheum. Dis* 58(Suppl. I):I32–I39.

Kournikakis, B., Mandeville, R., Brousseau, P., and Ostroff, G. 2003 Anthrax-protective effects of yeast beta 1,3 glucans. *Med Gen Med* 5(1):1.

Lasztity, R. 1996. *Wheat Proteins*. In *The Chemistry of Cereal Proteins* (2nd Ed.) CRC Press, New York, NY. 19–117.

Lewis, L.D., and Williams, J.A. 1990. Regulation of cholecystokinin secretion by food, hormones, and neural pathways in the rat. *Am J Physiol Gastrointest Liver Physiol* 258:G512–G518.

Lim, B.O., Yamada, K., Nonaka, M., Kuramoto, Y., Hung, P., and Sugano, M. 1997. Dietary Fibers Modulate Indices of Intestinal Immune Function in Rats. *J Nutr* 127(5):663–67.

Lopes, M.A., Larkins, B.A. 1993. Endosperm Origin, Development, and Function. Plant Cell 5:1383–99.

Lu, T.J., Pai, Y.Y., and Lii, C.Y. 1993. The susceptibility of A- and B-type wheat starch granules to bacterial alpha-amylase. Cereal Foods World. American Association of Cereal Chemists Annual Meeting 1999.

Lui, S., Willett, W.C., Manson, J.E., Hu, F.B., Rosner, B., and Colditz, G. 2003. Relation between changes in intakes of dietary fiber and grain products in weight and development of obesity among middle-aged women. *Am J Clin Nutr.* 78(5):920–27.

MacGregor, A.W., and Bhatty, R.S. 1993. Barley Chemistry and Technology. American Association of Cereal Chemists, St. Paul, Minn. 486 pages.

Mason, J.B., and Kodicek, E. 1973a. The chemical nature of the bound nicotinic acid of wheat bran: studies of partial hydrolysis products. *Cereal Chem* 50:637.

Mason, J.B. and Kodicek, E. 1973b. The identification of o-aminophenol and o-aminophenyl glucose in wheat bran. *Cereal Chem* 50:646.

Marlett, J.A., and Slavin, J.L. 1997. Position of the American Dietetic Association: Health implications of dietary fiber. *J Am Diet Assoc* 97:1157–59.

Mazur, W. 1998. Phytoestrogen contents in Foods. *Bailliere's Clin Endocrinol and Metabolism.* 12(4):729–42.

Mazur, W., and Adlercreutz, H. 1998. Natural and anthropogenic environment estrogens: the scientific basis for risk assessment. Anturally occurring estrogens in food. *J Pure and Applied Chem* 70(9):1759–76

McCallum, J.A., and Walker, J.R.L. 1991. Phenolic biosynthesis during grain development in wheat (Triticum aestivum L.) III. Changes in hydroxycinnamic acids during grain development. *J Cereal Sci.*13(2):161–172

McKeehen, J.D. 1988. Influence of phenolic acids on Fusarium-resistance in developing wheat kernels. PhD Dissertation.

McKeehen J.D., Busch, R.H., and Fulcher, R.G. 1999. Evaluation of wheat (Triticum aestivum L.) phenolic acids during grain development and their contribution to Fusarium resistance. *Journal of Agricultural and Food Chemistry.* 47(4):1476–1482.

McKeehen, J.D., and Fulcher, R.G. 1998. Wheat phenolic compounds and their potential role in Fusarium resistance. *Polyphenols Actualites* 17:7–10.

Mendall, M.A., Patel, P., Asante, M., Ballam, L., Morris, J., Strachan, D.P., Camm, A.J., and Northfield, T.C. 1997. Relation of serum cytokine concentrations to cardiovascular risk factors and coronary heart disease. *Heart* 78:273–77.

Milner, J.A. 2002. Functional Foods and Health: A U.S. Perspective. *Brit J Nutr* 88(Suppl 2):S151–S158.

Miller, S.S., Fulcher, R.G., Sen, A., and Arnason, J.T. 1995. Oat endosperm cell walls .1. Isolation, composition, and comparison with other tissues. *Cereal Chemistry.* 72(5):421–427.

Miller, S.S., and Fulcher, R.G. 1995. Oat endosperm cell walls Hot-water solubilization and enzymatic digestion of the wall. *Cereal Chemistry.* 72(5):428–432.

Miller, H.E., Rigelhof, F., Marquart, L., Prakash, A., and Kanter, M. 2000a. Whole-Grain Products and Antioxidants. *Cereal Foods World.* 45(2):59.

Miller, H.E., Rigelhof, F., Marquart, L., Prakash, A., Kanter, M. 2000b. Antioxidant content of whole grain breakfast cereals, fruits, and vegetables. *J Am Coll Nutr.* 9(13):312S–319S.

Mole, S., Rogler, J.C., and Butler, L. 1993. Growth reduction by dietary tannins: different effects due to different tannins. *Biochemical and Systematic Ecology* 21:667–677.

Morrison, W.R., Milligan, T.P., Azudin, M.N. 1984. A relationship between anylose and lipid contents of starches from diploid cereals. *J Cereal Sci* 2:257–71.

Nilsson, M., Aman, P., Harkonen, H., Hallmans, G., Bach Knudsen, K.E., Mazur, W. and Adlercreutz, H. 1997. Content of Nutrients and Lignans in Roller Milled Fractions of Rye. *J Sci Food Agric* 73:143–48.

Normen, L., Dutta, P., Lia, A., and Andersson, H. 2000. Soy sterol esters and beta-sitostanol ester as inhibitors of cholesterol absorption in human small bowel. *Am J Clin Nutr.* 2000 Apr;71(4):908–13.

Normen, A.L., Brants, H.A., Voorrips, L.E., Andersson, H.A., van den Brandt, P.A., and Goldbohm, R.A. 2001. Plant sterol intakes and colorectal cancer risk in the Netherlands Cohort Study on Diet and Cancer. *Am J Clin Nutr* 74(1):141–8.

Ofei, F., Hurel, S., Newkerk, J., Sowith, M., and Taylor, R. 1996. Effects of an engineered human anti-TNF-alpha antibody (CDP571) on insulin sensitivity and glycemic control in patients with NIDDM. *Diabetes.* 45(7):881–85.

Ohta, T., Yamasaki, S., Egashira, Y., and Sanada, H., 1994. Antioxidative Activity of Corn Bran Hemicellulose Fragments *J Agric Fd Chem.* 42:653–656.

Osborne, T.B. 1907. The proteins of the wheat kernel. Carnegie Institution, Washington, D.C.

Peterson, D.M., and Brinegar, A.C. 1986. Oat storage proteins.. In *Oats: Chemistry and Technology.* F.H. Webster (Ed.) pp 153–203. American Association Of Cereal Chemists, St. Paul, Minn.

Peterson, D.M., and Qureshi, A.A. 1993. Genotype and environmental effects on tocols of barley and oats. *Cereal Chem.* 70, 157–162.

Pietenen, P., Rimm, E.B., Korhonen, P., Hartman, A.M, Willett, W.C, Albanes, D, and Virtamo, J. 1996. Intake of dietary fiber and risk of coronary heart disease in a cohort of Finnish men. The Alpha-Tocopherol, Beta-Carotene Cancer Prevention Study. 94:2720–27.

Piironen, V., J. Toivo (1,3), and A.-M. Lampi (1). 2002. Plant Sterols in Cereals and Cereal Products. *Cereal Chem.* 79(1):148–154.

Platt, J., and Mensink, R.P. 2005. Food components and immune function. *Curr Opin Lipidol.* 16:31–37.

Poutanen K, Liukkonen K, and Adlercreutz H. 2002. Whole grains: Phytoestrogens and Health. Ch. 12, pp 259–268. In *Whole Grain Foods in Health and Disease.* L. Marquart, R.G. Fulcher and J.L. Slavin (Eds). American Association of Cereal Chemists, St. Paul, Minn.

Pussayanawin, V., Wetzel, D.L., and Fulcher, R.G. 1988. Fluorescence detection and measurement of ferulic acid in wheat milling fractions by microscopy and HPLC. *Journal of Agricultural & Food Chemistry.* 36(3):515–520.

Ramputh,A., Teshome, A., Bergvinson, D.J., Nozzolillo, C. and Arnason, J.T. 1999. Soluble phenolic content as an indicator of sorghum grain resistance to Sitophilus oryzae (Coleoptera: Curculionidae). *Journal-of-Stored-Products-Research* (United Kingdom). 35(1):57–64.

Rasper, V.F., and DeMan, J.M. 1980. Effects of granule size of substituted starches on the rheological character of composite doughs. *Cereal Chem.* 57(5):331–340.

Report of a Joint WHO/FAO Expert Consultation. 2003. Diet, Nutrition and the Prevention of Chronic Diseases, World Health Organization/Food and Agriculture Organization of the United Nations. WHO Technical Report Series 916. Geneva, Switzerland.

Rimm, E.B., Ascherio, A., Giovannucci, E., Spiegelman, D., Stampfer, M.J., and Willet, W.C. 1996. Vegetable, fruit and cereal fiber intake and risk of coronary heart disease among men. *JAMA* 275:447–51.

Robins, G., and Howdle, P.D. 2005. Advances in celiac disease. *Curr Opin Gastroenterol* 21:152–61.

Roe, D.A. 1973. *A Plague of Corn. The Social History of Pellagra.* Cornell University Press. 217 pp.

Rondini, L., Peyrat-Maillard, M.N., Marsset-Baglieri, A., Fromentin, G., Durand, P., Tome, D., Prost, M., and Berset, C. 2004. Bound Ferulic Acid from Bran is More Bioavailable than the Free Compound in Rats. *J Agric Food Chem* 52:4338–43.

Rooney Duke, T.K. 1996. Variation and distribution of barley cell wall polysaccharides and their fate during physiological processing (beta glucans, arabinoxylan) PhD dissertation.

Roubroeks, J.P., Skjak-Braek, G., Ryan, L., and Christensen, B.E. 2000. Molecular weight dependency on the production of the TNF stimulated by fractions of rye $(1{\rightarrow}3),(1{\rightarrow}4)$–betaᴅglucan. *Scand J Immunol* 52(6):584–7.

Schley, P.D., Field, C.J. 2002. The immune-enhancing effects of dietary fibres and prebiotics. *Brit J Nutr* 87(Supp s2):221–30.

Sen, A., Bergvinson, D., Miller, S.S., Atkinson, J., Fulcher, R.G., and Arnason, J.T. 1994. Distribution and microchemical detection of phenolic acids, flavonoids, and phenolic acid amides in maize kernels. *Journal of Agricultural and Food Chemistry.* 42(9):1879–83.

Sener, G., Toklu, H., Ercan, F., and Erkanli, G. 2005. Protective effect of beta-glucan against oxidative organ injury in a rat model of sepsis. *Int Immunopharmacol* 5(9):1387–96.

Serratos, J.A., Arnason, J.T., Nozzolillo, C., Lambert, J.D.H., Philogene, B.J.R., Fulcher, G., Davidson, K. Peacock, L., Atkinson, J., and Morand, P. 1987. Factors contributing to resistance of exotic maize populations to maize weevil Sitophilus zeamais. *Journal of Chemical Ecology.* 13(4):751–762.

Serratos, J.A., Blanco-Labra, A., Arnason, J.T., and Mihm, J.A. 1997. Genetics of maize grain resistance to maize weevil. Mihm, J.A. (Ed.). *Insect Resistant Maize: Recent Advances and Utilization*. Mexico, DF (Mexico). CIMMYT. 1997.

Shan, L., Molberg, O., Parrot, I., Hausch, F., Filiz, F., Gray, G.M., Sollid, L.M., and Khosla, C. 2002. Structural Basis for Gluten Intolerance in Celiac Sprue. *Science* 297:2275–79.

Shan, L., Marti, T., Sollid, L.M., Gray, G.M., and Khosla, C. 2004. Comparative biochemical analysis of three bacterial prolyl endopptidases: implications for coeliac sprue. *Biochem J* 383:311–18.

Shewry, P.R., and Mifflin, B.J. 1985. Seed storage proteins of economically important cereals. In: *Advances in Cereal Science and Technology* Y. Pomeranz (Ed). Pp. 183. American Association of Cereal Chemists. St Paul, Minn.

Shewry, P.R., and Tatham, A.S. 1990. The prolamin storage proteins of cereal seeds: structure and evolution. *Biochem J* 267:1–12.

Shopping for health 2001: Reaching out to the Whole Health Consumer. Food Marketing Institute, FMI publications, tenth annual report, Washington, D.C.

Slavin, J.L. 2002. Whole grains, dietary fiber and resistant starch. In: *Whole Grain Foods in Health and Disease*. L. Marquart, R.G. Fulcher and J.L. Slavin (Eds). American Association of Cereal Chemists, St. Paul, Minn.. p.283–300.

Slavin, J.L. 2005. Dietary fiber and body weight. *Nutrition* 21:411–18.

Sloan, E. 2002. The Top 10 Functional Food Trends: The Next Generation. *Food Technology* 56(4) pp32–57.

Sollid, L.M. 2002. Coeliac Disease: Dissecting a Complex Inflammatory Disorder. *Nature Rev Immun* 2:647–55.

Tilley, K.A., Benjamin, R.E., Bagorogoza, K.E., Okot-Kotber, B.M., Prakash, O., Kwen, H. 2001. Tyrosine crosslinks: Molecular basis of gluten structure and function. *J Agric Food Chem* 49:2627–32.

Topping, D.L., and Clifton, P.M. 2001. Short-Chain Fatty Acids and Human Colonic Function: Roles of Resistant Starch and Nonstarch Polysaccharides. *Physiological Reviews*, Vol. 81, No. 3, July 2001, pp. 1031–1064

USDA/GIPSA: United States Department of Agriculture's (USDA) Grain Inspection, Packers and Stockyards Administration (GIPSA). http://www.usda.gov/gipsa/reference-library/standards/standards.htm

Wang, L., Miller, R.A., and Hoseney, R.C. 1998. Effects of (1-3) (1–4)-β-D-Glucans of Wheat Flour on Breadmaking. *Cereal Chem.* 75(5):629–633.

Waniska, R.D., Poe J.H., and Bandyopadhyay, U. 1989. Effects of growth conditions on grain molding and phenols in sorghum caryopses *JCER SCI* 10:217–25

Waniska, R.D. 2000. Structure, phenolic compounds and antifungal proteins of sorghum caryopses. In: *Technical and institutional options for sorghum grain mold management*. P 72–106. Proceedings of an international conference, ICRISAT, May 18–19, Patancheru, India.

Watzl, B., Girrbach, S., and Roller, M. 2005. Inulin, oligofructose and immunomodulation. *Br J Nutr* 93(Suppl 1:S49–55.

Wende, G., and Fry, S.C. 1997a. Digestion by fungal glycanases of arabinoxylans with different feruloylated sidechains. *Phytochemistry*. Oxford. 45 (6):1123–1129.

Wende, G., and Fry, S.C. 1997b. 2-O-β-D-xylopyranosyl-(5-O-feruloyl)-L-arabinose, a widespread component of grass cell walls. *Phytochemistry* Oxford: 44 (6):1019–1030.

Wetzel, D.L., Pussayanawin, V., and Fulcher, R.G. 1988. Determination of ferulic acid in grain by HPLC and microspectrofluorometry. *Developments in Food Science* 17:409–428.

Willment, J.A., Marshall, A.S., Reid, D.M., Williams, D.L., Wong, S.Y., Gordon, S., and Brown, G.D. 2005. The human beta-glucan receptor is widely expressed and functionally equivalent to murine Dectin-1 on primary cells. *Eur J Immunol* 35(5):1539–47.

Woods, S.C. 2004. Gastrointestinal Satiety Signals I. An overview of gastrointestinal signals that influence food intake. *Am J Physiol Gastrointest Liver Physiol* 286:G7–G13.

Zangenberg, M., Hansen, H.B., Jorgensen, J.R., and Hellgren, L.I. 2004. Cultivar and year-to-year variation of phytosterol content in rye (Secale cereale L.). *J Agric Food Chem* 52(9):2593–7.

Zupfer J.M., Churchill, K.E., Rasmusson, D.C., and Fulcher, R.G. 1998. Variation in ferulic acid concentration among diverse barley cultivars measured by HPLC and microspectrophotometry. *Journal of Agricultural and Food Chemistry*. 46(4):1350–1354

9 Structure of Whole Grain Breads: Sensory Perception and Health Effects

Karin Autio, Kirsi-Helena Liukkonen, Hannu Mykkänen, Irene Katina, Katariina Roininen, and Kaisa Poutanen

Introduction

The glycemic indices of a number of starchy foods are provided in the literature. Starch in breads baked from refined flours generally evokes high metabolic responses (Holm and Björck 1992). The lowest glycemic index (G.I.) values (66 to 80) have been reported for pumpernickel-type breads containing intact kernels (Jenkins 1985, 1986; Wolever 1987, 1994). The intact botanical structure protects the encapsulated starch of the kernel against the hydrolysis (Brand 1990, Granfeldt 1992). Recent investigations have shown that as compared to white wheat breads, rye breads baked from fine flours showed equally high glycemic responses, but lower insulin responses in healthy subjects (Leinonen 1999, Juntunen 2003a). The fiber content does not predict the magnitude of the insulin response (Holt 1997, Juntunen 2003b). Protein-rich foods or protein added to a carbohydrate-rich meal can cause a rise in insulin secretion without increasing blood glucose concentrations (Nilsson 2004).

The characteristics of starch, per se, are also of crucial importance for glucose response. Amylose-rich starches are more resistant to amylolysis than waxy or normal starches. Native starches are hydrolyzed very slowly, and to a limited extent, by amylases (Björck 1995). As a result of gelatinization, the *in vitro* rate of amylolysis increases dramatically (Holm 1988). If amylose has leached out of the starch granule, it very frequently becomes retrograded and decreases starch digestibility (Slaughter 2000). The extent of retrogradation of amylose has been found to be of primary importance in determining the resistant starch (R.S.) content of starch (Cairns 1996).

There are several hundred publications examining the glycemic responses to various foods, and G.I. values have been collected in a review (Foster-Powel 2002). Most pasta products have low G.I. values, ranging from 50 to 70. Pasta has a dense, firm texture and requires a low degree of mastification before swallowing (Jenkins 1983, Read 1986). Meals composed of pasta delay gastric emptying in comparison to white bread. Great stomach motor activity and time is required to reduce the pasta particles to a size of 2 mm diameter, allowing them to pass through the pylorus (Mourot 1988). These results suggest that the macrostructure of food is also an important factor in relation to degradation of starch by α-amylase.

A greater variety of cereal-based products with a low glycemic load or index is needed, but the greatest challenge is the management of texture that is perceived to be good. Our objective has been to modify the textural characteristics, such as continuous bread matrix and mechanical properties of whole meal breads and endosperm rye bread, and to study their effects on sensory perception of texture, digestibility, and insulin response in healthy subjects.

Material and Methods

The following breads were studied (the formulas also are noted):

Regular white wheat bread: Commercial bread.

Regular white wheat bread (test bread): 1,000 grams of wheat flour, 690 grams of tap water, 15 grams of dried yeast, 15 grams of salt, 15 grams of sugar, 4.8 grams of bread improver, and 60 grams of margarine. The flour, water, and other ingredients were mixed 8 minutes. After the floor time of 15 minutes at 28°C (70% relative humidity [R.H.]), the dough was divided into 400-gram pieces that were molded and panned before proofing for 40 minutes at 37°C (70% R.H.). Loaves were baked at 220°C for 30 minutes and then cooled for 2 hours before further analysis.

60% whole meal oat bread: 900 grams of whole meal oat flour, 600 grams of white wheat flour, 105 grams of gluten, 1,275 grams of tap water, 45 grams of fresh yeast, 33 grams of salt, and 45 grams of margarine. The flour, water, and other ingredients were mixed for 7 minutes. The dough was divided into 400-gram pieces that were molded and panned before proofing for 60 minutes at 37°C (80% R.H.). The loaves were baked at 170°C for 30 minutes and then cooled for 2 hours before further analysis.

60% whole meal rye bread: 1,000 grams of whole meal rye flour, 700 grams of white wheat flour, 215 grams of gluten, 1,500 grams of tap water, 55 grams of fresh yeast, 40 grams of salt, and 25 grams of margarine. The flour, water, and other ingredients were mixed for 8 minutes. After the floor time of 30 minutes at 28°C (70% R.H.), the dough was divided into 400-gram pieces that were molded and panned before proofing for 55 minutes at 37°C (80% R.H.). Loaves were baked at 240°C for 5 minutes and at 220°C for 30 minutes, and then cooled for 2 hours before further analysis.

60% whole meal wheat bread: 1,000 grams of whole meal wheat flour, 700 grams of white wheat flour, 215 grams of gluten, 1,250 grams of tap water, 55 grams of fresh yeast, 30 grams of salt, and 25 grams of margarine. The flour, water, and other ingredients were mixed for 8 minutes. After the floor time of 30 minutes at 28°C (70% R.H.), the dough was divided into 400-gram pieces that were molded and panned before proofing for 60 minutes at 37°C (75% R.H.). Loaves were baked at 230°C for 20 minutes and then cooled for 2 hours before further analysis.

Sourdough endosperm rye bread without gluten: 900 grams of commercial rye endosperm flour, 731 grams of sourdough, 430 grams of water, 19 grams of fresh yeast, and 12.9 grams of salt. The sourdough was prepared from 380 grams of commercial endosperm flour, 0.4 grams of L62 (*L. brevis*), 0.4 grams of L73 (*L. plantarum*), 3.8 grams of fresh yeast, and 632 grams of water. The sourdough was fermented for 23 hours at 30°C. The endosperm flour, sourdough, water, fresh yeast, and salt were mixed 2 + 2 minutes. After the floor time of 45 minutes at 27°C (70% R.H.), the dough was divided into 400-gram pieces that were molded and panned before proofing for 50 minutes at 35°C (70% R.H.). The loaves were baked at 240°C for 10 minutes and at 220°C for 30 minutes. Loaves were cooled for 2 hours before further analysis.

Sourdough endosperm rye bread with gluten: This formula is identical to the previous one, except that 2.3% of the endosperm flour was replaced with gluten.

Endosperm rye bread (without sourdough and gluten): 1,775 grams of commercial rye endosperm flour, 28.2 grams of fresh yeast, 28.2 grams of salt, and 1,335 grams of water. The bread was mixed the same way the mixing was done according to the formula for the sourdough endosperm rye bread without gluten. To prepare this as flat bread, the same dough formula was mixed and then rolled on a dough mat to a thickness of 1 cm and round dough pieces of 120 grams were cut from the mat and proofed 45 minutes at 25°C (50% R.H.). The round flat bread was baked at 250°C for 10 minutes in a peel oven. The warm flat bread was cut in half and cooled for 2 hours before further analysis.

Structural Characterization of Bread

Crumb firmness and bread volume were measured on the baking day. Bread crumb firmness was determined as maximum compression force (40% compression, American Association of Cereal Chemists 1998, modified method 74-09) using the texture profile analysis (T.P.A.) test (TA-XT2 Texture Analyzer, Stable Micro Systems, Godalming, England). The results are means of the analyses of four replicate breads. The test bakings were repeated twice.

The bread volume was determined by rape seed displacement. The results are means of the analyses of four replicate breads. The test bakings were repeated twice.

The breads were studied under the microscope. For microscopy, several pieces were taken from the center of the bread crumb. Samples were embedded in agar gel and chemically fixed in 1% glutaraldehyde, dehydrated, and embedded in Historesin (Jung, Heidelberg, Germany) as recommended by the manufacturer. Sections measuring 4 μm thick were cut with a microtome (Leica Jung RM2055, Nussloch, Germany) and stained by 0.1 Light Green and Lugol solution and examined with a microscope (Olympus BH-2 microscope, Japan).

In Vitro *Digestibility by Particle Size*

The amount of available starch was measured with a specific enzymatic kit (Megazyme, Bray, United Kingdom). An equivalent amount of available starch (1 gram on the basis of analyzed data) from each bread was chewed for 15 seconds by four subjects. The masticated residues were then treated with pepsin to mimic stomach conditions (mixing, acid, pepsin, +37°C). After dilution, the particles were photographed and the particle size distribution was determined from all the masticated material by image analysis (Liukkonen et al. manuscript).

The study subjects were postmenopausal women with normal glucose tolerance. To determine the insulin index, the test products (refined wheat bread as a reference bread and different experimental breads) providing 50 grams of available carbohydrates were served in random order with breakfast. Fasting and eight postprandial blood samples (0 to 180 minutes) were collected for determination of plasma glucose and insulin concentrations. The area under the plasma insulin curve (A.U.C./180 min) was calculated from the postprandial curve above the fasting level. Insulin index values for the test products were calculated as the percentage of the A.U.C. for the reference product.

Sensory Attributes

A trained sensory panel at V.T.T. composed of ten assessors) generated sensory profiles of bread samples used in the study. The panel developed a texture glossary with detailed descriptions for the attribute evaluation. The glossary consisted of one odor, one flavor, two visual, and five texture attributes of the samples. The panel was familiarized with the attributes and their definitions during one training session. Each attribute was rated by placing a mark on an unstructured line scale (anchored from their ends) using a computerized data-collection system, Compusense 5 (Compusense Inc., Guelph, Canada). In addition, panelists were allowed to verbally describe the samples. Each assessor evaluated all samples twice. The samples were marked with three-digit random codes and presented in random order and were served on the odorless trays.

Results

In normal white wheat bread, the continuous dough matrix was formed of gluten (stained as green), and the starch granules were only slightly swollen (Figure 9.1a). No amylose leaching was observed. The microstructure of endosperm rye bread was very different. The starch granules were highly swollen and seemed to form the continuous phase (Figure 9.1b). A high amount of amylose was leached out. Due to the lack of gluten network, the breads were clearly less porous than gluten-based products.

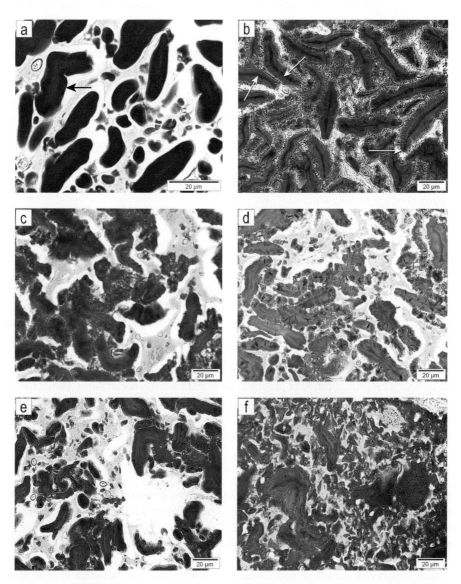

Figure 9.1.   (a) White wheat bread; arrow demonstrates starch granule; (b) white rye bread; arrows illustrate blue-stained amylose; (c) white wheat bread containing gluten; (d) 60% whole meal rye bread; (e) 60% whole meal wheat bread; and (f) 60% whole meal oat bread.

The continuous matrix of endosperm rye bread (containing gluten) was composed of both gluten- and starch-rich areas (Figure 9.1e). In all of the whole meal breads, the continuous phase was formed of a protein network like that in normal wheat bread (Figures 9.1d, 9.1e, and 9.1f). The 60% whole meal oat bread (Figure 9.1f) was less porous, and due to the compact structure starch granules, took more area than in the corresponding rye and wheat breads. The 6% wheat (Figure 9.1e) and rye (Figure 9.1d) whole meal breads were very porous and large areas of green-stained protein networks could be observed. The starch granule structure was, however, very different.

As shown in Table 9.1, white wheat bread had the highest volume and softest crumb structure. Both whole meal rye and wheat breads had high volume. The 60% whole meal wheat bread was twice as hard as normal endosperm wheat bread, but softer than the other 60% whole meal breads. Although the volume of whole meal oat bread was low, the crumb structure was acceptable. Endosperm rye bread had a very low porosity and hard texture.

A new method has been developed which evaluates particle size reduction of starchy foods at the stomach stage and predicts their insulin response *in vivo* (Liukkonen et al.). Recent studies in our own laboratory have shown that some foods, such as pasta and some breads, are swallowed partly in very large pieces, 2 mm to 20 mm in diameter (Liukkonen et al. manuscript). Table 9.2 shows the number of particles after *in vivo* chewing and subsequent *in vitro* incubation with stomach pepsin.

White wheat bread and 60% whole meal wheat bread broke down easily. The number of larger particles (greater than 3 mm) and their average size was low in both wheat breads, whereas sourdough white rye bread broke down to a clearly lower extent. Also, whole meal rye bread was digested at a much lower rate than the wheat breads (Liukkonen et al. manuscript.) Gastric emptying is affected by particle size (Thomsen 1994). The only exit from the stomach to the small intestine is the polyrus, which allows food pieces of less than 2 mm in diameter to exit. Gastric emptying half-time has been calculated for some food systems, including spaghetti (75 minutes) and mashed potato (35 minutes) (Mourot 1988). Gastric emptying half-time has shown to correlate with blood glucose and insulin values (Mourot 1988). Accessibility of salivary α-amylase to pasta starch is smaller than to wheat bread starch due to the more compact structure of pasta, which explains the slower hydrolysis and degradation of pasta in the mouth. Adding wheat flour gluten to sourdough whole meal or rye endosperm dough made the corresponding breads softer and more easily digestible, suggesting that bread texture has an important role.

The only bread product from which starch was digested at a slower rate than in normal wheat bread was white rye bread. A similar effect has been observed with whole meal rye breads (Leinonen 1999; Juntunen 2002, 2003). Mechanically, rye breads are clearly firmer than normal wheat breads. The specific loaf volume of white wheat bread is often 4 ml/gram

Table 9.1. Hardness and specific volume of breads.

Bread	Hardness (g)	Volume (g/ml)
White wheat bread	118	4.8
60% Whole meal oat bread	286	2.7
60% Whole meal wheat bread	264	4.2
60% Whole meal rye bread	322	3.9
Sourdough white rye bread, pan	386	2.4

Table 9.2. Number of particles over 3 mm in diameter after *in vivo* chewing and *in vitro* stomach phase.

Bread	Number of particles
White wheat bread	3±2
Whole meal wheat bread	7±4
Whole meal oat bread	95±62
Whole meal rye bread	29±2
Sourdough white rye bread, pan	81±36
Sourdough white rye bread, flat	217±39
Sourdough white rye bread with gluten, flat	73±23

to 5 ml/gram, whereas that in rye bread is typically between 2 ml/gram and 3 ml/gram or even lower. The matrix of wheat bread is much softer than that of rye bread. The maximum force in compression for rye breads can be four-fold to eight-fold that of normal wheat bread (Autio and Lähteenmäki 2001). Rye breads, even bread baked from rye white flour, clearly have lower specific volumes and they are clearly harder than all other breads baked from other cereals.

The insulin index was lowest for white rye bread, which had the hardest texture (Table 9.3). This is the only test bread that had an insulin index that was significantly lower than that of wheat bread. Previously, we have shown that 100% whole meal rye bread also gives as low insulin response as white rye bread (Juntunen 2003). Because no difference in glucose response was observed between the wheat and rye breads, our result indicates that less insulin is needed for regulation of blood glucose after ingesting a dose of 50 grams of starch from 100% rye breads. All breads containing 60% whole meal flour had an insulin index of about the same or slightly higher than normal white wheat bread. The addition of gluten to either whole meal or endosperm rye bread resulted in a higher insulin index.

Figure 9.2 shows the sensory profiles of breads containing 60% whole meal. 60% whole meal wheat and rye breads had higher volume and they were less dense than 60% whole meal oat bread. Of the whole meal breads, oat bread was lightest in color. No off-flavors were detected.

The sensory attribute intensities of the different flat white rye breads are shown in Table 9.4. Sourdough endosperm rye bread with gluten and endosperm rye bread without sourdough and gluten gave higher volume than sourdough white bread. Sourdough brought an off-flavor, which was not observed in products baked without sourdough.

Table 9.3. Insulinemic indices of breads.

Bread	Insulinemic index
Regular white wheat bread	100
60% Whole meal white bread	120
60% Whole meal oat bread	113
60% Whole meal rye bread	107
Sourdough endosperm rye bread, pan	71
Sourdough endosperm rye bread, flat	77
Flat sourdough endosperm rye bread with gluten	88

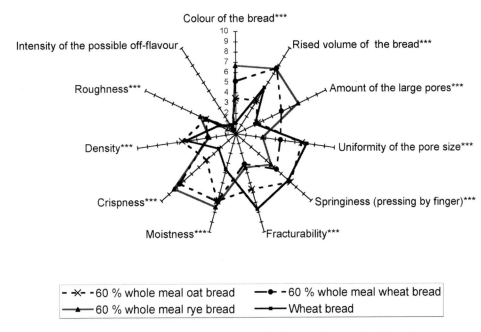

Figure 9.2. Sensory profiles of 60% whole meal breads in comparison to wheat bread.

Table 9.4. The sensory attribute intensities of different white rye breads.

	Sourdough endosperm rye bread	Sourdough endosperm rye bread + gluten	Endosperm rye bread
Intensity of the possible off-odor	2,6[b]	2,6[b]	0,3[a]
Uniformity of the pore size	6,1[b]	4,1[a]	4,3[a]
Doughy	2,8[ab]	4,6[bc]	5,6[c]
Springiness of the inside	7,6[a]	6,7[a]	7,4[a]
Crispness	3,8[a]	4,0[a]	3,4[a]
Toughness of the bottom	6,9[a]	7,3[a]	7,0[a]
Hardness of the bottom	6,7[b]	6,3[b]	7,0[b]
Volume of the bread	4,9[a]	5,6[ab]	5,8[ab]
Intensity of the possible off-flavor	1,7[b]	1,9[b]	0,2[a]
Desired texture quality	5,4[b]	4,7[ab]	4,4[a]

[a-c]*Means within columns followed by different superscripts are significantly different (p < 0.05)*

Conclusions

Our objective was to modify the textural characteristics, such as the continuous bread matrix and the mechanical properties of whole meal breads and endosperm rye bread, and study their effects on sensory perception of texture, instrumental hardness, and glucose and insulin responses in healthy subjects. The digestibility of the breads was determined by a new method based on particle size after *in vivo* chewing and the *in vitro* stomach phase. The results show that the appearance and sensory perception of breads containing whole meal flour can be improved by adding white wheat flour and/or gluten, which made the breads whiter, softer, and less dense. When gluten and/or wheat flour were added to endosperm rye bread, the above effect on the insulemic index (I.I.) was lost. The I.I. of all 60% whole meal breads was similar to white wheat bread. The conclusion from our studies is that the texture of the bread is more important than the whole meal or fiber content in producing beneficial insulin response.

References

Björck, I. 1995. Starch: nutritional aspects. In: *Carbohydrates in Food*, edited by Ann-Charlotte Eliasson, pp. 505–553. New York: Marcel Dekker.

Brand JC, Snow J, Nabhhan GP, Truswell, AS. 1990. Plasma glucose and insulin responses to traditional Pima Indian meals. *Am J Clin Nutr* 51: 416–420.

Cairns P, Morris VJ, Botham RL, Ring SG. 1996. Physicochemical studies on resistant starch *in vitro* and *in vivo*. *J Cereal Sci.* 23, 265–275.

Foster-Powell K, Holt SHA, Brand-Miller JC. 2002. International table of glycemic index and glycemic load values, 2002. *Am J Clin Nutr* 76, 5–56.

Granfeldt Y, Björck I, Drews A and Tovar J. 1992. An *in vitro* procedure based on chewing to predict metabolic response to starch in cereal and legume products. *Eur J Clin Nutr* 46, 649–660.

Guinard J-X, and Mazzucchelli R. 1996. The sensory perception of texture and mouthfeel. *Trends in Food Science and Technology* 7, 213–219.

Holm J, Lundquist I, Björck I, Eliasson A-C, and Asp N-G. 1988. Degree of starch gelatinization, digestion rate of starch in vitro, and metabolic responses in rats. *Am J Clin Nutr* 47, 1010–1016.

Holm J, Björck I. 1992. Bioavailability of starch in various wheat based bread products—evaluation of metabolic responses in healthy subjects and rate and extent of *in vitro* starch digestion. *Am J Clin Nutr 55,* 420–429.

Holt SHA, Miller JCB, and Petocz P. 1997. An insulin index of foods: the insulin demand generated by 1000-kJ portions of common foods. *Am J Clin Nutr* 66, 1264–1276.

Jenkins DJA, Wolever TMS, Kalmusky J, Giudici S, Giordano C, Wong GC, Bird JN, Patten R, Hall M, Buckley G, and Little JA. 1985. Low glycemic index carbohydrate foods in the management of hyperlipidemia. *Am. J. Clin. Nutr.* 42, 604–617.

Jenkins DJA, Wolever TMS, Jenkin AL, Giordano C, Giudici S, Thompson LU, Kalmusky J, Josse RG, and Wong G. 1986. Low glycemic response to traditionally processed wheat and rye products: bulgur and pumpernickel bread. *Am J Clin Nutr* 43, 516–520.

Juntunen KS, Laaksonen DE, Poutanen KS, Niskanen LK, and Mykkänen HM. 2003. High-fiber rye bread and insulin secretion and sensitivity in healthy postmenopausal women. *Am J Clin Nutr* 77, 385–391.

Juntunen K, Laaksonen DE, Autio K, Niskanen LK, Holst JJ, Savolainen KE, Liukkonen K-H, Poutanen K, and Mykkänen H. 2003. Structural differences between rye and wheat bread but not total fiber content may explain the lower postprandial insulin response to rye bread. *Am J Clin Nutr* 78, 957–64.

Leinonen K, Liukkonen K, Poutanen K, Uusitupa M, and Mykkänen, H. 1999. Rye bread decreases postprandial insulin response but does not alter glucose response in healthy Finnish subjects. *Eur. J. Clin. Nutr.* 53, 262–267.

Liukkonen K-H, Poutanen K, and Autio K. An *in vitro* particle size method for estimating particle size reduction in the digestion of starchy foods and for predicting insulin response (manuscript).

Mourot J, Thouvenot P, Couet C, Antoine JM, Krobicka A, Debry G. 1988. Relationship between the rate of gastric emptying and glucose and insulin responses to starchy foods in young healthy adults, *Am. J. Clin. Nutr.* 48 1035–1040.

Nilsson M, Stenberg M, Frid AH, Holts JJ, and Björck, I. 2004. Glycaemia and insulinemia in healthy subjects after lactose-equivalent meals of milk and other food proteins: the role of plasma amino acids and incretins. *Am. J. Clin. Nutr.* 80, 1246–1253.

Read NW, Welch I McL, Austen CJ, Barnish C, Bartlett CE, Baxter AJ, Brown G, Compton ME, Hume KE, Storie I, and Wordling J. 1986. Swallowing food without chewing: a simple way to reduce post-prandial glycaemia. *Brit J Nutr* 55, 43–47.

Slaughter SL, Ellis PR, and Butterworth PJ. 2002. An investigation of the action of porcine pancreatic alfa-amylase on native and gelatinised gels. *Biochimica et Biophysica acta* 1571, pp.55–63.

Wolever TMS, Jenkins DJA, Josse RG, Wong G, and Lee R. 1987. The glycemic index: similarity of values derived in insulin-dependent and non-insulin-dependent diabetic patients. *J. Am. Coll. Nutr.* 6, 295–305.

Wolever TMS, Katzman-Relle L, Jenkins AL, Vuksan V, Josse RG, and Jenkins DJA. 1994. Glycemic index of 102 complex carbohydrate foods in patients with diabetes. *Nutr. Res.* 14, 651–669.

10 Aleurone: Processing, Nutrition, Product Development, and Marketing

Bill Atwell, Walter von Reding, Jessica Earling, Mitch Kanter, and Kim Snow

Introduction

Before recorded history, people cultivated and consumed whole grains. They were likely consumed as is. Later it was discovered that if they were crushed and heated with water they could be made into simple pastes or porridges, which were more palatable. Eventually, leavened products such as bread were possible. These products were all hearty and dark colored because they contained the bran and germ and subsequently all the nutritional benefits of whole grains were realized.

As the centuries passed, crushing evolved to milling and people were able to separate the germ and bran from the endosperm. Off-flavors associated with the pigmented layers of the bran and the unstable oils of the germ were eliminated when the flour from the endosperm was used to make products. The flour with the bran and germ removed also was better able to retain gas and less dense bread could be produced.

The adoption of white bread as we know it occurred fairly recently, however. In the early 1900s most people were still consuming dark breads composed of whole grains, and they were still receiving all the benefits of whole grains. White bread was embraced by a major portion of the population soon after, and the segment quickly grew to be the largest one in the bakery category. As it did, deficiency diseases such as pellagra became more prevalent. Programs were then implemented to enrich flour and breads with B vitamins and iron, and the deficiency diseases declined radically.

Most of these essential nutrients that are located in the discarded fractions are in a layer removed with the bran known as aleurone. This highly nutritious layer contains extremely high levels of many vitamins and minerals and its removal from breads and other bakery products is almost exclusively the cause of the climbing rates of deficiency diseases. Aleurone also contains very significant levels of dietary fiber, phenolic acids, antioxidants, phytoestrogens, and sterols. Mounting evidence is currently being amassed by nutritionists on the benefits of these aleurone components on longer-term afflictions such as cancer, obesity, diabetes, and cardiovascular disease.

Aleurone also has a number of benefits that allow it to be incorporated into products more appealing to white bread consumers. A process has been patented to separate aleurone from the other bran layers. Aleurone is not a pigmented bran layer and subsequently the commercial product is lighter than the source bran. When mixed with white flour, as it is in product applications, it is lightened further. Breads made with aleurone-supplemented flour can be produced so they have all the nutritional benefits of whole grain bread but more closely resemble white bread. The pigments of the bran are associated with bitterness and consequently these breads also have a flavor profile similar to white bread. Children who inherently have especially sensitive palates prefer aleurone breads to whole wheat breads and their mothers are very favorably impressed with them as a means of delivering whole grain goodness to their children. This is a strong marketing concept and one that clearly delivers a major nutritional benefit to the consumer.

This chapter provides engineering, nutritional, food science, and marketing perspectives on aleurone. Individually and collectively, these discussions offer strong support that aleurone can provide all the healthy benefits of whole grain to consumers who traditionally prefer white bread. Clearly, returning this important wheat component to as many bakery products as possible is an important goal.

Wheat Aleurone Extraction and Process

The beneficial role of whole grain as part of a healthy eating pattern has been long established; there is no doubt about its benefit. The U.S. Department of Agriculture and medical associations thus recommend that consumers increase the intake of whole grain foods to protect against many chronic diseases.

The mechanisms by which whole grain acts are manifold, however they are not yet fully understood. It is most probable that protection comes from the combination of components in grain rather than from any isolated components. The physiologically most important substances are not evenly distributed over the kernel but are concentrated in the bran fractions, or more precisely, in the aleurone layers. In modern milling techniques, the aleurone layer of cereals is usually lost to human consumption because this layer is tightly bound to the pericarp (seed coat) and therefore is part of the bran fraction (Figure 10.1).

A new, patented pure mechanical industrial process isolates wheat aleurone cells; yield is good and the purity is high. Most of the nutritionally important substances of whole grain, such as dietary fiber (mainly arabinoxylans), vitamins, minerals, and phytonutrients (such as phenolic components), are concentrated in the aleurone cells. This innovative isolation

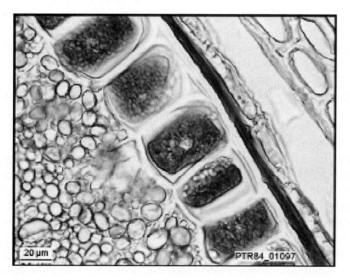

Figure 10.1. Aleurone cells.

Table 10.1.   Nutrient content of process fractions.

	Ash	Protein	Vitamins (Thiamin)	Minerals (Magnesia)	Fiber (TDF)
Whole Grain	2%	11%	480μ/100g	145mg/100g	10%
Wheat Bran	5%	15%	650μ/100g	590mg/100g	42%
Wheat Aleurone$_1$	8%	18%	870μ/100g	690mg/100g	48%
Wheat Aleurone$_2$	10%	21%	1150μ/100g	850mg/100g	43%

process enables recovery of the valuable aleurone layer from wheat bran to yield a light brown to yellowish free-flowing powder that can be used to enrich different food products.

The patented wheat aleurone process is purely mechanical. Wheat bran is used as a starting material to yield wheat aleurone cells in different grades (purities). Different nutrients and phytonutrients such as phenolic acids were increased during the process, as shown in Table 10.1.

Food safety will remain a very important issue as whole grain and whole grain components become more favorable. Pesticides and mycotoxins are reduced as a result of the wheat aleurone process, but further data from different bran are necessary to prove this in depth.

Bakery Product Development: The Aleurone Example

The benefits and hurdles in whole grain product development are very similar. To whole grain consumers, benefits include health, taste, texture, and appearance. However, a refined flour consumer may consider taste, texture, and appearance a hurdle. For the white bread consumer, health cannot be the only driver for consumption of whole grains. Product developers need to explore different opportunities to deliver whole grain nutrients in ways that a variety of consumers will enjoy.

Whole grains are typically associated with wheat. However, wheat is not the only grain that can be developed into products. Using different grains, in combination or alone, gives consumers different options for taste, texture, and appearance. Some examples of other grains to be developed may include corn, barley, rye, oats, triticale, spelt, and rice.

Wheat is the most cultivated grain in the world. Roughly three-quarters of all U.S. grain products are made from wheat flour. Wheat is used most in bread products because of its unique and functional bread-making properties. A whole grain wheat bread made with 100% whole wheat flour would yield a bread with a dense texture, a dry crumb, and perhaps a bitter flavor.

Corn is the number one field crop, leading in value and volume of production. Corn has a number of uses in food and industry. An example of a formulation for whole grain bread with corn uses 40% whole wheat flour, 36% whole grain corn grit, and 14% whole grain corn flour. Characteristics of this final product may include better volume, a yellowish appearance, and a mild and nutty flavor.

Barley is a minor cereal grain that is underused in food products. Barley is unique because of its high level of soluble fiber—it is actually higher than the β-glucan content in oats. Like most grains, barley can be milled into many different fractions, from flour to grits. Formulating a whole grain bread using barley may include a combination of 30% whole wheat flour, 39% whole grain crushed barley, and 19% whole grain barley flour. This bread may have a light texture, a moist crumb, and a sweeter flavor.

Barley and corn are good examples of ways to create whole grain bread products that are softer and perhaps more mild than whole wheat bread. But what if we want the opposite—a product that is more flavorful, dense, and darker than whole wheat? Rye is a very dark cereal grain that is known for its intense flavor. Currently, the U.S. only uses 25% of the annual rye crop for human food. As with other cereal grains, rye can take various forms such as flour, pearled, cut, and flaked. An example of a formulation using rye may include 42% whole wheat flour, 27% whole grain cut rye, and 18% whole grain rye flour. This bread would be very hearty, dense, and dark, and have a strong flavor.

The above breads are just examples of ways that we can alter sensory qualities to meet a specific need. We can make whole grain products that are dark, dense, and intense in flavor, or whole grain products that are lighter, softer, and milder in flavor.

For those segments of the population who consume white bread but don't find the above formulations acceptable, aleurone can be used to make bread with the health benefits of whole grains but with similar sensory characteristics of white bread.

Aleurone contains 45% to 50% total dietary fiber (T.D.F.), a concentrated source of essential vitamins including B_6, niacin, and E. It also is a concentrated source of important minerals such as potassium, magnesium, calcium, iron, and zinc. Aleurone contains most major antioxidants, and many phytochemicals. However, aleurone is a concentrated ingredient, not a whole grain ingredient. Can we use this ingredient to get the benefits of a whole grain? Cargill Incorporated asked Joanne Slavin and Gary Fulcher, at the University of Minnesota, to write a white paper to support the nutritional benefits of aleurone. They wrote:

> "In wheat, the majority of desirable "whole grain" components are concentrated in the aleurone layer, the primary component of bran which is a source of antioxidants, minerals, lysine-rich proteins, soluble and insoluble fiber, water- and fat-soluble vitamins, sterols, and lignans, among others. The aleurone layer is not only unique, it is the primary source of bioactive effects conferred by whole wheat products; indeed it is the core of whole wheat benefits."

The white paper supports the nutritional benefits of aleurone as an ingredient, but now it has to be incorporated into products to reap the whole grain benefits. Enriched white flour that has a 20% replacement with aleurone has similar nutritional characteristics as whole wheat flour (Table 10.2). Clearly, there are apparent differences between the nutritional profile of enriched white flour and whole wheat flour. There is noticeably higher fiber in whole wheat flour and a higher content of minerals. However, there are many similarities between whole wheat flour and the 20% aleurone blend. Fiber content, for example, is similar to whole wheat. Niacin is significantly higher in the aleurone flour. In fact, the aleurone layer is the most concentrated natural source of niacin. Most of the minerals also are similar or higher in the aleurone blend.

The nutritional similarities also translate into a final bread product (Table 10.3). The similarities provide a foundation for a new bread product with the nutritional benefits of whole wheat bread. Fiber is a good indicator of this similarity. Both the whole wheat bread and the aleurone bread are a good source of fiber.

Initial product development included bread made with a straight dough process. The objective was to make a bread using aleurone that is nutritionally equivalent to whole wheat bread. Formulation for white bread is fairly simple and straightforward (Table 10.4). Formulating a whole wheat bread requires the addition of vital wheat gluten, dough conditioners,

Table 10.2.   Nutritional comparison of white flour, whole wheat flour, and a 20% aleurone/80% white flour blend.

Nutritional Comparison		Enriched White Flour	Whole Wheat Flour	20% Aleurone Flour
Protein	%	12.20	14.20	13.40
Fiber	%	2.00	9.70	11.30
Insoluble	%	1.40	8.70	10.00
Soluble	%	0.60	1.00	1.30
Vitamins				
B_6	mg/100g	0.10	0.64	0.47
Niacin	mg/100g	3.92	2.19	9.21
Minerals				
Ca	mg/100g	16.30	30.60	37.20
Mg	mg/100g	29.40	138.00	156.00
Zn	mg/100g	0.71	2.65	2.24
K	mg/100g	109.00	333.00	406.00
Ash	%	0.48	1.50	1.83
Total Carbohydrates	%	72.10	62.10	61.50
Fat	%	1.63	2.52	2.66
Moisture	%	12.20	11.00	10.60
Whiteness (LAB)	L-Value	97.55	80.26	90.95

and increased absorptions. Aleurone bread made with the addition of 20% aleurone based on white flour is similar to whole wheat.

Indications of dough rheology, stability, and processability are measured by placing mixed dough into a farinograph (Figure 10.2). White bread dough has more stability after 15 minutes, which is to be expected. Whole wheat dough begins to break down after roughly 10 minutes, which is similar to aleurone dough. Texture was measured using a texture analyzer (TA-X2Ti). Texture measured on day 1 shows aleurone between white and whole

Table 10.3.   Nutritional comparison of white break, bread made with a 20% aleurone/80% white flour blend, and whole wheat bread.

Nutritional Comparison		White Bread	Aleurone Bread	Whole Wheat Bread
Serving Size		50g	50g	50g
Calories	kcal	140.00	110.00	130.00
Total Fat	g	1.00	1.50	1.50
Cholesterol	mg	0	0	0
Sodium	mg	250.00	230.00	220.00
Total Carbohydrate	g	27.00	23.00	25.00
Dietary Fiber	g	1.00	3.00	3.00
Insoluble	g	NA	2.85	NA
Soluble	g	NA	0.15	NA
Sugars	g	2.00	2.60	5.00
Protein	g	4.00	5.00	5.00
Niacin	mg	1.90	3.60	3.27
Calcium	mg	5.80	11.00	10.40
Iron	mg	1.50	1.80	1.20
Ash	%	0.80	1.00	1.20
Moisture	%	33.60	40.10	37.10

Table 10.4.   Straight dough bread formulations.

Ingredient	White		Whole Wheat		Aleurone	
	Bakers %	Dough %	Bakers %	Dough %	Bakers %	Dough %
Bread flour (11% to 13% protein)	100	56.1	0	0	100	43.9
Whole wheat flour	0	0	100	51.3	0	0
Aleurone	0	0	0	0	20.0	8.8
Vital wheat gluten	0	0	*3.0 to 4.5	1.5	*3.0 to 4.5	1.3
HFCS	10.0	5.6	10.0	5.1	10.0	4.4
Soybean oil	2.0	1.3	4.0	2.1	4.0	1.8
Salt	2.0	1.1	2.0	1.0	2.0	0.9
Dough conditioner	1.5	0.8	1.5	0.8	1.5	0.8
Yeast	3.0	1.7	4.5	2.3	4.5	2.0
Water	**60.0	33.4	**70.0	35.9	**84.0	36.8

*Dependent on protein level of bread flour
**Dependent of flour moisture and/or gluten level

wheat bread texture (Figure 10.3). However, day 4 shows the aleurone bread was less firm than whole wheat bread and just as soft as the white bread. Bread volumes indicate similarities between aleurone and whole wheat bread (Figure 10.4).

The next objective was to make bread that has similar characteristics as white bread based on taste, texture, and appearance. This may be achieved with a sponge dough process (Table 10.5). Sponge formulations for the white bread and aleurone bread are identical. Differences in formulation are apparent on the dough side. Again, as in the straight doughs, the aleurone

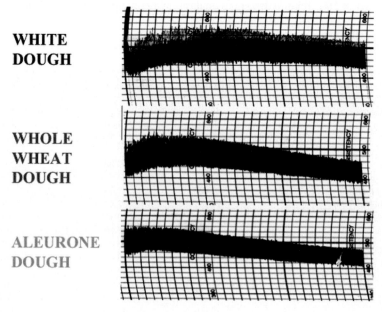

WHITE DOUGH

WHOLE WHEAT DOUGH

ALEURONE DOUGH

Figure 10.2.   Farinograph curves of straight doughs.

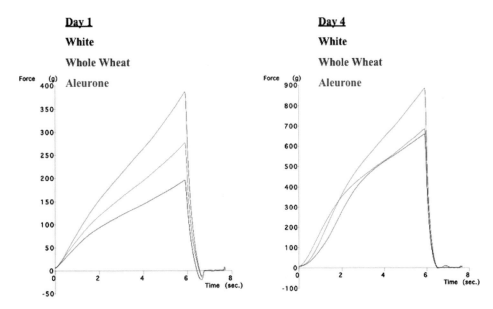

Figure 10.3. Texture analysis of straight doughs.

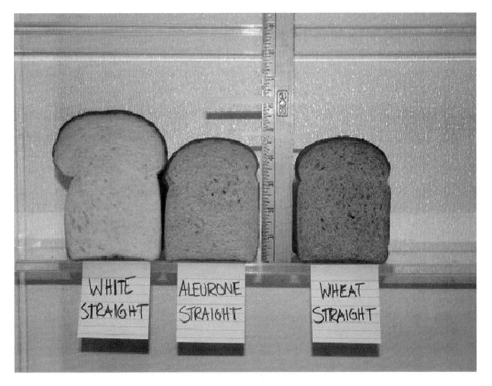

Figure 10.4. Appearance and volume of straight dough breads.

Table 10.5.   Sponge dough bread formulations.

Ingredient	White		Aleurone	
	Bakers %	Dough %	Bakers %	Dough %
Sponge				
Bread flour (11% to 13% protein)	60.0	33.33	60.0	25.61
Water	36.0	20.0	36.0	15.36
Yeast	3.0	1.67	3.0	1.28
Yeast food	0.05	0.28	0.05	0.21
Dough				
Bread flour (11% to 13% protein)	40.0	22.22	40.0	22.22
Vital wheat gluten	0	0	4.0	1.71
Aleurone	0	0	20.0	8.54
HFCS	12.0	6.67	15.0	6.4
Salt	2.0	1.11	2.0	0.85
Soybean oil	2.0	1.11	4.0	1.71
Ascorbic acid	60 ppm	0.003	60 ppm	0.002
Dough conditioners	0.05	0.28	1.0	0.42
Mono- and diglycerides	0	0	1.3	0.55
Yeast	0	0	1.5	0.64
Water	24.0	13.33	46.0	19.63

is incorporated at 20% based on the total flour. Additional vital wheat gluten, sweetener, mono- and diglycerides, dough conditioners, and additional absorption are added to the aleurone formula for optimization. Also, similar to the straight dough formulas, the white dough has longer stability than the aleurone dough (Figure 10.5). Interestingly, when it comes to texture of the final product, the aleurone bread is softer than the white bread on day 1 and remained softer after four days (Figure 10.6). The appearance is also very encouraging because the aleurone is very similar in volume to the white bread (Figure 10.7). In terms of texture and appearance, the sponge dough process was a success.

Whiteness is clearly an important factor in making the aleurone bread appear similar to white bread. A Hunter Colorimeter was used to obtain L-values as a measure of whiteness. The greater the L-value, the whiter the product (Table 10.6). Aleurone is clearly darker than the whole wheat flours, both red and white, as well as the unbleached white flour. This is expected because there is no starchy endosperm to lighten its color. The 20% aleurone blended with unbleached white flour is significantly whiter. The L-values also reflect in the finished product. The bread made with aleurone is similar to the white whole wheat bread as far as whiteness.

Taste is also very important. White flour is the base in aleurone bread. In addition, a majority of the bran is removed to isolate the aleurone. This may give the aleurone bread a less "wheaty" flavor. The long fermentation process of the sponge dough yields a flavor very close to white bread, whereas the bread made from straight dough has a flavor somewhere in between white and whole wheat bread.

We can further enhance nutrition by adding aleurone to whole wheat flour. Blending 25% aleurone with whole wheat flour increases fiber and other nutrients. Again, this formulation includes additional vital wheat gluten, dough conditioners, and absorption (Table 10.7). The final characteristics of this bread are similar to a whole wheat bread in which volume is decreased, texture is firmer, the color is darker, and the flavor is more like whole wheat.

WHITE DOUGH

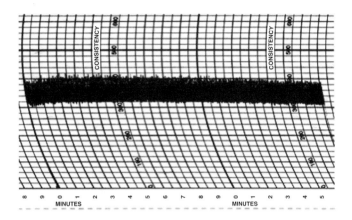

ALEURONE DOUGH

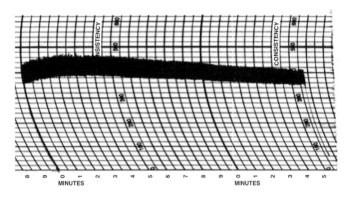

Figure 10.5. Farinograph curves of sponge doughs.

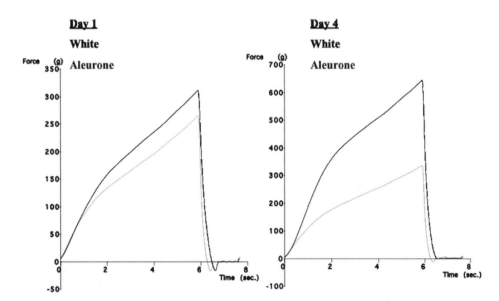

Figure 10.6. Texture analysis of sponge dough breads.

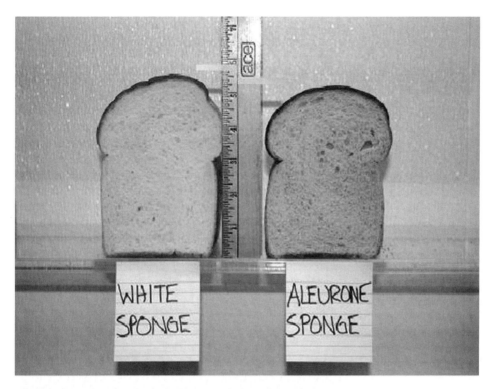

Figure 10.7. Appearance and volume of sponge dough breads.

Table 10.6. Whiteness of flours and breads.

	L-VALUES		
Ingredient	Ingredient Whiteness	20% Blend Whiteness	Bread Whiteness
Aleurone	73.27	90.95	83.3 straight/86.2 sponge
Whole Wheat Flour-Hard Red	80.26	—	75.6
Whole Wheat Flour-Hard White	84.21	—	84.9
Unbleached White Flour	97.55	—	96.5

Table 10.7. Aleurone and whole wheat bread formulation

Ingredients	Bakers %
Whole wheat flour	100
Aleurone	25.0
Vital wheat gluten	7.0 to 10.0
HFCS	12.0
Shortening	3.5
Salt	2.0
Mono and diglyceride	2.0
Dough conditioner	1.5
Yeast	4.0
Water	92.0

Other applications for aleurone that have been explored are artisan breads, buns, pizza crusts, snack foods, pasta, cereal, muffins, pie crust, and cookies. Replacing 20% of the white flour in any of these formulas with aleurone will yield the same nutritional outcome as the product made with 100% whole wheat flour but may have a closer taste, texture, and appearance to that of a product made with white flour.

Nutritional Benefits of the Aleurone Layer

The preponderance of data published in recent years strongly indicates that whole grain intake is inversely related to the risk of cancer, cardiovascular disease, obesity, and diabetes in various population groups (Anderson et al. 2000, Kritchevsky 1995, Liu et al. 2000, McKeown et al. 2002, Pereira et al. 2000, Porikos 1982). Further, historical data suggest that our understanding of various nutrient deficiency conditions (e.g., beriberi, pellagra) can be largely traced to the advent of milling processes in the late 1800s that made refined flours more appealing, less expensive, and more widely available to people, regardless of their socioeconomic status (Spiller 2002). More recently, the increased worldwide consumption of refined grain products has been questioned because of their implications on overall nutrition and health (Miller et al. 2002), prompting the U.S. Departments of Agriculture and Health and Human Services to alter their latest Food Guide Pyramid recommendations to specifically mention the increased daily consumption of whole grain products.

It has been well understood for some time that the bran layer of most grains (the portion of the grain that is generally removed and discarded during processing) is the most nutrient dense fraction of the whole grain. Bran contains a significant amount of insoluble and soluble fiber (Bacic et al. 1981), as well as the majority of the phenolic acids, lignans, and other antioxidants associated with the whole grain (Miller et al. 2002).

Despite our understanding of the nutritional benefits of consuming whole grains, and the recommendations of most credible nutrition groups and government agencies that we consume three or more servings of whole grains each day, whole grain intake in most Westernized countries is only about one serving per day (Albertson et al. 1995). There are historical as well as practical reasons why this is so, the most cogent being that the endosperm-rich (and bran-devoid) flours most often used today have better organileptic properties and better cooking/baking qualities than do whole grain alternatives. High-bran flours, for example, tend to have a negative effect on the flavor and color of most baked products (Shenoy et al. 2002), and they may impart strong bitter flavors on baked and extruded products as well (Fulcher et al. 2002). Consequently, it has become a challenge within the food industry to create grain-based flours and products that cook and taste like processed grains, but that retain the nutritional properties of whole grains. The aleurone layer of bran, long known as the most nutrient-dense bran fraction, may prove to be the grain component that drives the transformation from "taste or health" to "taste and health" in grain-based products.

The bran component of most grains contains upwards of seven different layers, the largest of which is the aleurone fraction. The aleurone fraction comprises as much as 75% of the dry weight of bran (Fulcher 1972). During the milling process, the aleurone layer is removed along with the pericarp, the testa, and other bran components.

Until recently, it was extremely difficult to isolate the aleurone layer from the remainder of the bran constituents, largely because extraction/separation techniques were inadequate to perform clean separations of the individual bran components. However, recent technological advances have made it possible to more cleanly extract the aleurone layer from other grain components. This will undoubtedly increase our understanding of the nutritional properties of the aleurone layer in the future. This is not to suggest, however, that our understanding of the aleurone fraction is non-existent. In fact, there are data dating back more than 150 years regarding the nutritional properties of aleurone.

Because of its role as a protective barrier in the intact grain kernel against penetration and damage by insects, fungi, etc., it is not surprising that a number of the protective compounds present in the bran fraction in general, and the aleurone layer in particular, serve as important nutritional sources as well (Fulcher et al. 2002). First described by Hartig in the 1850s, aleurone is a significant source of various B vitamins, and vitamin E, and numerous minerals, fibers, antioxidants, and phytosterols. More recent research conducted during the past thirty years has corroborated these findings (Fulcher et al. 1972, Collins 1986, and McKeehen et al. 1999) and suggest, as Fulcher stated, that "the nutritional properties of isolated aleurone layers are higher than those exerted by the intact, commercial bran fractions containing them."

A number of phenolic compounds with purported antioxidant activity have been identified in aleurone, most notably ferulic acid (Fulcher et al. 1972), as well as other lower molecular-weight phenolic esters (Collins 1986). These compounds most certainly serve a protective function within the grain kernel, and as far back as the 1930s were identified as potential preservatives to prolong the shelf life of dairy-based products, among other perishable food items (Peter and Musher 1937). More recently, physiological benefits have been ascribed to a number of these compounds as well. For example, Pascoe and Fulcher (unpublished observations) have suggested that they might serve as stimulators of the mammalian immune system. Additional antioxidants, including cinnamic acid derivatives, phytoestrogens (including lignans), and various tocopherols have also been identified in the aleurone fraction of some grains as well, most often in combination with various B vitamins.

Many grain-based B vitamins are almost exclusively sequestered within the aleurone fraction of the bran. Fulcher (1972) has indicated that niacin is contained entirely within the aleurone layer, and is accompanied by other water-soluble vitamins such as thiamine, folic acid, and riboflavin, as well as the fat-soluble tocopherols. The bioavailability of these aleurone-derived vitamins was in question for many years (Mason et al. 1973). However, a recent sixteen-week feeding study conducted by Fenech et al. (2005) indicated that daily consumption of bread made from aleurone flour was as effective as a high folate supplement in increasing red cell folate levels and decreasing plasma homocysteine levels in healthy men, indicating the bioavailability of aleurone-derived folate. Additional work is necessary to determine if other aleurone-derived B vitamins (and related compounds) are as bioavailable as folate.

Phytosterols, which have been demonstrated in numerous studies to be effective cholesterol-lowering compounds (Hendriks et al. 2003, N.C.E.P. Expert Panel 2001), have been identified in the aleurone layer of various grains (Piironen et Al. 2002). Primarily associated with soybean oil, phytosterols derived from wheat aleurone have recently been isolated in significant quantities (Buri et al. 2003). Further, the wheat aleurone sterol concentration has been shown to be about 25% greater than that contained in the bran fraction of the grain, and about 2.5-fold greater than that found in whole wheat fractions.

The aleurone layer of most grains may contain as much as 20% total protein (Peterson et al. 1985) and basic amino acids, especially lysine and arginine (Fulcher 1986). The high lysine content is appealing to feed processors, who seek to improve the lysine contents in livestock feed (Peterson et al. 1986); the arginine content in aleurone may have health implications for improving vascular dynamics and endothelial function (Cooke 2003). However, no research has been conducted to date that has specifically used aleurone as a source of arginine in endothelial function trials.

Marketing Aleurone

There is a lot of positive energy around whole grains, but there are still some distinct barriers for increasing consumer consumption, primarily information overload, perceived cost, and taste. According to the Shopping for Health 2004 Report, approximately 60% of consumers said there is too much conflicting information in coverage of nutrition issues and 30% said the confusion in part leads to an unhealthy diet. When it comes to taste, children are hardest to convert to whole grain products because many prefer white bread. To better understand the barriers and consumers, Cargill conducted some primary market research to explore consumer behavior in the bread category. We found that 60% of children and 38% of adults are still eating white bread, which suggests that barriers continue to exist in converting consumers to healthy bread products. We also confirmed that taste is a key driver in bread purchases that, in the case of whole grains, can often be the barrier to market entrance.

Clearly, there is an opportunity in the marketplace to develop products that have sensory attributes like those found in enriched products, but similar nutrient profiles to whole grains. These products would allow people permission to enjoy products with a taste profile they prefer and a nutrient profile they desire. Wheat aleurone is one ingredient that can meet these requirements. It can help fill this gap by providing nutrients similar to those found in whole wheat such as dietary fiber and concentrations of important vitamins, minerals, and antioxidants. Wheat aleurone, as an ingredient, provides an alternative to whole grains for consumers who are not willing to sacrifice taste for health.

To determine whether this message resonated with our target audience, we conducted market research on bread made with aleurone to see if it was appealing to both moms and kids. We found that 71% of moms believed their kids would eat it and that kids rated bread made with aleurone as an "8" on a 9-point scale, which was similar to white bread and significantly higher than whole wheat bread. These finding helped confirm that wheat aleurone would be a good alternative for whole wheat products in the marketplace.

References

Albertson, A.M. and Tobelmann, R.C. 1995. Consumption of grain and whole-grain foods by an American population during the years 1990 to 1992. *J. Am. Diet. Assoc.* 95:703.

Anderson, J.W., Hanna, T.J., Peng, X., and Kryscio, R. 2000. Whole grain foods and heart disease risk. *J. Am. Coll. Nutr.* 19 (Supple 3):291S.

Bacic, A., and Stone, B.A. 1981. Isolation and ultrastructure of aleurone cell walls from wheat and barley. *Aust. J. Plant Physiol.* 8:453.

Buri, R.C., von Reding, W., and Gavin, M.M. 2003. Isolation and characterization of aleurone from wheat bran. *Corp. Development Report, Buhler AG,* Uzwil, Switzerland.

Collins, F.W. 1986. Oat phenolics: structure, occurrence, and function. In *Oats: Chemistry and Technology,* F.H. Webster (ed.). Am. Assoc. of Cereal Chemists, St. Paul, Minn. p. 227.

Cooke, J.C. 2003. NO and angiogenesis. *Atheroscler.* Supple. Dec 4 (4):53.

Fenech, M., Noakes, M., Clifton, P., and Topping, D. 2005. Aleurone flour increases red cell folate and lowers plasma homocysteine substantially in man. *Br. J. Nutr. Mar.,* 93(3):353.

Fulcher, R.G. and Rooney Duke, T.K. 2002. Whole grain structure and organization: implications for nutritionists and processors. In *Whole Grain Food in Health and Disease,* Marquart, L., Slavin J.L., and Fulcher, R.G. (eds.) Am. Assn. Of Cereal Chemists, St. Paul, Minn. P. 9.

Fulcher, R.G., 1986. Morphological and chemical organization of the oat kernel. In *Oats: Chemistry and Technology.* F.H. Webster (ed.) Am. Assn. Of Cereal Chemists, St. Paul, Minn. P.47.

Fulcher, R.G., O'Brien T.P., and Lee, J.W. 1972. Studies on the aleurone layer I: Conventional and fluorescence microscopy of the cell wall with emphasis on phenol-carbohydrate complexes in wheat. *Aust. J. Biol. Sci.* 25(1):23.

Hartig, T. 1856. Weitere mittheilungen das klebermahl (aleurone) betreffend. *Bot. Zeit.* 14:257.

Hendriks, H.F., Brink, E.J., Meijer, G.W., Princin, H.M., Ntanios, F.Y. 2003. Safety of long-term consumption of plant sterol esters-enriched spread. *Eur. J. Clin. Nutr.* 142:681.

Kritchevsky, D. 1995. Epidemiology of fibre, resistant starch, and colorectal cancer. *Eur. J. Cancer Prev.,* 4:345.

Liu, S., Manson, J.E., Stampfer, M.J., Hu, F.B., Giovannucci, E., Colditz, G.A., Hennekens, C.H., and Willett, W.C. 2000. A prospective study of whole grain intake and risk of Type II diabetes in U.S. women. *Am. J. Public Health* 90:1409.

Mason, J.B. and Kodicek, E. 1973. The chemical nature of the bound nicotinic acid of wheat bran: studies of partial hydrolysis products. *Cereal Chem.* 50:637.

McKeehan, J.D., Busch, R.H., and Fulcher, R.G. 1999. Evaluation of wheat phenolic acids during grain development and their contribution to Fusarium resistance. *J. Agric. Food Chem.* 47(4):1476.

McKeown, N., Meigs, J., Lu, S., Wilson, P., and Jacques, P. 2002. Whole grain intake is favorably associated with metabolic risk factors for Type II diabetes and cardiovascular disease in the Framingham Offspring Study. *Am. J. Clin. Nutr.* 2002. Aug. 76(2):390.

Miller, G., Prakash, A., and Decker, E. 2002. Whole Grain Micronutrients. In *Whole Grain Foods in Health and Disease,* Marquart, L., Slavin, J.S., and Fulcher, R.G. (eds.), Am. Assoc. Cereal Chemists, St. Paul, Minn. P.243.

NCEP Expert Panel. 2001. Summary of the third report of the National Cholesterol Education Program (NCEP) expert panel on detection, evaluation, and treatment of high blood cholesterol in adults (adult treatment panel III). *J.A.M.A.* 285:2486.

Pereira, M., Jacobs, D., Pins, J., Raatz, S., Gross, M., Slavin, J., and Seaquist, E. 2000. The effect of whole grains on body weight and insulin sensitivity in overweight hyperinsulinemic adults. *Diabetes* 44 (Suppl.):A40.

Peters, F.N. and Musher, S. 1937. Oat flour as an antioxidant. *Indus. and Engineer.* Chem. 29:146.

Peterson, D.M. and Brinegar, A.C. 1986. Oat storage proteins: In *Oats: Chemistry and Technology.* F.H. Webster (ed.) Am. Assoc. Cereal Chem. St. Paul, Minn. P. 153.

Peterson, D.M., Saigo, R.H., and Holy, J. 1985. Development of oat aleurone cells and their protein bodies. *Cereal Chem.* 62:366.

Piironen, V., Toivo, J., and Lampi, A.M. 2002. Plant sterols in cereals and cereal products. *Cereal Chem.* 79(1):148.

Porikos, K.P., Hesser, M.F., and Van Itallie, T.B. 1982. Calorie regulation in normal weight men maintained on a palatable diet of conventional foods. *Physiol. Behav.* 29:293.

Shenoy, H.A. and Prakash, J. 2002. Wheat bran (triticum aestivum): composition, functionality and incorporation in unleavened bread. *J. Food Qual.* 25(3):197.

Spiller, G. 2002. Whole grains, whole wheat, and white flours in history. In *Whole Grain Foods in Health and Disease.* Marquart, L., Slavin, J.L., and Fulcher, R.G. (ed.) Am. Assoc. of Cereal Chemists, St. Paul, Minn., p. 1.

11   Active Components of Whole Grain Foods

Susan Cho and Carol J. Pratt

Introduction

The U.S. Department of Agriculture (2000, 2005) has recommended that Americans should consume a minimum of three servings of whole grain products daily. This recommendation was first made in the 1985 U.S.D.A. food guidance systems (Cronin 1985). The intent was to increase consumption of dietary fiber and key vitamins and minerals present in large quantities in whole grain foods. Increased consumption has been also recommended by the American Dietetic Association (A.D.A.) since 1994 (National Center for Nutrition and Dietetics 1994). Healthy People 2010, published in 2001, included the three-serving recommendation for whole grains in the national nutritional goals (U.S. Department of Health and Human Services 2001). It was recognized that whole grain consumers had significantly better nutrient profiles than non-consumers, including higher vitamins and minerals, and lower intakes of total fat, saturated fat, and sugar as a percentage of food energy. The U.S.D.A. Dietary Guidelines for Americans (2000, 2005) also have recommended daily consumption of a minimum of three servings of whole grain foods.

Despite numerous educational efforts to increase whole grain consumption, 90% of Americans do not meet the whole grain intake recommendation (Cleveland 2000). An average American consumes one serving of whole grain foods per day (Liu 2003). From a consumer perspective, identifying whole grain products is not always that simple. While consumers may be deceived by breads labeled "made with whole grain," consumers may not be aware of healthier choices among whole grain foods. This is partly due to inconsistencies and confusion involved in defining whole grain foods, the complexity involved in assessing whole grain food servings, and inconsistent ingredient labeling for whole grain foods. Given the lack of definition and inconsistent ingredient labeling, we reviewed the composition of bioactive nutrients as well as various epidemiological studies in relation to whole grain foods to suggest more physiologically relevant labeling standards.

Definition of Whole Grain Foods

Several reputable organizations have provided a definition of whole grains. A common feature of these definitions is that a whole grain food must contain the same relative proportions of endosperm, germ, and bran. According to the Wheat Foods Council, "Whole grain products are made with the whole kernel of grain," with nothing removed. The Whole Grains Council (W.G.C. 2004) has adopted a similar definition: "Whole grains or foods made from them contain all the essential parts and naturally-occurring nutrients of the entire grain seed. If the grain has been processed (e.g., cracked, crushed, rolled, extruded, lightly pearled and/or cooked), the food product should deliver approximately the same rich balance of nutrients that are found in the original grain seed." This W.G.C. definition has been crafted from the 1999 American Association of Cereal Chemists (A.A.C.C.) definition:

Table 11.1. Epidemiological studies which included more than 25% whole grain or bran cereals in the whole grain criteria to show the beneficial effects of whole grain foods.

Measurements in relation to whole grain intake	The name of the study, lead author, year of publication, and name of organization
Weight gain studies	
Weight gain over time	Nurses' Health Study, 12-year follow up. (Liu 2003, Harvard.)
Weight gain over time	Health Professionals Follow Up Study, 8-year follow up. (Koh-Benerjee 2004, Harvard.)
Heart disease risk	
Ischemic heart disease death in postmenopausal women	The Iowa Women's Health Study, 9-year follow up. (Jacobs 1998, Univ. of Minnesota.)
Coronary heart disease in women	Nurses' Health Study, 10-year follow up. (Liu 1999, Harvard.)
Coronary heart disease in men	Health Professionals Follow Up Study, 8-year follow up. (Hu 2000, Harvard.)
Cardiovascular disease and myocardial infarction	Nurses' Health Study, 6-year follow up. (Liu 2002, Harvard.)
Coronary artery disease	The Atherosclerosis Risk in Communities (ARIC) Study, 11-year follow up. (Steffen 2003, Univ. of Minnesota.)
Coronary heart disease	Health Professionals Follow Up Study, 14-year follow up. (Jensen 2004, Harvard.)
Ischemic stroke in women	Nurses' Health Study, 12-year follow up. (Liu 2000, Harvard.)
Diabetes/insulin sensitivity	
Type-2 diabetes mellitus	Health Professionals Follow Up Study, <12-year follow up. (Fung 2002, Harvard.)
Type-2 diabetes mellitus	Nurses' Health Study, 10-year follow up. (Liu 2000, Harvard.)
Type-2 diabetes mellitus	Framingham Offspring Study, Cross sectional study. (McKeown 2002, Tuft Univ.)

(*continued*)

"Whole grains shall consist of the intact, ground, cracked or flaked caryopsis, whose principal anatomical components—the starchy endosperm, germ and bran—are present in the same relative proportions as they exist in the intact caryopsis."

The currently authorized health claims for whole grains indicate that foods must contain 51% or more whole grain ingredient(s) by weight to be eligible for the claim (U.S. Food and Drug Administration 1999). In other words, eligible products for authorized whole grain health claims provide greater than 0.5 servings of whole grain per reference amount customarily consumed. For compliance purposes, the F.D.A. indicated that dietary fiber content of the food would be considered.

However, in major epidemiologic studies (Liu 1999, 2000, 2003; Jacobs 1998, 1999, 2000; Jensen 2004; Koh-Benerjee 2004; Steffen 2003a,b; Liese 2003), foods classified as whole grain products include cold breakfast cereals containing at least 25% whole grain or bran by weight, dark bread, popcorn, cooked oatmeal, wheat germ, and brown rice. Those epidemiological research studies include the Nurse's Health Study (Liu 1999, 2000, 2002, 2003) and Health Professionals Follow-Up Study (Koh-Benerjee 2004, Jensen 2004, Fung 2002, Hu 2000, Van Dam 2002) from the Harvard School of Public Health, the Iowa Women's Health Study (Jacobs 1999,

Table 11.1. Epidemiological studies which included more than 25% whole grain or bran cereals in the whole grain criteria to show the beneficial effects of whole grain foods. (*continued*)

Measurements in relation to whole grain intake	The name of the study, lead author, year of publication, and name of organization
Diabetes/insulin sensitivity (*continued*)	
Type-2 diabetes mellitus	Health Professionals Follow Up Study, <12-year follow up. (Van Dam 2002, Harvard.)
Type-2 diabetes mellitus	Finnish Mobile Clinic Health Exam Survey, 10-year follow up. (Montonen 2003, National Public Health Institute, Finland.)
Insulin sensitivity	The Insulin Resistance Atherosclerosis Study, 2- to 3-year follow up. (Liese 2003, Univ. of S. Carolina.)
Mortality risk	
Mortality	The Iowa Women's Health Study, 10-year follow up. (Jacobs 1999, Univ. of Minnesota.)
Mortality risk relative to a similar amount of refined grain fiber	The Iowa Women's Health Study, 12-year follow up. (Jacobs 2000, Univ. of Minnesota.)
Total mortality	The Atherosclerosis Risk in Communities (ARIC) Study, 11-year follow up. (Steffen 2003, Univ. of Minnesota.)
Cancer risk	
Colorectal cancer	A case-control study in Belgium. (Tuyns 1988. International Agency for Research on Cancer, France.)
Various types of cancer (oral cavity and pharynx, esophagus, stomach, colon, rectum, breast, ovary, prostate, liver, gallbladder, larynx, kidney, and others)	Whole grain intake and cancer: An expanded review and meta-analysis, Review of 40 studies published between 1984 and 1997. (Jacobs 1998, Univ. of Minnesota.)
Incident postmenopausal breast cancer	The Iowa Women's Health Study, 9-year follow up. (Nicodemus 2001, Univ. of Minnesota.)
Incident endometrial cancer and whether the association varied by use of hormone replacement therapy	The Iowa Women's Health Study, 12-year follow up. (Kasum 2001, Univ. of Minnesota.)

2000; Nicodemus 2001; Kasum 2001) and the Atherosclerosis Risk in Communities (A.R.I.C.) Study (Steffen 2003) from the University of Minnesota, the Insulin Resistance Atherosclerosis Study (Liese 2003) from the University of South Carolina, the Framingham Offspring Study (McKeown 2002) from Tufts University, and the Finnish Mobile Clinic Health Exam Survey (Montonen 2003) from the Finnish National Public Health Institute.

Table 11.1 describes epidemiological studies which included more than 25% whole grain or bran cereals in the whole grain criteria to show health benefits of whole grain foods. This definition is less stringent than the one used by the F.D.A., which specifies 51% whole grain by weight (F.D.A. 1999).

The U.S.D.A. has defined whole grain servings by using the Food Guide Pyramid. The database of Pyramid servings for foods included examples of whole grain ingredients. The Pyramid Servings Database contained servings per 100 grams for each food reported in the 1994-1996 Continuing Survey of Food Intakes by Individuals from thirty food groups and subgroups (three of which are grain, i.e., total grain, whole grain, and non-whole grain). Definitions of grain serving sizes were based on the Food Guide Pyramid and accompanying educational materials. Examples of a one-grain serving include: one slice of bread; one-half of a hamburger roll, one English muffin, one bagel, or one large croissant; and 1 ounce of ready-to-eat breakfast cereal (U.S.D.A. 1992, 2000).

When a food contained some whole grain and some non-whole grain ingredients, the recipe was used to determine the fraction of the grain servings from each. Raw wheat bran and oat bran were considered to be all whole grain in the pyramid. For example, wheat bran contains 3.53 servings of whole grain and zero servings of non-whole grain per 100 grams. These data are also reflected in U.S.D.A.-determined levels for whole grain in cereals containing wheat bran and oat bran. It is noteworthy that the U.S.D.A. did not consider rice bran as whole grain. Given the inconsistencies in whole grain criteria, consumers may not fully use a variety of whole grain foods available at the marketplace.

The Food Guide Pyramid was recently updated with the 2005 U.S.D.A. MyPyramid. The grains message states, "Make half your grains whole." Whole grains contain the entire grain kernel—the bran, germ, and endosperm—and are measured in ounce equivalents with suggested servings of one slice of bread, one cup of ready-to-eat cereal, or one-half cup of cooked rice, cooked pasta, or cooked cereal.

The U.S.D.A. Child Nutrition Program also recognizes whole grain, bran, and enriched grains when calculating fulfillment of grains/breads servings (U.S.D.A. 1997). These three grain "ingredients" are given equal weight for their contribution toward foods for the reimbursable meals program.

Nutrient Composition of Brans, Whole Grains, and Debranned Grains

The health-promoting effects of whole-grain consumption have been attributed in part to their dietary fiber, micronutrient, and phytochemical contents. From a botanical perspective, most whole grains, especially wheat, are composed of 15% bran, 5% germ, and 80% endosperm (Slavin, 2004). The bran component is a major source of bioactive compounds, such as dietary fiber, antioxidants, vitamins (including vitamin E, tocotrienols), minerals (including potassium, magnesium), and phytochemicals (including phytic acid, phenolic acids) (Truswell 2002). Thus, the intake of whole grains was positively associated with total intakes of dietary fiber ($r = 0.54$), magnesium ($r = 0.51$), folate ($r = 0.45$), vitamin E ($r = 0.40$), and vitamin B_6 ($r = 0.45$), which are important constituents of whole grains (McKeown 2003).

Nutrient Composition of Wheat Bran, Whole Wheat, and White Wheat Flour

Table 11.2 summarizes dietary fiber and selective micronutrient contents in wheat bran, whole wheat, and debranned white flour. Dietary fiber content in the bran component is 3.5 times higher than in whole grain kernels. Whole grain wheat has 4.5 times higher fiber content than debranned white wheat flour. The energy content of wheat bran was significantly lower than that of whole grain wheat or white flour. With the combination of high-fiber content and low-energy density, bran foods may promote weight management (Burton-Freeman 2000, Yao and Roberts 2001). High-fiber content in wheat bran and whole grain wheat may promote satiation (lower meal energy content) and satiety (longer duration between meals) due to its bulk and relatively low energy density, leading to decreased energy intake.

With the exception of selenium, the mineral content of wheat bran is 2.1 to 3 times higher than whole wheat flour, which has two to four times higher mineral content than debranned white flour. Thus, the mineral content of wheat bran is five to twenty-eight times higher than that present in white flour. In addition, the vitamin E content of wheat bran is almost twice

Table 11.2.   Nutrient compositions of wheat bran, whole grain wheat, and white wheat flour (per 100 grams).

	Wheat bran	Whole wheat flour	White wheat flour*	Bran/whole grain	Bran/white flour	Whole grain/ white flour
Proximates						
Energy, Kcal.	216	339	364	0.64	0.59	0.91
Fiber, g	42.8	12.2	2.7	3.5	15.8	4.5
Minerals						
Calcium, mg	73	34	15	2.1	4.9	2.3
Iron, mg	10.6	3.9	1.2	2.7	8.8	3.2
Magnesium, mg	611	138	22	4.4	27.8	6.3
Phosphorus, mg	1013	346	108	2.9	9.4	3.2
Potassium, mg	1182	405	107	2.9	11.0	3.8
Zinc, mg	7.3	2.9	0.7	2.5	10.4	4.1
Copper, mg	1.0	0.38	0.14	2.6	6.9	2.6
Manganese, mg	11.5	3.8	0.68	3.0	16.9	5.6
Selenium, ug	77.6	70.7	33.9	1.1	2.3	2.1
Vitamins						
Thiamin, mg	0.52	0.45	0.12	1.17	4.4	3.7
Riboflavin, mg	0.58	0.22	0.04	2.7	144.2	53.8
Niacin, mg	13.6	6.4	1.25	2.1	10.9	5.1
Pantothenic acid, mg	2.2	1.0	0.44	2.2	5.0	2.3
Vitamin B_6, mg	1.3	0.34	0.04	3.8	29.5	7.7
Folate, ug	79	44	26	1.8	3.0	1.7
Vitamin E, mg	1.49	0.82	0.06	1.8	24.8	13.7

*Debranned

Data source: U.S.D.A. National Nutrient Database for Standard Reference, Release 17. 2004.

that of whole wheat flour and almost twenty-five times greater than debranned white wheat flour. Martinez-Tome (2004) reported that antioxidant capacity of wheat bran is twenty-fold that of white wheat flour.

The data support that bran fractions are concentrated sources of these micronutrients and bran components appear to provide health benefits of whole grain foods. These micronutrients, in addition to dietary fiber, provide various health benefits. For example, potassium plays a key role in risk reduction of hypertension (Caulin-Glaser 2000, He and MacGregor 2003). Potassium intake also may play an important role in carbohydrate intolerance (He and MacGregor 2003). A reduced serum potassium level increases the risk of lethal ventricular arrhythmias in those at risk of heart failure or left ventricular hypertrophy (i.e. patients with ischemic heart disease). Furthermore, increasing potassium intake may help prevent these conditions. Magnesium is critical in risk reduction of heart disease (Mu 2005).

Epidemiologic data suggest that people with high calcium intake have a lower prevalence of being overweight or obese and having insulin resistance syndrome (Schrager 2005, Soares 2004, Loos 2004). High calcium intake depresses levels of parathyroid hormone and 1,25-hydroxy vitamin D. These decreased hormone levels lead to decreases in intracellular calcium, inhibiting lipogenesis and stimulating lipolysis. High dietary calcium intakes also increase excretion of fecal fat (Schrager 2005).

Nutrient Composition of Rice Bran, Whole Grain Brown Rice, and White Rice

Table 11.3 compares the nutrient content in rice bran, whole grain brown rice, and debranned white rice. With the exception of selenium, the mineral content in rice bran is 2.5-fold to 12-fold that of whole grain brown rice. The vitamin contents in bran are three to eight times higher than those present in whole grains, and whole grain rice contains two to eleven times higher vitamin content than debranned white grains. With the exception of selenium, the mineral and vitamin content of rice bran are up to two- to thirty-one-fold and six- to forty-four-fold those of debranned white rice, respectively.

Nutrient Composition of Oat Bran and Oat Flour

Table 11.4 lists nutrient compositions of oat bran and partially debranned oat flour. The energy content of oat bran is 39% lower than that of oat flour. The content of iron, magnesium, phosphorus, and potassium in oat bran is 26% to 38% higher than that of partially debranned oat flour. With the exception of niacin, the content of B vitamins and vitamin E in oat bran is 27% to 86% higher than that in partially debranned oat flour.

Nutrients and Antioxidant Content in Rye Bran

Liukkonen (2003) confirmed that sterols, folates, tocopherols and tocotrienols, alkylresorcinols, lignans, phenolic acids, and total phenolics are concentrated in the bran layers of the

Table 11.3. Nutrient compositions of rice bran, whole grain brown rice, and white rice (per 100 grams).

	Rice bran	Brown rice	White rice*	Bran/whole grain	Bran/white rice	Whole grain/ white rice
Proximates						
Energy, Kcal	316	370	365	0.85	1.01	0.87
Fiber, g	21.0	3.5	1.3	6.0	16.1	2.7
Minerals						
Calcium, mg	57	23	28	2.5	2.0	0.82
Iron, mg	18.5	1.5	0.8	12.3	23.1	1.9
Magnesium, mg	781	143	25	5.5	31.2	5.7
Phosphorus, mg	1677	333	115	5.0	19.3	2.9
Potassium, mg	1486	223	115	6.7	12.9	1.9
Zinc, mg	6.0	2.0	1.1	3.0	5.4	1.8
Copper, mg	0.73	0.28	0.22	2.6	3.3	1.3
Manganese, mg	14.2	3.7	1.1	3.8	12.9	3.4
Selenium, ug	15.6	23.4	15.1	0.64	1.03	1.6
Vitamins						
Thiamin, mg	2.75	0.40	0.07	6.9	39.3	5.7
Riboflavin, mg	0.284	0.09	0.05	3.2	5.7	1.8
Niacin, mg	34.0	5.1	1.6	6.7	21.2	3.2
Pantothenic acid, mg	7.4	1.5	1.0	4.9	7.4	1.5
Vitamin B_6, mg	4.1	0.51	0.16	8.0	25.6	3.2
Folate, ug	63	20	8	3.2	7.9	2.5
Vitamin E, mg	4.9	1.2	0.11	4.1	44.5	10.9

*Debranned
Data source: U.S.D.A. National Nutrient Database for Standard Reference, Release 17. 2004.

Table 11.4. Nutrient compositions of oat bran and oat flour (partially debranned) (per 100 grams)

	Oat bran	Oat flour, partially debranned	Bran/oat flour
Proximates			
Energy, Kcal	246	404	0.61
Fiber, g	15.4	6.5	2.4
Minerals			
Calcium, mg	58	55	1.05
Iron, mg	5.4	4.0	1.85
Magnesium, mg	235	144	1.63
Phosphorus, mg	734	452	1.62
Potassium, mg	566	371	1.53
Zinc, mg	3.1	3.2	0.97
Copper, mg	0.403	0.44	0.92
Manganese, mg	5.63	4.02	1.4
Selenium, ug	45.2	34	1.33
Vitamins			
Thiamin, mg	1.17	0.69	1.69
Riboflavin, mg	0.22	0.12	1.76
Niacin, mg	0.934	1.47	0.64
Pantothenic acid, mg	1.49	0.20	7.45
Vitamin B_6, mg	0.165	0.12	1.32
Folate, ug	52	32	1.62
Vit E, mg	1.01	0.7	1.44

Data source: U.S.D.A. National Nutrient Database for Standard Reference, Release 17. 2004.

rye grain, and are only present at low levels in the flour endosperm. Adom (2005) studied antioxidant activities of different fractions of whole wheat. In whole grain wheat flour, the bran/germ fraction contributed 83% of the total phenolic content, 79% of the total flavonoid content, 51% of the total lutein, 78% of the total zeaxanthin, 42% of the total beta-cryptoxanthin, and 85% to 94% of the antioxidant activities. On average, bran/germ fractions of whole grain wheat had four-fold more lutein, twelve-fold more zeaxanthin, and two-fold more β-cryptoxanthin than the endosperm fractions. Total phenolic content of bran/germ fractions (2,867 to 3,120 umol of gallic acid equiv/100 grams) was fifteen- to eighteen-fold higher than that of respective endosperm fractions. Ferulic acid content in bran/germ fractions (1,005 to 1,130 μmol/100 grams) was five to seven times higher than the endosperm fractions. Antioxidant activities of bran/germ samples (7.1 to 16.4 μmol of vitamin C equiv/gram and 1,785 to 4,669 μmol of vitamin E equiv/gram) were thirteen- to eighty-nine-fold higher than that of the respective endosperm samples. The results showed that the bran/germ are concentrated sources of bioactive compounds.

Antioxidant Content in Sorghum Bran

Awika (2004) also found that sorghum bran had three to four times higher anthocyanin (a functional compound in sorghum) contents than the whole grains. These findings provide information necessary for evaluating contributions to good health and disease prevention from whole grain consumption.

Active Components of Whole Grain Foods in Weight Gain Reduction

Recent studies from Harvard suggest that bran parts of whole grains are active components in whole grains. Koh-Benerjee (2004) demonstrated the importance of bran components in weight gain reduction by using the Health Professionals' Follow-up Study (H.P.F.S.) database. H.P.F.S. is a prospective investigation of 27,082 male health professionals aged 40 to 75 years at baseline in 1986. Detailed dietary information was obtained in 1986, 1990, and 1994 through the use of a semi-quantitative food frequency questionnaire (F.F.Q.) developed by Willett and colleagues. Daily intakes of whole grain, bran, and germ were derived from a detailed 131-item semi-quantitative food frequency questionnaire with information on daily servings of brown rice, breakfast cereals, breads, and pasta. The whole grain percentage for each food was multiplied by the gram weight per serving to obtain the grams of whole grain content per recommended amount customarily consumed. They also calculated separate measures of intake of bran and germ added to products during processing or by participants during cooking or food preparation.

In this study, all participants tended to gain weight over the eight-year follow-up period and the mean weight gain was 1.9 kg $\pm$ 5.2 kg. After adjustments for various confounding factors, an increase in whole grain intake was inversely associated with weight gain over the eight-year period and a dose response was observed. For every 20 gram/day increment in whole grain food intakes, weight gain in eight years was reduced by 0.25 kg. Bran that was added to the diet or obtained from fortified cereals further reduced the risk of weight gain in a dose response manner and weight gain was reduced by 0.36 kg for every 20 gram/day increment in bran intake. The men in the highest tertile of changes in bran intake gained 15% less than did the men in the lowest tertile over eight years (p for trend = 0.01).

Cereal fiber was more strongly associated with weight gain reduction and, for every 20 gram/day increase in cereal fiber intake, weight gain reduction was reduced by 0.81 kg. The germ fraction did not show any association with weight gain reduction (Koh-Benerjee 2004). These epidemiology data supported the previous findings (Liukkonen 2003, Adom 2005) that bran components are concentrated sources of fiber and micronutrients in the whole grains, which provide various health benefits. In the small intestine, soluble fiber may blunt postprandial glycemic and insulinemic responses (Jenkins 2002, Nizami 2004) that are linked to reductions in the rate of return of hunger and subsequent energy intake in several previous studies (Slavin 2005). Dietary fiber consumption generally has been inversely associated with body weight and body fat (King 2005, Liu 2003).

The study also investigated the impact of using different definitions of whole grains. Whole grain intakes were more strongly associated with weight gain reduction when more than 25% bran cereals were included in the whole grain category. When whole grain intakes as defined by the FDA-authorized health claim criteria (excluding more than 25% bran cereals), the men in the lowest quintile of changes in whole grain intake gained 1.64 kg, whereas the men in the highest quintile gained 1.03 kg, resulting in 0.61 kg difference in long-term weight gain between the two groups. However, when the researchers' broader definition of whole grain (including more than 25% bran cereals) was used, whole grain intake provided a greater protection; long-term weight gain was reduced by 0.9 kg in the men in the highest quintile of changes in whole grain consumption as compared to the men in the lowest quintile of changes.

For every 100 gram/day increase in whole grain consumption, weight reduction over eight years was 1.05 kg and 1.42 kg, when the F.D.A.-accepted definition and the researchers' definition were employed, respectively. The data indicate that the current FDA whole grain criteria may not adequately capture all of the health benefits associated with whole grain foods because bran cereals are excluded from the definition.

Active Components of Whole Grain Foods in Heart Disease Risk Reduction

Jensen (2004) evaluated the association between new quantitative measures of whole grain, bran, and germ intake and risk of coronary heart disease (C.H.D.) in a prospective population study of 42,850 male health professionals free of baseline cardiovascular disease (C.V.D.), cancer, and other chronic disease. During fourteen years of follow-up, 1,818 incident cases of C.H.D. were documented. In a model including intake of whole grain, added bran, added germ, and established C.V.D. risk factors, a relative risk (R.R.) of 0.82 (95% C.I.: 0.70-0.96) between the fifth (median = 42.4 grams/day) and the first quintile (median = 3.6 grams/day) of whole grains was determined. Thus, individuals in the highest quintile of whole grain intake had an 18% lower risk of C.H.D. than those in the lowest quintile of intake. Each 20-gram increment in whole grain intake reduced the risk of C.H.D. by 0.94 (0.87 to 1) (p, trend = 0.01). In the same model, intake of added bran [R.R. = 0.70 (95% C.I.: 0.60 to 0.82) for median of 11.1 grams/day vs. no bran intake] was inversely associated with a reduced risk of C.H.D. Thus, people with the highest intake of added bran may have a 30% lower risk of C.H.D. than do people with negligible amounts of bran intake. Added germ was not associated with C.H.D. risk.

This study supports the previous findings on the beneficial association of whole grain intake and C.H.D., and suggests that the bran component could be a key factor in this relation. Bran may contain the most bioactive compounds including dietary fiber. In the C.A.R.D.I.A. study (Ludwig 1999), fiber consumption further predicted insulin levels, ten-year weight gain, and other C.V.D. risk factors including blood pressure and cholesterol levels. Fiber may regulate body weight through its intrinsic effects and hormonal responses.

Active Components of Whole Grain Foods in Risk Reduction of Diabetes and Metabolic Syndrome

In the Framingham Offspring Study, with 2,941 subjects (McKeown 2002), the inverse association between whole grain intake and fasting insulin was observed among overweight participants. The association between whole-grain intake and fasting insulin (207 pmol/L and 198 pmol/L for the highest compared with the lowest quintile category, respectively; $P = 0.002$) was attenuated after adjustment for intake of magnesium (206 pmol/L and 202 pmol/L, respectively; N.S.) or dietary fiber (205 pmol/L and 201 pmol/L, respectively; N.S.). Insoluble fiber, as opposed to soluble fiber, showed stronger attenuation effects. The study also found that people who ate more fiber from cereals were less likely to develop the metabolic syndrome. Liu (2000) also found that fiber and magnesium intakes attenuate the association between whole grain intake and the risk of type 2 diabetes. These data indicate that cereal fiber and magnesium in whole grain foods may protect against the development of type 2 diabetes by improving insulin sensitivity.

Brans and aleurone layers of whole grains are concentrated sources of dietary fiber which are associated with magnesium. Dietary fiber concentrated in bran components modulate insulin sensitivity by slowing absorption of carbohydrates and may blunt postprandial glycemic and insulinemic responses (Jenkins 2002).

Diets low in glycemic load and high in dietary fiber may increase plasma adiponectin concentrations in diabetic patients. Adiponectin may improve insulin sensitivity, reduce inflammation, and ameliorate glycemic control. Magnesium is another component in whole grains that may improve insulin sensitivity, because magnesium deficiency promotes insulin resistance in humans (McCarty 2005). Supplemental magnesium has been found to improve the insulin sensitivity of elderly or diabetic people. Magnesium-rich diets as well as above-average serum magnesium levels are associated with reduced diabetes risk and with greater insulin sensitivity (Lopez-Ridaura 2004, Salmeron 1997). Higher magnesium intake was also associated with increased plasma adiponectin (Qi 2005). There could be synergistic effects between dietary fiber and magnesium.

Conclusions

The whole grain foods criteria for the authorized FDA health claim should be expanded to include added bran as well as breakfast cereals containing at least 25% bran by weight. Whole grain products should be redefined as foods containing 51% or more whole grain(s) or 25% or more bran by weight. This conclusion is supported by the fact that there is a preponderance of original research associating whole grain consumption with health benefits (e.g., reduced risk of various chronic diseases including heart disease, diabetes, insulin sensitivity, weight gain, various types of cancers, mortality, etc.) including foods that contain 25% or more bran by weight in the whole grain category. Given the fact that the bran component is the concentrated source of active compounds in the whole grain kernel, consumer education should promote increased consumption of bran-rich foods.

References

Adom, K.K. 2005. Phytochemicals and antioxidant activity of milled fractions of different wheat varieties. *J Agric Food Chem* 23;53(6):2297–306.

American Association of Cereal Chemists (A.A.C.C.). 1999. aaccnet.org/definitions/wholegrain.asp

Awika, J.M. 2004. Properties of 3-deoxyanthocyanins from sorghum. *J Agric Food Chem* 52(14):4388–94.

Burton-Freeman, B. 2000. Dietary fiber and energy regulation. *J Nutr* 130(2Suppl):272S–275S.

Caulin-Glaser, T. 2000. Primary Prevention of Hypertension in Women. *J Clin Hypertens* (Greenwich). 2(3):204–209.

Cleveland, L.E. 2000. Dietary intake of whole grains. *J Am Coll Nutr* 19:331S–338S.

Cronin F.J. 1985. Developing the Food Guidance System for "Better Eating for Better Health," A Nutrition Course for Adults. U.S. Department of Agriculture Human Nutrition Information Service. Administrative Report no. 377.

Fung, T.T. 2002. Whole grain intake and the risk of type-2 diabetes: A prospective study in men. *Am J Clin Nutr* 76(3):535–40.

He, F.J. 2003. Potassium: more beneficial effects. *Climacteric* 6 Suppl 3:36–48.

Hu, F.B. 2000.Prospective study of major dietary patterns and risk of coronary heart disease in men. *Am J Clin Nutr* 72(4):912–21.

Huerta, M.G. 2005. Magnesium Deficiency Is Associated With Insulin Resistance in Obese Children. *Diabetes Care* 28(5):1175–1181.

Jacobs, D.R. Jr. 1998. Whole grain intake may reduce the risk of ischemic heart disease in postmenopausal women: The Iowa Women's Health Study. *Am J Clin Nutr* 68(2):248–57.

Jacobs, D.R. Jr. 1998. Whole grain intake and cancer: An expanded review and meta-analysis. *Nutr Cancer* 30(2):85–96.

Jacobs, D.R. Jr. 1999. Is whole grain intake associated with reduced total and cause-specific death rates in older women? The Iowa Women's Health Study. *Am J Pub Health* 89(3):322–9.

Jacobs, D.R. 2000. Fiber from whole grains, but not refined grains, is inversely associated with all-cause mortality in older women: The Iowa Women's Health Study. *J Am Coll Nutr* 19(3 Suppl):326S–330S.

Jenkins, D.J. 2002. Soluble fiber intake at a dose approved by the U.S. Food and Drug Administration for a claim of health benefits: serum lipid risk factors for cardiovascular disease assessed in a randomized controlled crossover trial. *Am J Clin Nutr* 75:834–9.

Jensen, M.K. 2004. Intake of whole grains, brans, and germ and the risk of coronary heart disease in men. *Am J Clin Nutr* 80:1492–9.

Kasum, C.M. 2001. Whole grain intake and incident endometrial cancer: The Iowa Women's Health Study. *Nutr Cancer* 39(2):180–6.

King, D.E. 2005. Fiber and C-reactive protein in diabetes, hypertension, and obesity. *Diabetes Care* 28(6):1487–9.

Koh-Benerjee, P. 2004. Changes in whole grain, bran, and cereal fiber consumption in relation to 8-y weight gain in men. *Am J Clin Nutr* 80:1237–45.

Lau, C. 2005. Dietary Glycemic Index, Glycemic Load, Fiber, Simple Sugars, and Insulin Resistance: The Inter99 study. *Diabetes Care* 28(6):1397–1403.

Liese, A.D. 2003. Whole grain intake and insulin sensitivity: The Insulin Resistance Atherosclerosis Study. *Am J Clin Nutr* 78(5):965–71.

Liu, S. 1999. Whole grain consumption and risk of coronary heart disease: Results from the Nurses' Health Study. *Am J Clin Nutr* 70(3):412–9.

Liu, S. 2000. A prospective study of whole-grain intake and risk of type 2 diabetes mellitus in U.S. women. *Am J Public Health* 90:1409-15.

Liu, S. 2000. Whole grain consumption and risk of ischemic stroke in women: A prospective study. *J.A.M.A.* 284(12):1534–40.

Liu S. 2002. A prospective study of dietary fiber intake and risk of cardiovascular disease among women. *J Am Coll Cardiol* 39(1):49–56.

Liu, S. 2003. Relation between changes in intakes of dietary fiber and grain products and changes in weight and development of obesity among middle-aged women. *Am J Clin Nutr* 78(5):920–7.

Liukkonen, K.H. 2003. Process-induced changes on bioactive compounds in whole grain rye. *Proc Nutr Soc.* 62(1):117–22.

Loos, R.J. 2004. Calcium intake is associated with adiposity in Black and White men and White women of the HERITAGE Family Study. *J Nutr.* 134(7):1772–8.

Lopez-Ridaura, R. 2004. Magnesium intake and risk of type 2 diabetes in men and women. *Diabetes Care* 27(1):134–40.

Ludwig, D.S. 1999. Dietary fiber, weight gain, and cardiovascular disease risk factors in young adults. *J.A.M.A.* 282(16):1539-46

Martinez-Tome, M. 2004. Evaluation of antioxidant capacity of cereal brans. *J Agric Food Chem* 52:4690–9.

McCarty, M.F. 2005. Magnesium may mediate the favorable impact of whole grains on insulin sensitivity by acting as a mild calcium antagonist. *Med Hypotheses.* 64(3):619–27.

McKeown, N.M. 2002. Whole-grain intake is favorably associated with metabolic risk factors for type 2 diabetes and cardiovascular disease in the Framingham Offspring Study. *Am J Clin Nutr* 76(2):390–8.

Montonen, J. 2003. Whole-grain and fiber intake and the incidence of type-2 diabetes. *Am J Clin Nutr* 77(3):622–9.

Mu, J.J. 2005. Reduction of blood pressure with calcium and potassium supplementation in children with salt sensitivity: a 2-year double-blinded placebo-controlled trial. *J Hum Hypertens.* 19(6):479–83.

National Center for Nutrition and Dietetics. 1994. Nutrition Fact Sheet, Whole-Grain Goodness 3 Are Key. *J Am Diet Assoc* 94 inside back page.

Nicodemus, K.K. 2001. Whole and refined grain intake and risk of incident postmenopausal breast cancer (United States). *Cancer Causes and Control* 12(10):917–25.

Nizami, F. 2004. Effect of fiber bread on the management of diabetes mellitus. *J Coll Physicians Surg Pak* 14(11):673–6.

Qi, L. 2005. Dietary glycemic index, glycemic load, cereal fiber, and plasma adiponectin concentration in diabetic men. *Diabetes Care* 28(5):1022–8.

Salmeron, J. 1997. Dietary fiber, glycemic load, and risk of N.I.D.D.M. in men. *Diabetes Care* 20(4):545–50.

Schrager S. 2005. Dietary calcium intake and obesity. *J Am Board Fam Pract* 18(3):205–10.

Slavin J. 2004. Whole grains and human health. *Nutr Res Rev* 17:99–110.

Slavin, J.L. 2005. Dietary fiber and body weight. *Nutrition* 21(3):411–8.

Soares, M.J. 2004. Higher intakes of calcium are associated with lower BMI and waist circumference in Australian adults: an examination of the 1995 National Nutrition Survey. *Asia Pac J Clin Nutr* 13(Suppl):S85.

Steffen, L.M. 2003. Associations of whole-grain, refined-grain, and fruit and vegetable consumption with risks of all-cause mortality and incident coronary artery disease and ischemic stroke: the Atherosclerosis Risk in Communities (A.R.I.C.) Study. *Am J Clin Nutr.* 78(3):383–90.

Truswell, A.S. 2002. Cereal grains and coronary heart disease. *Eur J Clin Nutr* 56:1–14.

Tuyns et al. 1998. Colorectal cancer and the consumption of foods: A case-control study in Belgium. *Nutr Cancer* 11(3):189–204.

U.S. Department of Agriculture, U.S. Department of Health and Human Services. 1992 and 2000. The Food Guide Pyramid. Home and Garden Bull. 252, U.S. Government Printing Office, Washington, D.C.

U.S. Department of Agriculture, U.S. Department of Health and Human Services. 2005. MyPyramid, U.S. Government Printing Office, Washington, D.C.

U.S. Department of Agriculture. 2004. National Nutrient Database for Standard Reference, Release 17.

U.S. Department of Agriculture. 1997. U.S.D.A. Food and Consumer Service Instruction 783–1, Revision 2 for Grains/Breads Requirement for the Food-Based Menu Planning Alternatives.

U.S. Department of Health and Human Services. 2000 and 2005. Dietary Guidelines for Americans.

U.S. Department of Health and Human Services, Office of Disease Prevention and Health Promotion. 2001. Healthy People 2010: Objectives for Improving Health. U.S. Government Printing Office, Washington, D.C.

U.S. Food and Drug Administration. A food labeling guide. 1999 Health claim notification for whole grain foods. Docket 99p–2209. www.cfsan.fda.gov/label.html.

Van Dam, R.M. 2002. Dietary patterns and risk for type-2 diabetes mellitus in U.S. men. *Ann Intern Med* 5;136(3):201–9.

Wheat Foods Council. 2005. Grains of truth about Whole-Grain Products and Enriched Products. http://www.wheatfoods.org. Parker, Colo.

Whole Grains Council. 2004. Web site:wholegrainscouncil.org. Boston, Mass.

Yao, M. and Roberts, S.B. 2001. Dietary energy density and weight regulation. *Nutr Rev* 59(8 Pt 1):247–58.

12 White Wheat: Biochemical and Sensory Characteristics of Bread

Scott R. Frazer

Introduction

While it has been well-documented that whole-grain products are a healthier option than foods made from processed flour, there has been slow acceptance of these products. The main complaints about whole wheat bread are due to its darker color, harsher texture, and "grainy" or bitter taste. There have been numerous attempts to disguise those features with various ingredients and innovative bread formulas, but few efforts have been made to simply select whole wheat flours that minimize these negative characteristics.

In an effort to make a superior-quality whole wheat flour, we have developed analytical methods to choose wheat supplies that make bread and other products that are light in color, acceptable in texture, and mild in taste. Twenty-five wheat samples of different varieties were milled and baked into bread. Analyses were run on the wheat, flour, and bread to determine what testing should be conducted to choose the best wheat for making whole wheat flour. Analytical data were correlated with sensory data to determine the method to best evaluate taste.

Wheat Samples

All wheat samples were obtained from the Cargill Bake Lab. Wheat varieties included Hard Red Spring (H.R.S.), Hard Red Winter (H.R.W.), Hard White Winter (H.W.W.), and Hard White Spring (H.W.S.). All wheat samples were run through a Whisper Mill™ wheat grinder twice. The resulting flour was then baked into bread using a standard straight-dough formula.

Instrumental Analyses

Flour analysis consisted of protein analysis (combustion), moisture (oven analysis), and ash (furnace). Average particle size was determined on a Cilas 1064 Particle Size Analyzer.

Procedure for Texture Analysis of Whole Wheat Breads

A TA-XT2i texture analyzer from Texture Technologies (Scarsdale, N.Y.) was used to conduct texture analysis of the bread. One pup loaf of whole wheat bread was used for texture analysis. The loaf was sliced with a commercial slicer. Two end pieces from each end of the loaf were discarded and each remaining slice tested. A 1-inch square piece of the bread was cut out from the very center of each slice and was tested by the texture analyzer probe. All loaves were sliced on day 1, and texture analysis was conducted on days 1, 4, and 7 after the day of the bake. The pup loaves were stored in moisture-impermeable plastic bags at room temperature. A separate sample from the middle of the pup loaf was removed such that moisture analysis could be accomplished on the same day as the texture analysis.

Procedure for Luminosity Analysis of Whole Wheat Breads

Luminosity (L) values were collected on all wheat, flour, and bread samples, using a Minolta CR-310 Chromameter. For wheat and flour analysis, the hand-held probe was pushed beneath the surface of the sample and a reading taken. To analyze bread, two separate slices were removed from the middle portion of the loaf and placed on the bench top. The probe from the chromameter was placed on the middle of each slice and pushed down such that the bread was compressed under the probe. Readings were taken on each slice and averaged to give a final "L" value for that loaf.

Procedure for Bread Volume Analysis of Whole Wheat Breads

Two pup loaves of each flour sample were run on a BVM-L500 Bread Volume Measurer from TexVol Instruments (Viken, Sweden). The results were averaged to give a final bread loaf volume.

Free Phenolics Analysis: Gas Chromatographic Method

Gas Chromatography with a Flame Ionization Detector (G.C./F.I.D.) analysis was used to determine the presence of free phenolic acids in flours and breads. One gram of vacuum-dried flour or bread crumbs was shaken with 8 mL of methanol for 1.5 hours, and 1.5 mL of the supernatant extract was evaporated to dryness in a G.C. vial. The dried extracts were silylated to form trimethyl silane (T.M.S.) ethers. The derivatization used N,O,-bis-(trimethylsilyl) trifluoroacetoamide (B.S.T.F.A.), 1% trimethylchlorosilane (1.0 mL), and pyridine (0.5 mL). After addition of these components the sealed injection vials were sonicated for ten minutes followed by twenty minutes in a 70°C oven. The TMS ethers were analyzed by cool on-column (C.O.C.) injection onto a D.B.-5 column (30 m × 0.25 mm × 0.25 μm) with hydrogen as the carrier gas. Two-point calibration curves were established using phenolic standards cinnamic acid, vanillic acid, protocatchuic acid, syringic acid, p-coumaric acid, ferulic acid, and caffeic acid at concentrations of approximately 600 ppm and 60 ppm in MeOH.

Lipid Oxidation Products Analysis

Twenty-five grams of a representative sample of bread were weighed into a 125-ml round-bottom flask with 80 ml of saturated sodium chloride solution. The bread was macerated in a polytron for approximately twenty to thirty seconds. Five μl of internal standard (50 ppm ethyl benzene-D10) was added and the flask purged with helium at 35°C for thirty minutes. The purge gas was passed through a tenax T.A. (ca. 200 mg) and two Twisters (polydimethylsiloxane phase) absorption columns. Absorbed compounds were then thermally desorbed (35°C to 220°C) onto a cryofocused inlet (−100°C) and then onto a DB-5MS capillary column for separation and into an H.P. 5973N mass spectrometer for detection. A number of lipid oxidation products were identified. However, since hexanal was one of the major, and most well-known, of these, it was chosen to correlate with taste scores.

Sensory Evaluation

An internal panel of associates within the Cargill Bake Lab (Minnetonka, Minnesota) conducted the sensory evaluation. These associates mill wheat, analyze flour, and bake and score bread on a daily basis. Five breads were scored in each sensory session. Testers were asked to score the test breads on a scale of 0 to 10 to indicate the level of whole wheat taste, bitterness, aftertaste, and mouth feel. Three "calibration" breads were provided in each session. White flour bread was provided as the "0" level of each of these taste attributes. The most bitter Hard Red Spring (H.R.S.) wheat that we could obtain was provided as the "10" level of each taste attribute. Finally, a 50/50 mixture of white flour and the HRS flour was provided to represent a "5" taste level. Based on these standards, each taster was asked to score the four taste attributes of each bread sample. These attributes were averaged to give a final taste score.

Results and Discussion

A total of twenty-five wheat samples were milled, baked into bread, and analyzed. The goal of this project was to determine if analytical measurements of wheat, flour, and Bake Lab test loaves could be used to select the best wheat lots for milling into whole wheat flour. Luminosity, texture, and taste were all measured. Results were as follows.

Crumb Color: Luminosity

Wheat, flour, and bread crumb luminosities are plotted in Figure 12.1 for comparison. There was good correlation between the three luminosities. The correlation (R^2) of flour luminosity to wheat luminosity was 0.75. The correlation (R^2) of bread luminosity to wheat

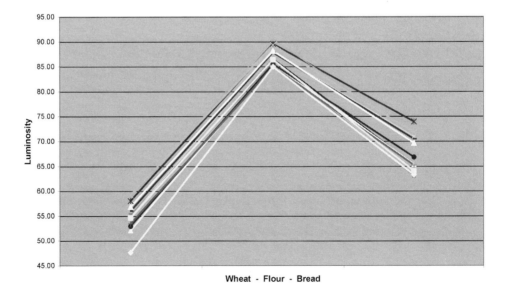

Figure 12.1. Wheat-flour-bread luminosity: 25-bread study.

luminosity was 0.50. This data was encouraging in that it indicates that bread whiteness can be predicted to some extent from wheat luminosity. Wheat luminosity could potentially be used as a screen to determine which wheat samples will be baked into test loaves for further analysis.

Crumb Texture

Crumb texture can, of course, only be measured by actually baking bread and measuring hardness (or another texture feature) on a texture analyzer. Texture however, is a characteristic of bread that is known to change drastically over time. A plot of hardness of bread at one, four, and seven days after bake is provided in Figure 12.2. Again, we see very little crossover of these plot lines. Correlation (R^2) of bread hardness at four days compared to one day was 0.92. The correlation (R^2) of bread hardness at seven days compared to one day was 0.83.

This hardening process can be attributed to starch retrogradation. To determine if moisture loss may have had a role in this staling process, moisture measurements were taken on a number of the bread samples over seven days. The average moisture loss was only about 3%, which we do not consider enough to significantly affect bread hardness.

This indicates that bread texture at seven days, or, if you wish, the point in time one expects the consumer will be eating this bread, can be predicted from the texture of the bread one day after baking. Thus, test loaves can be baked in a test lab and the wheat used to bake that bread can be accepted or rejected based on the one-day texture of the bread.

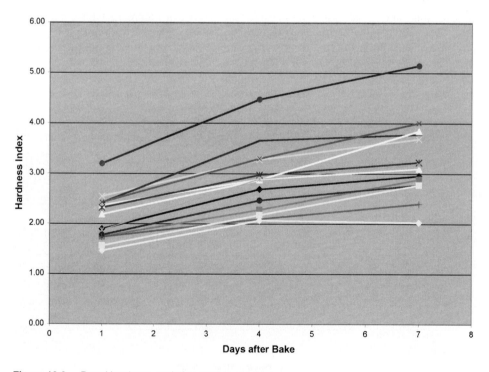

Figure 12.2. Bread hardness evolution over seven days.

We found that crumb hardness is not dependent on wheat type as much it is on loaf volume. A larger loaf volume, which depends on vital wheat gluten levels and other ingredients, provides a much softer bread texture after the bake. Figure 12.3 gives a plot of this relationship for the twenty-five bread samples. Conceivably, texture could be predicted from loaf volume, farinograph data, or even from gluten protein levels in the flour. However, the prediction would not be as accurate and the bread texture analysis is a fairly easy test to run.

Taste Assessment

All breads were tasted by a panel and given scores for the level of whole wheat taste, bitterness, aftertaste, and hardness. However, to have a sitting panel available every day to select superior breads (and thus wheat lots) is rather impractical. The bitterness and grainy taste of whole wheat bread comes from a number of components. While it is probably impractical to try to measure every one of those taste components, we attempted to measure two that are regarded as likely sources of whole wheat bitterness—lipid oxidation products and phenolics.

Hexanal is one of the main breakdown products of the oxidation of polyunsaturated fats. Figure 12.4 shows the correlation of hexanal concentration and taste scores of our bread samples. The R^2 correlation for this plot is only 0.17, so no significant correlation is noted. However, the two samples with the highest hexanal levels and high bitterness (taste) scores were from bagged storage wheat that was several years old. It may be possible that the effects of lipid oxidation products on the taste properties of bread are not significant, unless, perhaps, the wheat or flour samples are old or have been exposed to severe conditions.

A comparison plot of total bread phenolics and the average taste panel bitterness scores is given in Figure 12.5. The R^2 correlation for this relationship is 0.48. Given the

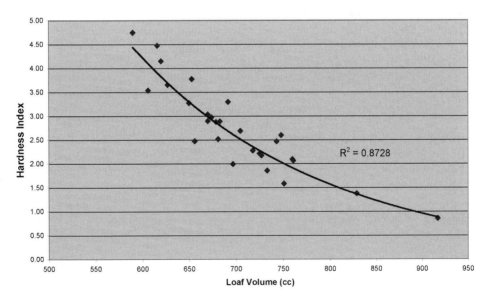

Figure 12.3. Bread hardness vs. loaf volume.

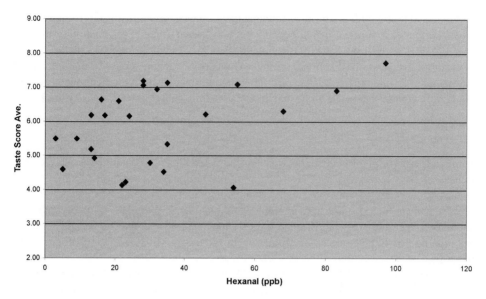

Figure 12.4. Taste score vs. hexanal (ppb).

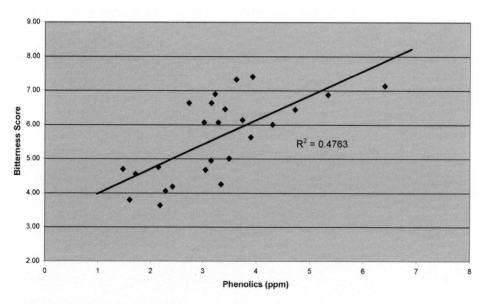

Figure 12.5. Bitterness vs. phenolics.

high standard deviations in our sensory taste results (and even in the free phenolics assay), a low correlation coefficient was not unexpected.

Comparisons also were made between total phenolics and other taste aspects, including overall taste score average. All correlations were worse than that attained for bitterness. Obviously, an R^2 correlation of 0.48 is not conclusive. Also, the levels of free phenolic acids analyzed were lower than what would be expected to affect taste (Maga 1973), though the levels we found were in line with other work (Sosulski 1982). More work to improve our supporting data needs to be done.

Conclusions

It appears that certain analyses could be run on test bakes of different wheat samples to determine which would be more desirable for making whole wheat flour. Since wheat luminosity is predictive of bread whiteness, it would be relatively easy to use wheat luminosity as a screening tool. If the wheat luminosity was not high enough to meet the desired specifications for bread luminosity, that wheat would be eliminated from consideration. Other analyses of the wheat or flour, such as protein levels, would also be part of this initial screening process.

Any wheat that makes it through the initial screen would be milled and baked into test loaves of bread. Texture analysis would be accomplished to determine if the bread is of a soft enough texture to be acceptable at the time it is eaten by the consumer. This can be assessed by correlating the bread texture one day after baking with bread texture at later dates.

If the wheat being considered passes the initial color screen and one-day texture analysis, an assessment of taste, possibly using an analysis of phenolics levels, could be run. Efforts are under way to identify the taste components of whole wheat breads to gain greater accuracy and understanding of taste assessments through analytical means.

References

Chang, C.Y. and Chambers, E. 1992. Flavor characterization of breads made from Hard Red Winter wheat and Hard White Winter wheat. *Cereal Chemistry* 69(5):556–559.

Maga, J.A. and Lorenz, K. 1973. Taste threshold values for phenolic acids which can influence flavor properties of certain flours, grains and oilseeds. *Cereal Science Today* 18(10):326–328.

Sosulski, F., Krygier, K., and Hogge, L. 1982. Free, esterified, and insoluble-bound phenolic acids. 3. Composition of phenolic acids in cereal and potato flours. *J. Agric. Food Chem* 30:337–340

13 Barley β-glucan and Wheat Arabinoxylan Soluble Fiber Technologies for Health-promoting Bread Products

Isabel Trogh, Christophe Courtin, and Jan Delcour

Introduction

The health benefits of foods with elevated dietary fiber, and especially soluble dietary fiber, have increased consumer awareness in those products. Soluble dietary fiber lowers serum cholesterol levels, a risk factor for coronary heart disease, and reduces postprandial blood glucose levels in humans, which is of potential benefit to diabetics. In general, insoluble dietary fiber has a high water-holding capacity which increases and softens fecal bulk. It also reduces transit time of fecal material through the large intestine (Manthey 1999; American Association of Cereal Chemists 2001, 2003). For individuals between 19 and 50 years of age, the recommended daily intake of total dietary fiber is 38 grams for men and 25 grams for women (American Association of Cereal Chemists 2003).

The cereal non-starch polysaccharides arabinoxylan (AX) and mixed-linkage (1-3),(1-4)-β-D-glucan, further referred to as β-glucan, are dietary fiber components and minor constituents in cereal grains. Both are present in water-extractable and water-unextractable forms. Water-unextractable AX (WU-AX) and β-glucan can be solubilized by enzymes. The total AX content varies between 4% and 10% in barley kernels (Oscarsson 1996, Andersson 1999) and between 4% and 8% in wheat (Hong 1989, Saulnier 1995). The total β-glucan content in barley grain is 3% to 11% (Bhatty 1992, Oscarsson 1996, Andersson 1999) compared to only 0.5% to 1% in wheat grain (Lineback and Rasper 1988, Wood 1991).

Nevertheless, both components are major constituents of cereal cell walls. In barley, the cell walls of the aleurone and starchy endosperm have been reported to contain 71% and 20% AX respectively (MacGregor and Fincher 1993), and 26% and 75% β-glucan respectively, while in wheat these contents have been stated to be 65% and 70% AX and 29% and 20% β-glucan, respectively (Fincher and Stone 1986). Because wheat and barley respectively contain significant levels of AX and β-glucan, they can be a valuable source of dietary fiber (American Association of Cereal Chemists 2001).

Bread is a staple food, and, therefore, in principle an ideal carrier of total and soluble dietary fiber. Considerable research into the milling and bread-making quality of wheat has been carried out because bread is most commonly produced from wheat flour (Pomeranz 1988, Hoseney 1994).

In contrast, the milling performance of barley and the characterization of barley milling streams have received relatively little research attention. This is in part due to the limited use of barley as a food ingredient, but also due to the hulled character of regular barley, which hampers the milling process (Newman and Newman 1991). However, today, hull-less barley is available. Like wheat, hull-less barley kernels lose their hull during threshing, making pearling unnecessary and resulting in benefits for food uses (easy to mill, no loss of nutrients due to pearling). In addition, hull-less barley contains higher β-glucan levels than wheat or hulled barley (Bhatty 1986, 1999; Klopfenstein 1988; Newman 1989).

Hull-less Barley Milling and Constituents

Milling Process

Andersson (2003) milled four hull-less barley (*Hordeum vulgare* L.) samples using a Bühler MLU 202 laboratory mill and characterized the resulting milling fractions with emphasis on health-promoting components such as AX, β-glucan, and antioxidants. To determine milling conditions, hull-less barley kernels of one sample were conditioned to moisture contents of 14.3%, 16.3%, and 17.8%. With increasing moisture content, bran yields increased at the expense of the flour yields, whereas the yields of the shorts remained fairly constant. The ash content of the flour fraction was similar for all three conditioning levels (0.7%) (Andersson 2003). Based on these results, all hull-less barley samples were conditioned to 14.3% moisture content before milling to obtain good yields of flour fractions with low ash contents.

The yield of the shorts fraction (47% to 56%) was highest for all hull-less barley samples, whereas that of the bran was lowest (5% to 8%). For the flour fractions, the yield varied between 37% and 48% (Table 13.1). The hull-less barley flour yields are low partly because it was impossible to adjust the sifting time of the mill, designed for wheat milling (Bhatty 1997). Although the resulting hull-less barley flours were somewhat darker and grayer than wheat flours, the former contained relatively low levels of bran particles (Andersson 2003).

The ash and protein contents (Table 13.1) were highest in the bran and lowest in the flour fractions, while the starch content was highest in the flour fractions. The highest total AX and β-glucan levels were obtained in the bran and shorts fractions respectively, which corresponds with the physical location in the kernel of both components, while the lowest levels were found in the flour fractions. Furthermore, the water-extractability of AX (at 4°C) and β-glucan (at 38°C) were highest in the flour and shorts fractions, respectively. The lower temperature used for AX extraction than that used for β-glucan extraction probably accounted at least partly for the lower AX extractability levels.

Besides being rich in AX and β-glucan, hull-less barley also is a source of antioxidants. The contents of flavanoids, tocopherols, and tocotrienols were highest in the bran fractions and lowest in the flour fractions (Table 13.1). These components are situated in the outermost layers of barley kernels (Bhatty 1993a).

In addition, α-amylase, β-glucanase, endoxylanase, and endoxylanase inhibitor activities were lower for the flour than for the shorts and bran fractions of hull-less barley. Low activities of cell-wall-degrading enzymes may benefit the production of products with high molecular weight soluble fiber components (Andersson 2003).

Because of their significance in cereal-based processes, the dietary fiber components β-glucan and AX are further discussed in detail.

β-glucan

β-glucan is a heterogeneous group of polymers with a general structure consisting of long, linear chains of β-(1-4)- and β-(1-3)-linked D-glucopyranosyl residues. On average, about 30% of the glucose residues are connected by β-(1-3)- and 70% by β-(1-4)-bonds. The

Table 13.1. Milling yields and chemical compositions of the milling fractions of hull-less barley samples[a].

Hull-less barley	Yield[b]	Ash	Protein	Starch	Arabinoxylan	β-Glucan	Flavanoid	Tocopherol	Tocotrienol
Sample 1									
Flour	48	0.8	10.3	79.3	1.5	2.1	74	5	9
Bran	5	4.5	19.7	54.8	10.6	3.6	536	17	69
Shorts	47	3.0	17.6	40.5	7.7	4.6	360	14	48
Whole meal	100	1.9	14.1	64.6	4.9	3.5	214	9	29
Sample 2									
Flour	45	0.9	11.5	75.8	1.5	1.6	112	5	8
Bran	7	4.9	18.5	48.2	12.1	3.0	605	14	44
Shorts	49	3.3	18.7	34.8	8.0	4.2	517	13	48
Whole meal	100	2.4	15.6	60.3	5.5	3.0	336	8	25
Sample 3									
Flour	37	0.9	11.4	77.0	1.2	2.0	108	7	10
Bran	7	3.3	20.2	51.8	8.3	4.7	509	14	62
Shorts	56	2.3	16.9	43.9	6.3	5.8	389	13	40
Whole meal	100	1.9	15.2	59.2	4.6	4.4	283	10	31
Sample 4									
Flour	39	1.0	9.7	76.1	1.3	2.0	94	8	10
Bran	8	4.2	16.1	51.2	10.6	4.2	433	11	48
Shorts	54	2.9	15.1	38.1	7.1	5.8	378	12	45
Whole meal	100	2.2	13.1	60.7	5.1	4.2	275	10	32

[a]Data from Andersson et al. (2003).
[b]Yield, ash, protein, starch, arabinoxylan and β-glucan contents are expressed in % dry matter (dm); flavanoid content is expressed in ppm; and tocopherol and tocotrienol contents are expressed in μg/g dm.

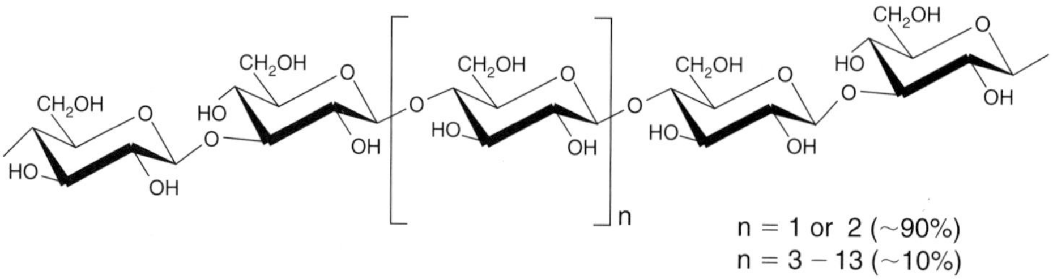

$$n = 1 \text{ or } 2 \ (\sim 90\%)$$
$$n = 3 - 13 \ (\sim 10\%)$$

Figure 13.1. Schematic representation of the structure of β-glucan. The linear β-glucan chain is mainly (about 90%) made up of blocks of cellotriosyl and cellotetraosyl units, separated by single β-(1-3)-linkages. Approximately 10% of the chain consists of blocks of four to fifteen consecutive β-(1-4)-linked D-glucopyranosyl residues.

β-glucan chain is mainly (about 90%) made up by blocks of cellotriosyl and cellotetraosyl units, separated by single β-(1-3)-linkages (Figure 13.1). Approximately 10% of the chain consists of blocks of four to fifteen consecutive β-(1-4)-linked glucose residues (Fincher and Stone 1986; Wood 1991, 1994; Saulnier 1994).

The β-(1-3)-linkages interrupt the extended, ribbon-like shape of β-(1-4)-linked glucose molecules, inducing kinks in the chain. This makes the β-glucan chains more flexible, more soluble, and less inert than cellulose, which solely has β-(1-4)-linkages and is often found in ordered (semi-)crystalline structures (Fincher and Stone 1986, MacGregor and Fincher 1993). In solution, β-glucan molecules take the shape of worm-like chains (Roubroeks 2000).

A main property of β-glucan is its high viscosity forming potential, which depends on its conformation, molecular weight, and concentration (Bengtsson 1990, Wood 1991, Böhm and Kulicke 1999, Izydorczyk 2000). Several studies showed that β-glucan can lower cholesterol and blood glucose levels, probably because of its highly viscous properties (Klopfenstein 1988, McIntosh 1993, Yokoyama 1997, Hecker 1998, Cavallero 2002). According to the U.S. Food and Drug Administration (FDA), consumption of about 3 grams/day of β-glucan soluble dietary fiber lowers blood cholesterol levels (1997).

Limited information is available in the literature on the impact of β-glucan on dough and bread making. Several researchers suggest that added β-glucan can improve dough characteristics (Bhatty 1986, Fincher and Stone 1986, Wang 1998, Izydorczyk 2001). Wang (1998) observed no effect on bread loaf volume by addition of β-glucan to the recipe, while Knuckles (1997a) and Cavallero (2002) noted a decrease in loaf volume. More research is thus needed to identify and clarify the impact of β-glucan in bread making.

In contrast to hull-less barley AX, β-glucan from hull-less barley has already been examined intensively (Bhatty 1993b, 1995; Knuckles and Chiu 1999; Izydorczyk 2000). An efficient method recently was developed to determine the molecular weight and structure of cereal β-glucan (Rimsten 2003). A calibrated high-performance size-exclusion chromatography system with Calcofluor detection was used. Because the method was based on the specific binding of Calcoflour to β-glucan, the β-glucan population of crude extracts from cereal raw materials and foods can be analyzed without any further purification steps. Andersson (2004) used this method to determine the molecular weight distribution of hull-less barley β-glucan. The distribution was mono-modal and similar for all flour, shorts, bran, and whole-meal fractions of different hull-less barley samples. For flour and bran fractions, the average molecular weight of β-glucan ranged from 155×10^4 to 164×10^4 and from

154×10^4 to 173×10^4, respectively, for the different hull-less barleys. Shorts (169×10^4 to 188×10^4) and whole-meal β-glucans (173×10^4 to 183×10^4) had somewhat higher values. The β-glucan cellotriosyl to cellotetraosyl ratio was similar among the hull-less barley samples and milling fractions. It varied from 1.53 to 1.77, with β-glucan from shorts generally having slightly lower values than bran or flour (Andersson 2004).

Arabinoxylan

In general, AX consist of a backbone of β-(1-4)-linked D-xylopyranosyl residues (xylose) to which α-L-arabinofuranosyl residues (arabinose) can be linked at the *O*-2 and/or *O*-3 positions (Perlin 1951, Viëtor 1992, Vinkx and Delcour 1996). Ferulic acid can be coupled to the *O*-5 position of arabinose through an ester linkage (Smith and Hartley 1983). Thus, unsubstituted, *O*-2 or *O*-3, and *O*-2,*O*-3 substituted xylose residues are the different structural elements of AX (Figure 13.2). Depending on the tissues in which the AX are located, they can bear additional substitutents such as uronic acids, mostly glucuronic acid or its 4-methyl ether derivative, at position *O*-2 of xylopyranosyl residues, and p-coumaric acid at some arabinofuranosyl units.

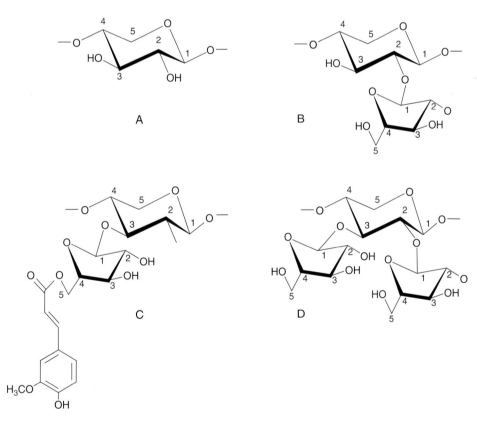

Figure 13.2. Structural elements of arabinoxylan. A: unsubstituted D-xylopyranosyl residue (xylose), B: xylose residue substituted at the *O*-2 position with L-arabinofuranose (arabinose), C: xylose residue substituted at the *O*-3 position with arabinose, and D: xylose residue substituted at the *O*-2 and *O*-3 position with arabinose. Structure C shows the link of ferulic acid to the *O*-5 position of an arabinose residue.

The structure and physico-chemical properties of AX affect their functionality in bread making. Water-extractable AX (WE-AX) form highly viscous aqueous solutions, whereas water-unextractable AX (WU-AX) have strong water-holding capacity. In bread making, WU-AX are detrimental, while WE-AX and solubilized AX have positive effects on dough and bread characteristics such as loaf volume and crumb structure (Rouau 1994; Courtin 1999, 2001).

AX also are important from a nutritional point of view. Lu (2000a,b) showed that AX reduce the postprandial blood glucose and insulin responses in humans. In addition, there are indications that AX can lower blood cholesterol levels because of their highly viscous properties (Bourdon 1999, Rieckhoff 1999), and that both AX and β-glucan have prebiotic effects (Charalampopoulos 2002, Crittenden 2002, Gråsten 2003).

To supplement the scarce data on the isolation and structural characterization of hull-less barley WE-AX and WU-AX (Dervilly-Pinel 2001, Izydorczyk 2003), Trogh (2004a, 2005a) developed procedures for the purification of WE-AX and WU-AX from hull-less barley flour. WU-AX were characterized following alkali-solubilization with saturated barium hydroxide. The isolation procedures include inactivation of endogenous enzymes by boiling the flour under reflux in 80% ethanol, removal of protein with silica gel, and removal of β-glucan, arabinogalactan-peptide, and starch fragments by enzyme or solvent precipitation.

The AX content of WE-AX samples isolated from different hull-less barley flours ranged between 84.8% and 91.8%, while the arabinose to xylose ratio, a measure for the degree of substitution of the AX backbone, varied between 0.57 and 0.63 (Table 13.2). On average, the levels of unsubstituted, O-2, O-3, and O-2,O-3 substituted xylose residues in the purified hull-less barley WE-AX samples were 62%, 8.9%, 8.2%, and 21%, respectively. The average peak molecular weight of the purified WE-AX ranged between 73×10^4 and 25×10^4 (Trogh 2004a). The small structural differences between the purified hull-less barley WE-AX samples are probably due to genetic and/or environmental factors. In addition, no distinct differences in arabinose to xylose ratio and apparent peak molecular weight were observed between hull-less and hulled barley flour WE-AX samples, while significant differences in xylose substitution levels were found. On average, the levels of unsubstituted xylose residues were higher for hulled compared to hull-less barley flour WE-AX, while those of O-2 and O-3 monosubstituted xyloses were lower (Trogh 2004b).

For the same hull-less barley flour (sample 2), the alkali-solubilized AX obtained after alkaline treatment of partially purified WU-AX (Trogh 2005a) had a higher arabinose to xylose ratio and contained higher levels of O-2 mono- and O-3 monosubstituted xyloses and lower levels of unsubstituted xylose residues than WE-AX (Table 13.2). Alkali-solubilized AX were thus generally more (mono) substituted with arabinose than WE-AX, irrespective of the hull-less or hulled character of the flour. Furthermore, proton nuclear magnetic resonance showed that both O-3 mono- and O-2,O-3 disubstituted xylose residues occurred isolated and/or next to O-2,O-3 disubstituted xylose residues in the AX chain of the different hull-less and hulled barley flour WE-AX and alkali-solubilized AX samples. Alkali-solubilized AX from hull-less and hulled barley flour had a higher apparent peak molecular weight (markedly higher than 78.8×10^4) than WE-AX from the same flour (Trogh 2004b).

Fractionation of barley flour alkali-solubilized AX by stepwise ethanol precipitation resulted in structurally different AX fractions (Viëtor 1992, Trogh 2004b). Apart from the remaining $F_{80+\%}$ fraction (23.8%), the AX content of the other hull-less barley flour alkali-solubilized AX fractions exceeded 80% (Table 13.2). The arabinose to xylose ratio of the AX fractions increased from 0.42 to 1.25 with increasing ethanol concentration (from 0 to

Table 13.2. Arabinoxylan (AX) contents (% dm), arabinose to xylose ratios (A/X), and xylose substitution levels (%) of purified water-extractable AX (WE-AX) and alkali-solubilized AX (AS-AX) isolated from hull-less barley flour samples[a].

Purified AX	AX	A/X	Un[b]	*O*-2 Mono	*O*-3 Mono	Di
WE-AX from						
Sample 1	91.8	0.63	59.1	10.0	9.0	21.9
Sample 2	90.9	0.62	61.1	8.3	7.5	23.1
Sample 3	84.8	0.57	64.7	8.2	5.7	21.4
Sample 4	86.3	0.55	62.8	9.0	10.6	17.6
AS-AX from						
Sample 2	85.8	0.71	51.5	13.4	12.2	22.9
$F_{0-20\%}$[c]	80.6	0.42	70.2	5.1	13.0	11.7
$F_{20-30\%}$	90.3	0.44	69.5	5.5	11.9	13.1
$F_{30-40\%}$	90.3	0.48	67.8	6.5	10.3	15.5
$F_{40-50\%}$	91.9	0.56	62.6	10.0	8.9	18.5
$F_{50-60\%}$	93.7	0.71	54.2	11.5	8.4	25.9
$F_{60-70\%}$	95.4	0.96	33.6	21.1	16.0	29.2
$F_{70-80\%}$	82.5	1.25	n.d.[d]	n.d.	n.d.	n.d.

[a]Data from Trogh et al. (2004a) and Trogh (2004b).
[b]Un, *O*-2 Mono, *O*-3 Mono and Di: percentages of total xylose occurring as un-, *O*-2 mono-, *O*-3 mono- and *O*-2,*O*-3 disubstituted xylose residues.
[c]$F_{0-20\%}$, $F_{20-30\%}$, $F_{30-40\%}$, $F_{40-50\%}$, $F_{50-60\%}$, $F_{60-70\%}$, and $F_{70-80\%}$: arabinoxylan fractions obtained after ethanol precipitation (0-20%, 20%-30%, 30%-40%, 40%-50%, 50%-60%, 60%-70% and 70%-80%, respectively) of alkali-solubilized arabinoxylans.
[d]n.d.: not determined.

80%). This increase in arabinose to xylose ratio was reflected in the levels of un- and *O*-3 monosubstituted xyloses, which decreased, and of *O*-2 mono- and *O*-2,*O*-3 disubstituted xyloses, which increased (Trogh 2004b).

Endoxylanase and Endoxylanase Inhibitor

Endo-(1-4)-β-D-xylanases, further referred to as endoxylanases (E.C. 3.2.1.8), are the main AX degrading enzymes. They strongly impact AX structure and functionality because they hydrolyze internal β-(1-4)-linkages between xylose residues in the AX backbone, reduce the molecular weight of AX molecules, and ultimately form (arabino) xylo-oligosaccharides. Based on amino acid sequences and structural similarities, endoxylanases are mainly classified in two glycoside hydrolase families, namely families 10 and 11 (Henrissat 1991, Coutinho and Henrissat 1999). Cereals probably produce only endoxylanases from family 10 (Simpson 2003), while fungal and bacterial endoxylanases belong to both families (Coutinho and Henrissat 1999).

In general, endoxylanases can hydrolyze WU-AX, resulting in a reduced water-holding capacity of WU-AX and the release of solubilized AX, and, consequently, in an increased viscosity of the aqueous phase. The viscosity decreases when solubilized AX and native WE-AX are degraded to AX fragments with low molecular weight (Petit-Benvegnen 1998, Courtin 2001).

Endoxylanase functionality depends *inter alia* on the biochemical properties of the enzyme (e.g. pH and temperature optima), and its substrate specificity and selectivity. Endoxylanases differ in their mode of action toward substrates. This is evident by the variety and size of hydrolysis products obtained. The literature mentions differences in pattern of hydrolysis or substrate specificity between endoxylanases from glycoside hydrolase families 10 and 11. Endoxylanases of family 10 are less specific and more catalytically versatile, and release shorter fragments than those of family 11 (Jeffries 1996, Biely 1997). Furthermore, Trogh (2005a) showed that the enzymic degradability of hull-less barley flour alkali-solubilized AX is strongly affected by the arabinose to xylose ratio of the AX substrate.

More specifically, the enzymic degradability of AX and specific endoxylanase activity decreased with increasing arabinose to xylose ratio of the hull-less barley flour AX substrates, implying that endoxylanases are sterically hindered by arabinose substituents. In addition, lower molecular weight fragments were obtained when these substrates were incubated with an endoxylanase of family 10 than with one of family 11, indicating that the former enzyme has a lower substrate specificity toward hull-less barley flour AX than the latter (Trogh 2004b, 2005a).

Endoxylanases also vary in substrate selectivity, i.e. in their relative activity toward WU-AX and WE-AX/solubilized AX. Some enzymes preferentially degrade WE-AX and solubilized AX and leave WU-AX rather unharmed (Moers 2003), while others preferentially hydrolyze WU-AX. In bread making, endoxylanases with a higher relative activity toward WU-AX than toward WE-AX and solubilized AX are beneficial (Courtin 2001, Courtin and Delcour 2002).

The functionality of endoxylanases currently used in bread making also is influenced by wheat endogenous endoxylanase inhibitors (Debyser 1999, Sibbesen and Sørensen 2001, Trogh 2004c). In wheat, two types of endoxylanase inhibitors with different structures and specificities have been identified, i.e. *Triticum aestivum* L. endoxylanase inhibitor (TAXI) (Debyser and Delcour 1998, Debyser 1999, Gebruers 2001) and endoxylanase inhibiting protein (XIP) (McLauchlan 1999, Flatman 2002). Affinity chromatography with immobilized endoxylanase allowed to purify TAXI-type and XIP-type inhibitors from different cereals (Gebruers 2002, Goesaert 2003a,b).

TAXI-type inhibitors are basic, non-glycosylated proteins with a molecular weight of approximately 40×10^3 and occur in two different molecular forms (A and B). Form A is a polypeptide chain of about 40×10^3 with intramolecular disulfide bridges. Presumably following proteolytic modification, form A is converted into form B, which consists of disulfide-linked subunits of about 30×10^3 and 10×10^3 (Figure 13.3). In general, TAXI-type proteins inhibit fungal and bacterial endoxylanases of glycoside hydrolase family 11, but not those of family 10. They form a reversible tightly binding 1:1 complex with family 11 endoxylanases. TAXI proteins show structure homology with aspartic proteases, but possess no protease activity (Debyser and Delcour 1998; Gebruers 2001, 2004; Fierens 2003; Goesaert 2003a; Sansen 2004).

TAXI can be further classified into the TAXI I and TAXI II subfamilies with similar structures and N-terminal amino acid sequences but different endoxylanase specificities (Gebruers 2001). TAXI I-type inhibitors occur in wheat, rye, durum wheat, and barley, whereas TAXI II-type inhibitors have only been found in wheat and durum wheat but not in rye or barley. While multiple TAXI-type isoforms occur in wheat and rye, a single isoform is predominantly present in barley and durum wheat (Goesaert 2003a).

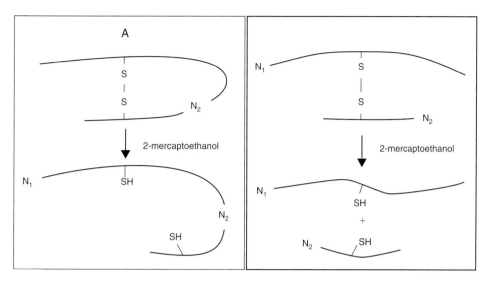

Figure 13.3. Structural model for the two molecular forms (A and B) of TAXI-type endoxylanase inhibitors. A: non-proteolytically modified form, which results after reduction (with 2-mercaptoethanol) in a polypeptide, with a molecular weight of about 40×10^3 and N-terminal amino acid sequence N_1. B: proteolytically modified form, which gives after reduction two polypeptides with molecular weight of about 30×10^3 and about 10×10^3 and N-terminal amino acid sequences N_1 and N_2, respectively (modified from Debyser 1999).

XIP-type inhibitors are basic, glycosylated proteins with a molecular weight of about 29×10^3. In contrast to TAXI-type proteins, they occur in only one molecular form. Furthermore, there is no sequence homology between the N-terminal amino acid sequences of TAXI-type and XIP-type inhibitors. In general, only fungal endoxylanases of both glycoside hydrolase families 10 and 11 are inhibited by XIP-type inhibitors, while no activity is found against bacterial endoxylanases. Based on amino acid sequence homology and X-Ray crystallographic analysis, XIP proteins have been classified into glycoside hydrolase family 18, to which chitinases also belong. However, they do not have chitinase activity. The kinetics of inhibition are competitive and reversible. XIP-type inhibitors have been purified from wheat, rye, durum wheat, barley, and maize, and multiple XIP-type isoforms occur in the different cereals (McLauchlan 1999, Elliott 2002, Flatman 2002, Goesaert 2003b, Payan 2003). Because neither TAXI-type nor XIP-type inhibitors inhibit cereal endogenous endoxylanases, they probably play a role in plant defense rather than in the regulation of the activity of plant endoxylanases (Fierens 2003, Bellincampi 2004, Juge 2004, Gebruers 2004). Igawa (2005) obtained different expression profiles for XIP-I and TAXI-I genes, suggesting that both inhibitors have distinct roles in plant defense.

To overcome the impact of endoxylanase inhibition sensitivity on endoxylanase functionality in biotechnological processes, uninhibited endoxylanases have been developed by site-directed mutagenesis of a wild type endoxylanase of *Bacillus subtilis* (from family 11), which is sensitive to inhibition by TAXI but not by XIP (Sibbesen and Sørensen 2001). Wheat flour dough and bread-making experiments with different dosages of the wild type and uninhibited endoxylanases clearly showed the impact of endoxylanase inhibition sensitivity on endoxylanase functionality, as higher bread loaf volumes were obtained with lower dosages of the uninhibited enzyme than with its inhibited wild type counterpart. This coincided with differences in AX hydrolysis. At similar endoxylanase dosages and at the same stage during dough and bread-making, solubilization of WU-AX was much higher for the uninhibited endoxylanase than for the wild type enzyme, although the former endoxylanase had a lower substrate selectivity for WU-AX than the latter. Because of inhibition, the wild type endoxylanase solubilized most of the WU-AX during mixing, whereas with the uninhibited enzyme, the rate of solubilization decreased less with increasing processing time (Trogh 2004c). According to Courtin (1999, 2001), the endoxylanase-induced increase in bread loaf volume is mainly due to transformation of WU-AX into solubilized AX. The fact that higher bread loaf volumes were obtained with the uninhibited than with the inhibited endoxylanase is probably due to the higher solubilization levels obtained with the uninhibited enzyme.

Taken together, the data clearly demonstrated that endoxylanases, which *in vitro* are inhibited by endoxylanase inhibitors and still are active in the bread-making process, as demonstrated by their functional (bread volume) enhancing effect, gradually lose their activity in the process. It follows that much lower dosages of uninhibited endoxylanases are needed. In conclusion, the functionality and performance of endoxylanases in biotechnological processes is not only affected by biochemical properties, substrate specificity, and substrate selectivity of the enzyme, but also by its inhibition sensitivity (Trogh 2004c).

Hull-Less Barley Bread Making

Because hull-less barley flour is a good source of health-promoting components (Andersson 2003) and bread is a staple food product, incorporating hull-less barley flour in bread products would be an ideal tool to produce breads with increased levels of the dietary fiber components AX and β-glucan. Therefore, Trogh (2004d) developed a technology to produce such bread products with good consumer acceptability.

Laboratory-scale Bread-making Experiments

Dough and Bread Characteristics

Doughs and breads were prepared with composite flour, consisting of 60% wheat flour and 40% hull-less barley flour and endoxylanase. The composite flour doughs in which wheat flour was replaced with hull-less barley flour were weaker than wheat flour doughs. In addition, the loaf volume of the control composite flour bread (100-gram scale; straight dough bread-making procedure) decreased to 68% of that of the control wheat flour bread (Trogh 2004d). The decrease in loaf volume when hull-less barley flour was added was already observed earlier (Bhatty 1986, Berglund 1992, Gill 2002). The negative effect on loaf volume could mainly be ascribed to dilution of gluten in the composite flour recipe, but may also have been due to the higher level of dietary fiber components and the addition of barley proteins, which disturbed the formation of a visco-elastic gluten network (Trogh 2004d).

Because previous research has already shown the power of AX and endoxylanase technologies in improving wheat flour bread-making characteristics (Rouau 1994; Courtin 1999, 2001; Courtin and Delcour 2002), endoxylanase was added to significantly increase loaf volume of wheat/hull-less barley flour breads. Thus, the negative effect on loaf volume was to a large extent overcome by use of an endoxylanase preferentially transforming detrimental WU-AX into solubilized AX and consequently resulting in an increased viscosity of aqueous dough and bread extracts. Because much lower dosages of uninhibited than inhibited endoxylanase are needed to reach similar loaf volumes (Trogh 2004c), an uninhibited endoxylanase was used in the bread-making experiments described here. For both flours, loaf volume increased with increasing endoxylanase dosages (Figure 13.4). At the highest endoxylanase dosage used, loaf volume increased with 8.8% and 20.1% for breads made with wheat and composite flour, respectively (Trogh 2004d). The better response of composite flour to endoxylanase addition is in line with the general observation that endoxylanases are more functional with weaker flour than stronger flour (McCleary 1986, Rouau 1994).

Wheat and composite flour breads both had homogeneous but different crumb structures, irrespective of the endoxylanase dosages (Figure 13.4). The crumb structure was denser, whereas the crumb color of the composite flour breads was slightly darker than that of the wheat flour breads (Trogh 2004b). The latter could be explained by the fact that hull-less barley flours were more gray than wheat flours (Andersson 2003).

Wheat flour + endoxylanase

A

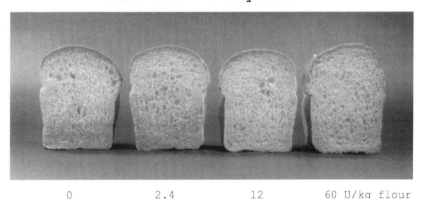

0	2.4	12	60 U/kg flour

Composite flour + endoxylanase

B

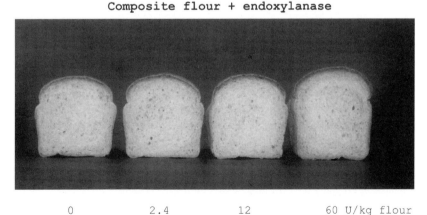

0	2.4	12	60 U/kg flour

Figure 13.4. Cross-section of bread loaves made with wheat flour (A) and composite flour consisting of 60% wheat flour and 40% hull-less barley flour (B) and different dosages of uninhibited endoxylanase (Trogh 2004b).

AX Population in Dough and Bread Samples

As expected, the endoxylanase affected the AX population of doughs and breads made with wheat and composite flour. For both flours, solubilization of WU-AX increased with increasing endoxylanase dosage and was very high during fermentation. As a result, the bread soluble dietary fiber content markedly increased. At each stage during bread making (mixing, fermentation, baking), solubilization of WU-AX led to the formation of high and intermediate molecular weight AX fragments (greater than 10×10^4) at low endoxylanase dosage, resulting in an increase in viscosity. When the highest enzyme dosage was used, WU-AX were further solubilized and WE-AX and/or solubilized AX were markedly degraded during fermentation and baking, leading to a decrease in molecular weight and viscosity (Trogh 2004d). These data indicate the importance of using an optimal endoxylanase dosage to achieve a good balance between AX solubilization and AX molecular weight, which is relevant for viscosity-related health benefits (e.g. cholesterol-lowering effect).

Furthermore, the maximum solubilization was higher for dough and bread samples made with wheat flour than for those made with composite flour (Trogh 2004d). This may partly be due to the fact that hull-less barley flour WU-AX, partially present as bran particles in composite flour, are less liable to solubilize than wheat endosperm cell wall WU-AX (Maes and Delcour 2002, Maes 2004) on the one hand, and to the limited degradability of hull-less barley flour AX by endoxylanases on the other hand (Trogh 2004b).

In addition, the lower solubilization levels obtained for bread samples made with wheat and composite flour (63% and 40%, respectively) than for dough samples after fermentation (82% and 49%, respectively) indicate that part of the solubilized AX become unextractable during baking, probably due to physical inclusion or chemical cross-linking of AX with themselves or with other bread components (Geissmann and Neukom 1973, Elofsson 2000, Oudgenoeg 2001).

β-glucan Population in Dough and Bread Samples

In contrast to Kanauchi and Bamforth (2001), who reported that some endoxylanases increase the solubility of β-glucan from cell walls of barley endosperm by hydrolysis of accompanying AX, Trogh (2004d) showed that added endoxylanase did not affect the extractability and molecular weight of β-glucan, implying that AX and β-glucan are not entangled. These researchers reported that the extractability of β-glucan increases from about 46% before mixing to 75% after mixing and then decreases during further processing. On average, the extractability of β-glucan was 48% after proofing and 43% after baking. The increase in extractability during mixing may be due to increased solubility of β-glucan because solubility generally increases with time, temperature, and pH (Åman and Graham 1987, Knuckles 1997b) and/or activation of endogenous β-glucanases. The decrease in extractability during fermentation and baking probably implies that extractable β-glucan, that was partly enzymically degraded, associated with each other or with other components to form unextractable aggregates. The β-glucan extractability was clearly affected by the bread-making process and not influenced by endoxylanase addition (Trogh 2004d).

The molecular weight distribution profiles showed that β-glucan was degraded during bread making, especially during fermentation, resulting in a strong decrease in β-glucan molecular weight, irrespective of the endoxylanase dosage used (Figure 13.5).

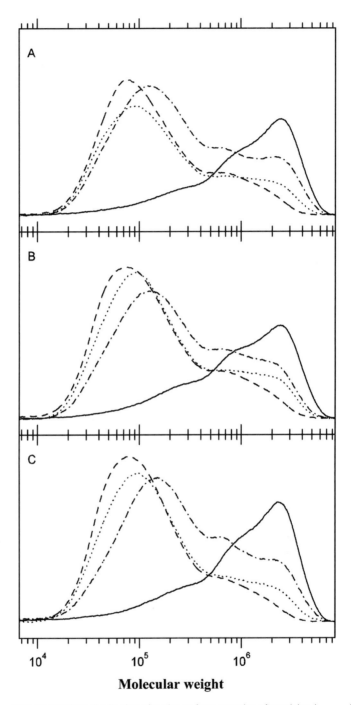

Figure 13.5. Molecular weight distribution of β-glucan from samples after mixing (————), before first punch (or 52 min. fermentation) (— · — ·), after proofing (or 126 min. fermentation) (·······), and after baking (— — —) for composite flour consisting of 60% wheat flour and 40% hull-less barley flour, without (A) and with a low (B) and high dosage (C) of uninhibited endoxylanase (Trogh et al. 2004d).

At similar stages during bread making, similar molecular weight distribution profiles were obtained for β-glucans from doughs and breads made with or without endoxylanase. In both cases, three populations of β-glucan, with a different distribution for samples taken after mixing and before the first punch, were noticed in the profiles (Figure 13.5). For the samples withdrawn before the first punch, all β-glucan populations had shifted to lower molecular weight compared to samples after mixing. After proofing and baking, there were only two significant populations of β-glucan that had shifted further to lower molecular weight. The molecular weight of β-glucan of bread was the lowest. Because the molecular weight distribution of β-glucan is mono-modal for hull-less barley flour fractions, the observed poly-modal distribution of β-glucan in composite flour dough and bread samples was probably due to the non-random action of endogenous β-glucanases, present in the hull-less barley and/or wheat flours, during processing (Andersson 2004, Trogh 2004d). The above examples show the importance of the preferential use of flours with low β-glucan hydrolyzing activities and/or of reduced processing times to obtain soluble β-glucans of high molecular weight and viscosity.

AX and β-glucan Contents of Bread Samples

Table 13.3 lists the total and soluble AX and β-glucan content of wheat and composite flour breads without or with endoxylanase (highest dosage).

The total AX content was higher for the composite flour breads (1.92%) than for the wheat flour breads (1.45%) because of the higher total AX content in composite flour (Trogh 2004d). The WE-AX contents were 0.33% and 0.37%, respectively, for control wheat and composite flour breads. The soluble AX contents increased strongly upon use of endoxylanase because of conversion of WU-AX into solubilized AX. Thus, the endoxylanase not only contributes positively to loaf volume, it also can be used to significantly increase the soluble AX levels. The total and soluble β-glucan contents and the sum of total AX and β-glucan contents were much higher for the composite flour than for the wheat flour breads because of the hull-less barley flour addition (Table 13.3).

It follows from the above examples that consumption of e.g. 100-gram composite flour bread supplemented with endoxylanase would result in an estimated intake of 3.1 grams total

Table 13.3. Total and soluble arabinoxylan (AX) and β-glucan contents (% dm) of wheat flour (WF) and composite flour (CF) (consisting of 60% wheat flour and 40% hull-less barley flour) breads (100-gram scale) without or with endoxylanase[a].

	WF bread (control)	WF bread + endoxylanase	CF bread (control)	CF bread + endoxylanase
Total AX	1.4	1.4	1.9	1.9
Soluble AX	0.3	1.0	0.4	0.9
Total β-glucan	0.3	0.3	1.2	1.2
Soluble β-glucan	0.2	0.2	0.5	0.5
Total (AX + β-glucan)	1.7	1.7	3.1	3.1
Soluble (AX + β-glucan)	0.5	1.2	0.9	1.4

[a]Data from Trogh et al. (2004d).

of AX and β-glucan and 1.4 grams of soluble AX and β-glucan compared to 1.7 grams and 0.5 gram, respectively, for 100 grams of wheat flour bread (Trogh 2004d). Hence, the combined use of hull-less barley flour and endoxylanase allows for production of bread with total AX and β-glucan levels 1.8 times those of wheat flour bread, and with soluble AX and β-glucan levels 2.8 times those of the corresponding wheat flour bread. These data imply a potential positive contribution to recommended daily total dietary fiber levels (between 25 grams/day and 38 grams/day) (American Association of Cereal Chemists 2003) and soluble dietary fiber levels (about 3 grams/day of β-glucan soluble dietary fiber) (FDA 1997).

Large-scale Bread-making Experiments

Trogh (2005b) showed that industrial-scale breads with increased levels of total and soluble dietary fiber components AX and β-glucan could be prepared. Two types of breads, i.e. Swedish tea cake (a round, flat, sweet bread) and regular bread baked in pans, were produced (straight-dough procedure) on an industrial scale with a mixture of 70% wheat flour and 30% hull-less barley flour and endoxylanase (Figure 13.6).

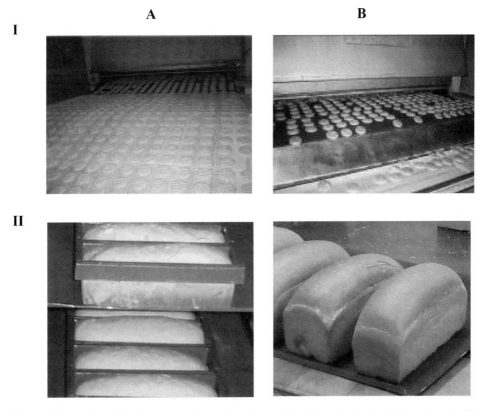

Figure 13.6.   Industrial-scale produced fermented dough (A) and bread samples (B) from tea cake (I) and regular "pan baked" bread (II), both made with a mixture of 70% wheat flour and 30% hull-less barley flour and uninhibited endoxylanase (Trogh et al. 2005b).

The recipe and process of both bread types were slightly adapted from those used on laboratory scale (e.g. 30% instead of 40% hull-less barley flour, extra baking aids, other fermentation, and baking times) to obtain doughs that were manageable during the entire industrial-scale bread-making process. The resulting composite flour breads had loaf volumes which were similar to or higher than those of the control wheat flour breads and had a fine and homogeneous crumb structure. Also, they remained softer over a longer period of time than wheat flour breads (Trogh 2005b).

In accordance with the laboratory-scale bread-making experiments, hull-less barley flour increased bread total AX and bread total and soluble β-glucan levels, but decreased bread loaf volume. However, the detrimental effect on loaf volume was largely overcome by the use of endoxylanase technology, which at the same time increased bread soluble AX level (Trogh 2004d).

Consumer acceptability studies carried out in Sweden showed that the new types of bread had a distinct but very enjoyable taste, which was typical for added hull-less barley flour. In a large group taste session, 75% of the panelists preferred the tea cake prepared with 70% wheat flour and 30% hull-less barley flour over the traditional product made with 100% wheat flour, while 81% indicated that they would buy the new tea cake if it was available on the market (Trogh 2005b). It is therefore possible to produce and introduce tasty, consumer acceptable bread products with increased levels of the health promoting dietary fiber components AX and β-glucan. This would imply a positive contribution to daily recommended dietary fiber levels on the one hand, and a likely beneficial effect on human health on the other hand.

Conclusions

Hull-less barley is a good source of health-promoting constituents such as the dietary fiber components AX and β-glucan, and especially their soluble forms.

Hull-less barley flour can be successfully incorporated in bread-making in both laboratory-scale and industrial-scale trials. Hull-less barley flour addition increased bread total and soluble β-glucan as well as bread total AX levels, but decreased bread loaf volume. However, the negative effect on loaf volume was to a large extent neutralized by applying appropriate endoxylanase technologies. The endoxylanase not only improved loaf volume of wheat flour and composite flour breads, it also had a potential nutritional impact because it increased the soluble AX content of the bread samples and, hence, the soluble dietary fiber level due to the conversion of WU-AX into solubilized AX. The combined use of hull-less barley flour and endoxylanase technologies results in consumer-acceptable breads containing increased levels of total and soluble dietary fiber. Indeed, a daily consumption of 100-gram wheat/hull-less barley flour bread produced with the developed technology would typically result in an intake of 3.1 grams of total and 1.4 grams of soluble AX and β-glucan, implying a potential positive contribution to recommended daily total and soluble dietary fiber levels.

Acknowledgements

This work was conducted with financial support from the Commission of the European Communities, specifically the RTD programme "Quality of Life and Management of Living Resources," QLK1-2000-00324, "SOLFIBREAD: Barley β-glucan and wheat arabinoxylan soluble fibre technologies for health promoting bread products." It does not necessarily reflect its views and in no way anticipates the commission's future policy in this area. This study was also carried out within the framework of research project GOA/03/10 financed by the Research Fund K.U.Leuven.

References

Åman P, Graham H. 1987. Analysis of total and insoluble mixed-linked $(1\rightarrow3),(1\rightarrow4)$- β-D-glucans in barley and oats. *Journal of Agricultural and Food Chemistry* 35:704–709.

American Association of Cereal Chemists. 2001. Report of the Dietary Fiber Definition Committee. The definition of dietary fiber. *Cereal Foods World* 46:112–126.

American Association of Cereal Chemists. 2003. Report by the AACC Dietary Fiber Technical Committee. All dietary fiber is fundamentally functional. *Cereal Foods World* 48:128–132.

Andersson AAM, Arnö E, Grangeon E, Fredriksson H, Andersson R, Åman P. 2004. Molecular weight and structure units of $(1\rightarrow3,1\rightarrow4)$-β-glucans in dough and bread made from hull-less barley milling fractions. *Journal of Cereal Science* 40:195–204.

Andersson AAM, Courtin CM, Delcour JA, Fredriksson H, Schofield JD, Trogh I, Tsiami AA, Åman P. 2003. Milling performance of North European hull-less barleys and characterization of resultant millstreams. *Cereal Chemistry* 80:667–673.

Andersson AAM, Elfverson C, Andersson R, Regnér S, Åman, P. 1999. Chemical and physical characteristics of different barley samples. *Journal of the Science of Food and Agriculture* 79:979–986.

Bellincampi D, Camardella L, Delcour JA, Desseaux V, D'Ovidio R, Durand A, Elliot G, Gebruers K, Giovane A, Juge N, Sørensen JF, Svensson B, Vairo D. 2004. Potential physiological role of plant glycoside inhibitors. *Biochimica et Biophysica Acta* 1696:213–221.

Bengtsson S, Åman P, Graham H, Newman CW, Newman RK. 1990. Chemical studies on mixed-linked β-glucans in hull-less barley cultivars giving different hypocholesterolaemic responses in chickens. *Journal of the Science of Food and Agriculture* 52:435–445.

Berglund PT, Fastnaught CE, Holm ET. 1992. Food uses of waxy hull-less barley. *Cereal Foods World* 37:707–714.

Bhatty RS. 1986. Physiochemical and functional (breadmaking) properties of hull-less barley fractions. *Cereal Chemistry* 63:31–35.

Bhatty RS. 1992. β-Glucan content and viscosities of barleys and their roller-milled flour and bran products. *Cereal Chemistry* 69:469–471.

Bhatty RS. 1993a. Nonmalting uses of barley, in: Barley: Chemistry and Technology, MacGregor AW, Bhatty RS, editors, American Association of Cereal Chemists, Inc., St. Paul, Minn. pp 355–417.

Bhatty RS. 1993b. Extraction and enrichment of $(1\rightarrow3),(1\rightarrow4)$- β-D-glucan from barley and oat brans. *Cereal Chemistry* 70:73–77.

Bhatty RS. 1995. Laboratory and pilot plant extraction and purification of β-glucans from hull-less barley and oat brans. *Journal of Cereal Science* 22:163–170.

Bhatty RS. 1997. Milling of regular and waxy starch hull-less barleys for the production of bran and flour. *Cereal Chemistry* 74:693–699.

Bhatty RS. 1999. The potential of hull-less barley: review. *Cereal Chemistry* 76:589–599.

Biely P, Vrsanska M, Tenkanen M, Kluepfel D. 1997. Endo-β-1,4-xylanase families: differences in catalytic properties. *Journal of Biotechnology* 57:151–166.

Böhm N, Kulicke W-M. 1999. Rheological studies of barley $(1\rightarrow3)(1\rightarrow4)$- β-glucan in concentrated solution: investigation of the viscoelastic flow behaviour in the sol-state. *Carbohydrate Research* 315:293–301.

Bourdon I, Yokoyama W, Davis P, Hudson C, Backus R, Richter D, Knuckles B, Schneeman BO. 1999. Postprandial lipid, glucose, insulin, and cholecystokinin responses in men fed barley pasta enriched with β-glucan. *American Journal of Clinical Nutrition* 69:55–63.

Cavallero A, Empilli S, Brighenti F, Stanca AM. 2002. High $(1\rightarrow3,1\rightarrow4)$- β-glucan barley fractions in bread making and their effects on human glycemic response. *Journal of Cereal Science* 36:59–66.

Charalampopoulos D, Wang R, Pandiella SS, Webb C. 2002. Application of cereals and cereal components in functional foods: a review. *International Journal of Food Microbiology* 79:131–141.

Courtin CM, Delcour JA. 2002. Arabinoxylans and endoxylanases in wheat flour bread-making. *Journal of Cereal Science* 35:225–243.

Courtin CM, Gelders GG, Delcour JA. 2001. Use of two endoxylanases with different substrate selectivity for understanding arabinoxylan functionality in wheat flour breadmaking. *Cereal Chemistry* 78:564–571.

Courtin CM, Roelants A, Delcour JA. 1999. Fractionation-reconstitution experiments provide insight into the role of endoxylanases in bread-making. *Journal of Agricultural and Food Chemistry* 47:1870–1877.

Coutinho PM, Henrissat B. 1999. Carbohydrate-active enzymes server at URL: http://afmb.cnrs-mrs.fr/cazy/CAZY/index.html.

Crittenden R, Karppinen S, Ojanen S, Tenkanen M, Fagerström R, Mättö J, Saarela M, Mattila-Sandholm T, Poutanen K. 2002. *In vitro* fermentation of cereal dietary fibre carbohydrates by probiotic and intestinal bacteria. *Journal of the Science of Food and Agriculture* 82:781–789.

Debyser W, Delcour JA. 1998. Inhibitors of xylanolytic and β-glucanolytic enzymes. *European Patent Application* WO 98/49278.

Debyser W, Peumans WJ, Van Damme EJM, Delcour JA. 1999. *Triticum aestivum* xylanase inhibitor (TAXI), a new class of enzyme inhibitor affecting breadmaking performance. *Journal of Cereal Science* 30:39–43.

Debyser W. 1999. Arabinoxylan solubilisation during the production of Belgian white beer and a novel class of wheat proteins that inhibit endoxylanases. *PhD dissertation*, Katholieke Universiteit Leuven, Leuven, Belgium.

Dervilly-Pinel G, Rimsten L, Saulnier L, Andersson R, Åman P. 2001. Water-extractable arabinoxylan from pearled flours of wheat, barley, rye and triticale. Evidence for the presence of ferulic acid dimers and their involvement in gel formation. *Journal of Cereal Science* 34:207–214.

Elliot GO, Hughes RK, Juge N, Kroon PA, Williamson G. 2002. Functional identification of the cDNA coding for a wheat endo-1,4- β-D-xylanase inhibitor. *FEBS Letters* 519:66–70.

Elofsson U, Eliasson A-C, Wahlgren M, Loosveld A-MA, Courtin CM, Delcour JA. 2000. Adsorption studies of interaction between water-extractable nonstarch polysaccharides and prolamins in cereals. *Cereal Chemistry* 77:679–684.

FDA (Food and Drug Administration). 1997. Food labeling: Health claims; Oats and coronary heart disease; Rules and Regulations. *Federal Register* 62:3584–3601.

Fierens K, Brijs K, Courtin CM, Gebruers K, Goesaert H, Raedschelders G, Robben J, Van Campenhout S, Volckaert G, Delcour JA. 2003. Molecular identification of wheat endoxylanase inhibitor TAXI-I, member of a new class of plant proteins. *FEBS Letters* 540:259–263.

Fincher GB, Stone BA. 1986. Cell walls and their components in cereal grain technology, in: *Advances in Cereal Science and Technology*, volume VIII, Pomeranz Y, editor, American Association of Cereal Chemists, Inc., St. Paul, Minn., pp 207–295.

Flatman R, McLauchlan WR, Juge N, Furniss C, Berrin J-G, Hughes RK, Manzanares P, Ladbury JE, O'Brien R, Williamson G. 2002. Interactions defining the specificity between fungal xylanases and the xylanase-inhibiting protein XIP-I from wheat. *Biochemical Journal* 365:773–781.

Gebruers K, Brijs K, Courtin CM, Fierens K, Goesaert H, Rabijns A, Raedschelders G, Robben J, Sansen S, Sørensen JF, Van Campenhout S, Delcour JA. 2004. Properties of TAXI-type endoxylanase inhibitors. *Biochimica et Biophysica Acta* 1696:213–221.

Gebruers K, Brijs K, Courtin CM, Goesaert H, Proost P, Van Damme J, Delcour JA. 2002. Affinity chromatography with immobilised endoxylanases separates TAXI- and XIP-type endoxylanase inhibitors from wheat (*Triticum aestivum* L.). *Journal of Cereal Science* 36:367–375.

Gebruers K, Debyser W, Goesaert H, Proost P, Van Damme J, Delcour JA. 2001. *Triticum aestivum* L. endoxylanase inhibitor (TAXI) consists of two inhibitors, TAXI I and TAXI II, with different specificities. *Biochemical Journal* 353:239–244.

Geissmann T, Neukom H. 1973. On the composition of the water soluble wheat flour pentosans and their oxidative gelation. *Lebensmittel-Wissenschaft und Technologie* 6:59–62.

Gill S, Vasanthan T, Ooraikul B, Rossnagel B. 2002. Wheat bread quality as influenced by the substitution of waxy and regular barley flours in their native and cooked forms. *Journal of Cereal Science* 36:239–251.

Goesaert H, Gebruers K, Brijs K, Courtin CM, Delcour JA. 2003a. TAXI type endoxylanase inhibitors in different cereals. *Journal of Agricultural and Food Chemistry* 51:3770–3775.

Goesaert H, Gebruers K, Brijs K, Courtin CM, Delcour JA. 2003b. XIP-type endoxylanase inhibitors in different cereals. *Journal of Cereal Science* 38:317–324.

Gråsten S, Liukkonen K-H, Chrevatidis A, El-Nezami H, Poutanen K, Mykkänen H. 2003. Effects of wheat pentosan and inulin on the metabolic activity of fecal microbiota and on bowel function in healthy humans. *Nutrition Research* 23:1503–1514.

Hecker KD, Meier ML, Newman RK, Newman CW. 1998. Barley β-glucan is effective as a hypocholesterolaemic ingredient in foods. *Journal of the Science of Food and Agriculture* 77:179–183.

Henrissat B. 1991. A classification of glycosyl hydrolases based on amino acid sequence similarities. *Biochemical Journal* 280:309–316.

Hong BH, Rubenthaler GL, Allan RE. 1989. Wheat pentosans. I. Cultivar variation and relationship to kernel hardness. *Cereal Chemistry* 66:369–373.

Hoseney RC. 1994. *Principles of Cereal Science and Technology*, second edition, Hoseney RC, editor, American Association of Cereal Chemists, Inc., St. Paul, Minn..

Igawa T, Tokai T, Kudo T, Yamaguchi I, Kimura M. 2005. A wheat xylanase inhibitor gene, Xip-I, but not Taxi-I, is significantly induced by biotic and abiotic signals that trigger plant defense. *Bioscience, Biotechnology, and Biochemistry* 69:1058–1063.

Izydorczyk MS, Hussain A, MacGregor AW. 2001. Effect of barley and barley components on rheological properties of wheat dough. *Journal of Cereal Science* 34:251–260.

Izydorczyk MS, Jacobs M, Dexter JE. 2003. Distribution and structural variation of nonstarch polysaccharides in milling fractions of hull-less barley with variable amylose content. *Cereal Chemistry* 80:645–653.

Izydorczyk MS, Storsley J, Labossiere D, MacGregor AW, Rossnagel BG. 2000. Variation in total and soluble β-glucan content in hull-less barley: effects of thermal, physical, and enzymic treatments. *Journal of Agricultural and Food Chemistry* 48:982–989.

Jeffries TW. 1996. Biochemistry and genetics of microbial xylanases. *Current Opinion in Biotechnology* 7:337–342.

Juge N, Payan F, Williamson G. 2004. XIP-I, a xylanase inhibitor protein from wheat: a novel protein function. *Biochimica et Biophysica Acta* 1696:203–211.

Kanauchi M, Bamforth CW. 2001. Release of β-glucan from cell walls of starchy endosperm of barley. *Cereal Chemistry* 78:121–124.

Klopfenstein CF. 1988. The role of cereal beta-glucans in nutrition and health. *Cereal Foods World* 33:865–869.

Knuckles BE, Chiu M-CM. 1999. β-Glucanase activity and molecular weight of β-glucans in barley after various treatments. *Cereal Chemistry* 76:92–95.

Knuckles BE, Hudson CA, Chiu MM, Sayre RN. 1997a. Effect of β-glucan barley fractions in high-fiber bread and pasta. *Cereal Foods World* 42:94–99.

Knuckles BE, Yokoyama WH, Chiu MM. 1997b. Molecular characterisation of barley β-glucans by size-exclusion chromatography with multiple-angle laser light scattering and other detectors. *Cereal Chemistry* 74:599–604.

Lineback DR, Rasper VF. 1988. Wheat carbohydrates, in: *Wheat: Chemistry and Technology*, third edition, volume 1, Pomeranz Y, editor, American Association of Cereal Chemists, Inc., St. Paul, Minn., pp 277–372.

Lu ZX, Gibson PR, Muir JG, Fielding M, O'Dea K. 2000b. Arabinoxylan fiber from a by-product of wheat flour processing behaves physiologically like a soluble, fermentable fiber in the large bowel of rats. *Journal of Nutrition* 130:1984–1990.

Lu ZX, Walker KZ, Muir JG, Mascara T, O'Dea K. 2000a. Arabinoxylan fiber, a byproduct of wheat flour processing, reduces the postprandial glucose response in normoglycemic subjects. *American Journal of Clinical Nutrition* 71:1123–1128.

MacGregor AW, Fincher GB. 1993. Carbohydrates of the barley grain, in: *Barley: Chemistry and Technology*, MacGregor AW, Bhatty RS, editors, American Association of Cereal Chemists, Inc., St. Paul, Minn., pp 73–130.

Maes C, Delcour JA. 2002. Structural characterisation of water-extractable and water-unextractable arabinoxylans in wheat bran. *Journal of Cereal Science* 35:315–326.

Maes C, Vangeneugden B, Delcour JA. 2004. Relative activity of two endoxylanases towards water-unextractable arabinoxylans in wheat bran. *Journal of Cereal Science* 39:181–186.

Manthey FA, Hareland GA, Huseby DJ. 1999. Soluble and insoluble dietary fiber content and composition in oat. *Cereal Chemistry* 76:417–420.

McCleary BV. 1986. Enzymatic modification of plant polysaccharides. *International Journal of Biological Macromolecules* 8:349–354.

McIntosh GH, Le Leu RK, Kerry A, Goldring M. 1993. Barley grain for human food use. *Food Australia* 45:392–394.

McLauchlan WR, Garcia-Conesa MT, Williamson G, Roza M, Ravestein P, Maat JA. 1999. A novel class of protein from wheat which inhibits xylanases. *Biochemical Journal* 338:441–446.

Moers K, Courtin CM, Brijs K, Delcour JA. 2003. A screening method for endo-β-1,4-xylanase substrate selectivity. *Analytical Biochemistry* 319:73–77.

Newman RK, Newman CW, Graham H. 1989. The hypocholesterolemic function of barley β-glucan. *Cereal Foods World* 34:883–886.

Newman RK, Newman CW. 1991. Barley as a food grain. *Cereal Foods World* 36:800–805.

Oscarsson M, Andersson R, Salomonsson A-C, Åman P. 1996. Chemical composition of barley samples focusing on dietary fibre components. *Journal of Cereal Science* 24:161–170.

Oudgenoeg G, Hilhorst R, Piersma SR, Boeriu CG, Gruppen H, Hessing M, Voragen AGJ, Laane C. 2001. Peroxidase-mediated cross-linking of a tyrosine-containing peptide with ferulic acid. *Journal of Agricultural and Food Chemistry* 49: 2503–2510.

Payan F, Flatman R, Porciero S, Williamson G, Juge N, Roussel A. 2003. Structural analysis of xylanase inhibitor protein I (XIP-I), a proteinaceous xylanase inhibitor from wheat (*Triticum aestivum*, var. Soisson). *Biochemical Journal* 372: 399–405.

Perlin AS. 1951. Structure of the soluble pentosans of wheat flours. *Cereal Chemistry* 28:382–393.

Petit-Benvegnen M-D, Saulnier L, Rouau X. 1998. Solubilization of arabinoxylans from isolated water-unextractable pentosans and wheat flour doughs by cell-wall-degrading enzymes. *Cereal Chemistry* 75:551–556.

Pomeranz Y. 1988. *Wheat: Chemistry and Technology*, third edition, volume I and II, Pomeranz Y, editor, American Association of Cereal Chemists, Inc., St. Paul, Minn..

Rieckhoff D, Trautwein EA, Mälkki Y, Erbersdobler HF. 1999. Effects of different cereal fibers on cholesterol and bile acid metabolism in the Syrian golden hamster. *Cereal Chemistry* 76:788–795.

Rimsten L, Stenberg T, Andersson R, Andersson A, Åman P. 2003. Determination of β-glucan molecular weight using SEC with calcofluor detection in cereal extracts. *Cereal Chemistry* 80:485–490.

Rouau X, El-Hayek M-L, Moreau D. 1994. Effect of an enzyme preparation containing pentosanases on the bread-making quality of flours in relation to changes in pentosan properties. *Journal of Cereal Science* 19:259–272.

Roubroeks JP, Mastromauro DI, Andersson R, Christensen BE, Åman P. 2000. Molecular weight, structure and shape of of oat $(1{\to}3),(1{\to}4)$-β-D-glucan fractions obtained by enzymatic degradation with lichenase. *Biomacromolecules* 1:584–591.

Sansen S, De Ranter CJ, Gebruers K, Brijs K, Courtin CM, Delcour JA, Rabijns, A. 2004. Structural basis for inhibition of Aspergillus niger xylanase by Triticum aestivum xylanase inhibitor-I. *Journal of Biological Chemistry* 279:36022–36028.

Saulnier L, Gévaudan S, Thibault J-F. 1994. Extraction and partial characterisation of β-glucan from the endosperms of two barley cultivars. *Journal of Cereal Science* 19:171–178.

Saulnier L, Peneau N, Thibault J-F. 1995. Variability in grain extract viscosity and water-soluble arabinoxylan content in wheat. *Journal of Cereal Science* 22:259–264.

Sibbesen O, Sørensen JF. 2001. Enzyme. *Patent application*, WO 01/66711 A1.

Simpson DJ, Fincher GB, Huang AHC, Cameron-Mills V. 2003. Structure and function of cereal and related higher plant $(1{\to}4)$-β-xylan endohydrolases. *Journal of Cereal Science* 37:111–127.

Smith MM, Hartley RD. 1983. Occurrence and nature of ferulic acid substitution of cell-wall polysaccharides in graminaceous plants. *Carbohydrate Research* 118:65–80.

Trogh I, Courtin CM, Andersson AAM, Åman P, Sørensen JF, Delcour JA. 2004d. The combined use of hull-less barley flour and xylanase as a strategy for wheat/hull-less barley flour breads with increased arabinoxylan and $(1{\to}3,1{\to}4)$-β-D-glucan levels. *Journal of Cereal Science* 40:257–267.

Trogh I, Courtin CM, Delcour JA. 2004a. Isolation and characterization of water-extractable arabinoxylan from hull-less barley flours. *Cereal Chemistry* 81:576–581.

Trogh I, Courtin CM, Goesaert H, Andersson AAM, Åman P, Fredriksson H, Pyle DL, Sørensen JF, Tsiami AA, Delcour JA. 2005b. From hull-less barley and wheat to soluble dietary fiber enriched bread (SOLFIBREAD). *Cereal Foods World*, submitted for publication.

Trogh I, Croes E, Courtin CM, Delcour JA. 2005a. Degradability of structurally different alkali-solubilized arabinoxylan fractions isolated from hull-less barley flour. *Journal of Agricultural and Food Chemistry*, submitted for publication.

Trogh I, Sørensen JF, Courtin CM, Delcour JA. 2004c. Impact of inhibition sensitivity on endoxylanase functionality in wheat flour breadmaking. *Journal of Agricultural and Food Chemistry* 52:4296–4302.

Trogh I. 2004b. Arabinoxylans, endoxylanases and endoxylanase inhibition sensitivity in hull-less barley flour and bread-making. *PhD dissertation*, Katholieke Universiteit Leuven, Leuven, Belgium.

Viëtor RJ, Angelino SAGF, Voragen AGJ. 1992. Structural features of arabinoxylans from barley and malt cell wall material. *Journal of Cereal Science* 15:213–222.

Vinkx CJA, Delcour JA. 1996. Rye (*Secale cereale* L.) arabinoxylans: a critical review. *Journal of Cereal Science* 24:1–14.

Wang L, Miller RA, Hoseney RC. 1998. Effects of $(1{\to}3)(1{\to}4)$-β-D-glucans of wheat flour on breadmaking. *Cereal Chemistry* 75:629–633.

Wood PJ, Weisz J, Blackwell BA. 1991. Molecular characterization of cereal β-D-glucans. Structural analysis of oat β-D-glucan and rapid structural evaluation of β-D-glucans from different sources by high-performance liquid chromatography of oligosaccharides released by lichenase. *Cereal Chemistry* 68:31–39.

Wood PJ, Weisz J, Blackwell BA. 1994. Structural studies of $(1{\to}3),(1{\to}4)$-β-D-glucans by ^{13}C-nuclear magnetic resonance spectroscopy and by rapid analysis of cellulose-like regions using high-performance anion-exchange chromatography of oligosaccharides released by lichenase. *Cereal Chemistry* 71:301–307.

Yokoyama WH, Hudson CA, Knuckles BE, Chiu M-CM, Sayre RN, Turnlund JR, Schneeman BO. 1997. Effect of barley β-glucan in durum wheat pasta on human glycemic response. *Cereal Chemistry* 74:293–296.

14 Modulating Glycemia with Cereal Products

Inger Björck, Elin Östman, and Anne Nilsson

Introduction

There is currently a global increase in the prevalence of obesity and disorders related to insulin resistance. In particular, the development of type 2 diabetes (T2D) is referred to as a pandemic (World Health Organization 2003). Recent epidemiological data suggest that a whole grain diet protects against disorders associated with the insulin resistance syndrome (I.R.S.), such as T2D (Fung et al. 2002) and cardiovascular disease (C.V.D) (Jensen et al. 2004, McKeown et al. 2002). Furthermore, there is substantial epidemiologic evidence that dietary fiber (D.F.) and whole grains are associated with a decreased risk of some cancers (Kushi et al. 1999).

The mechanisms for the benefits of a whole grain diet remain to be elucidated, and the key product feature is not known. A variety of food factors have been implicated, such as D.F. and a range of potentially bioactive components present in whole grain, e.g. magnesium (Song et al. 2004), vitamin E (Kushi et al. 1996), and betaine (Olthof et al. 2003). Parallel to the epidemiological evidence of a protective role of a whole grain diet, accumulating observational data also suggest that foods with a low glycemic index (G.I.) reduce the risk of insulin resistance, as measured by the homeostasis model assessment of insulin resistance (HOMA-IR) (McKeown et al. 2004) as well as a reduced risk of C.V.D (Liu et al. 2000) and T2D (Salmeron et al. 1997a,b). Furthermore, data are available from interventions (Slabber et al. 1994) and mechanistic studies (Frost et al. 1996) supporting metabolic benefits of a low G.I. diet as manifested by reducing C.V.D risk factors in subjects with hyperlipidemia (Jenkins et al. 1987), T2D (Järvi et al. 1999), or obesity (Ebbeling et al. 2003).

According to Wolever (1990), there is a significant inverse relation between total D.F. and G.I. ($r = 0.461$, $p < 0.05$) if a wide range of carbohydrates is included. It should be noted that certain whole grain products on the market have a low G.I., e.g. bulgur, pumpernickel, barley, and certain rice varieties. However, the importance of the lente features, *per se*, for the long term benefits of a low G.I. diet, was specifically studied in T2D subjects in work by Järvi et al. (1999) using a cross-over design. The test diets were identical with respect to macronutrient composition and type and amount of D.F., and the differences in G.I. were achieved by altering the structure of the starchy foods. The decrease in fructosamine and L.D.L.-cholesterol was significantly more pronounced after the low-G.I. diet and plasminogen activator inhibitor-1 (P.A.I.-1) activity was normalized (-54%, $P < 0.001$), whereas it remained unchanged on the high-G.I. diet (Järvi et al. 1999). This study indicates that the low-G.I. features improved glycemic control and importantly reduced established risk factors for cardiovascular complications in T2D. A mechanism could not simply be assigned to the presence of D.F. or associated components.

Although there is a lack of agreement regarding the impact of the G.I. concept in relation to satiety and weight regulation (Pawlak et al. 2002, Raben 2002), recent studies have indicated that a low-G.I. diet facilitates weight loss in overweight children (Warren et al. 2003) and adolescents (Ball et al. 2003). Recent case-control studies also suggest a protective role against certain cancers, e.g. ovarian (Augustin et al. 2003), breast (Augustin et al. 2001), and colorectal (Franceschi et al. 2001, Higginbotham et al. 2004). It is probably mediated by the lower insulinemia associated with low-G.I. foods. Possibly, some components of the insulin-like growth factor (IgF) axis may be the link between G.I. and cancer (Biddinger and Ludwig 2005, Brand-Miller et al. 2005). It has been suggested that the hormone-related cancers also could be included in the I.R.S. (Barnard et al. 2002).

Taken together, there is strong evidence supporting a preventive potential of the two food concepts, low-G.I. and whole grain, respectively, to diseases related to insulin resistance and certain cancers. However, despite this growing body of knowledge there is shortage of low-G.I. alternatives, particularly among cereal foods. An extended list of low-G.I. whole grain cereal foods is necessary to exploit the synergistic potential of such products.

Tailoring Acute Glycemia and Insulinemia

Most common breads and, in particular, flour-based breads, are characterized by a high G.I. There is, however, substantial evidence that the G.I. of bread products can be modulated by use of certain food factors. Parallel to increasing the knowledge base concerning food factors affecting glycemia and hormonal responses, it is also important to develop analytical tools for assessing the key product features to be used for quality assurance during industrial production. There follows a discussion of some food factors and analytical tools that might be used to tailor low-G.I. whole grain products. It should be noted that the glycemic response needs to be measured in human subjects according to recommended procedures, and that the analytical tools suggested for prediction of glycemia are relevant only in the context of the specific cereal food system used.

Organic Acids

Baking bread in the presence of lactic acid reduces G.I. and the insulinemic index (I.I.) (Liljeberg et al. 1995). During baking, the presence of lactic acid seems to create macromolecular interactions between starch and cereal protein, which serves as a barrier to amylolysis (Östman et al. 2002). In addition, lactic acid has been shown to promote retrogradation of starch. The G.I. of sourdough bread processed using a homofermentative lactic acid starter culture, or bread with added lactic acid, can thus be predicted from measurement of the rate of in vitro starch hydrolysis (Liljeberg et al. 1995).

Acetic acid is the major acid formed upon spontaneous sourdough fermentation. The addition of acetic acid in the form of vinegar to a high-G.I. bread meal reduces the glycemic response in a linear dose-dependent manner (Östman et al. 2005b). Higher levels of acetic acid also are associated with lower insulinemic excursions and increased post-meal ratings of satiety. The mechanism is a reduced rate of gastric emptying (Liljeberg and Björck 1998). In a given food system, analysis of acetic acid may be one tool for quality assurance of the glycemic response to fermented cereal products or test meals containing this acid. However, methods that predict the rate of digestion fail to detect the possible glycemic effect of acetic acid.

Degree of Gelatinization

The enzyme availability of native starch is low, and the maintenance of starch crystallinity in the finished product provides another food factor for design of low-G.I. products. Flaking of cereals under commercial conditions results in a comparatively low degree of gelatinization, ranging from about 24% to 40%. Despite these low figures, the G.I. of commercial barley, oat, and wheat flakes typically falls above 90 (Granfeldt et al. 2000). The degree of gelatinization must be kept very low, or below 12%, to achieve a significant reduction in G.I.s (Granfeldt and Björck, unpublished observation). Extremely mild conditions for pre-heating and flaking could thus be used to obtain low G.I. muesli products, and measurement of the degree of starch gelatinization provides a tool for quality assurance of the glycemic effect.

Retrogradation

A high crystallinity of starch also can be induced during processing. In one study, whole grain barley flours with different amylose contents were subjected to different baking conditions, i.e. conventional baking or pumpernickel baking conditions (Liljeberg et al. 1996). The pumpernickel baking includes an extended holding temperature at 100°C, which is the wet temperature in the bread that specifically promotes amylose retrogradation. This favors a slower enzymatic digestion, and hence a lower G.I. Consequently, the use of high amylose genotypes and specific baking conditions can be used to design low-G.I. bread, and the G.I. can be predicted by measuring the rate of in vitro starch hydrolysis (Liljeberg et al. 1996).

Soluble Fiber

An established method to lower glycemia involves enrichment with soluble D.F. (Würsch and Pi-Sunyer 1997). In this context it is important to emphasize the need for quality assurance of relevant viscous properties. In a recent study with flat bread (Östman et al. 2005c), Prowashonupana (PW) flour was included in mixtures with white wheat at the levels 0, 35%, 50% and 75% PW. At the 50% level two commercial batches of PW were used, both containing elevated levels of β-glucans (14%). A bread product with 50% common barley flour, with less than 3% β-glucans, was also included.

In addition to measuring G.I. and I.I. in healthy subjects, a simple consistometer was used to measure fluidity of the corresponding in vitro enzymatic digestas. The digestas were prepared by incubating the products with enzymes at simulated in vivo conditions. Enclosure of PW lowered fluidity of the digesta, and lowered G.I. and I.I. in a dose-dependent manner ($r = 0.9782$, $P = 0.0007$). Enclosure of common barley was much less effective due to the lower β-glucan content. However, the β-glucan content per se is a very poor predictor of G.I., and enclosure of 50% PW from another batch failed to lower glycemic properties despite an almost identical content of β-glucans. The high fluidity indicates that the β-glucans in that particular batch of PW had depolymerized.

This study shows that the G.I. of bread containing different levels of β-glucans can be predicted with good accuracy by measuring fluidity in this in vitro system and a physiological product characteristic such as fluidity, rather than the analyzed content of β-glucans, should be used for quality assurance of the glycemic effect.

The "Rye Factor"

The food factors described above consistently lower glycemia and insulinemia in the cereal products. Consequently, in the absence of food factors reducing the rate of glucose delivery to the blood, cereal products produce high G.I.s and high I.I.s.

There are exceptions though, and whole grain rye products (bread and flaked rye kernels) display low I.I.s (below 70), even at high glycemic responses (Figure 14.1). That is, the rate

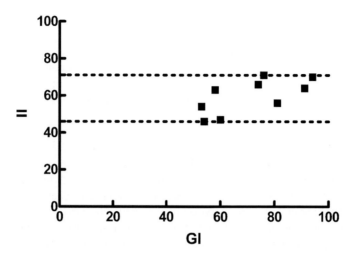

Figure 14.1. Relation between G.I. and I.I. for nine whole grain rye products (bread and flakes). Correlation equation: I.I. = 35.3 +0,340 G.I. Pearsons correlation test: r = 0.6251, p = 0.072.

of glucose delivery to the blood does not appear to be the major determinant of insulinemia to rye products. Possibly some component in whole grain rye improves insulin economy. The metabolic effects of these comparatively modest insulinemic responses to whole grain rye products remain to be elucidated.

Modulating Glycemia at a Second Meal

Breakfast to Lunch Perspective

The glucose and insulin responses were measured in healthy subjects at a standardized lunch meal served four hours after a test breakfast with white wheat bread or pasta (Liljeberg and Björck 2000). Glucose and insulin excursions to the standardized lunch were significantly reduced with the pasta breakfast. Because these two test breakfasts had similar nutrient composition, the improved glucose tolerance seen with pasta from breakfast to lunch appears to be related to the low-G.I. features, per se. The suggested cause of such a second meal effect is that a prolonged absorptive phase following breakfast favors a more efficient suppression of free fatty acids, thus improving insulin sensitivity at the time of the next meal (Wolever et al. 1995).

In fact, the pasta breakfast was able to postpone the "in-between-meal" fasting state (Liljeberg and Björck, 2000), which adds further evidence to the suggested mechanism. In addition, the pasta breakfast lowered triglyceride levels at the subsequent standardized lunch meal (Liljeberg and Björck 2000), also indicating the importance of lente features for reducing risk factors for C.V.D.

Overnight Perspective

In a recent study (Nilsson, Granfeldt, Östman, and Björck unpublished observation), test meals based on wheat and barley were served at two levels of G.I. (53 to 54 and 100) and differing in content of resistant starch (R.S.) and D.F. (3.6 to 20.5 grams R.S. + D.F./portion).

Despite similar and low G.I., the incremental area under the curve (I.A.U.C., 0 to 120 min) for blood glucose in response to the standardised breakfast was significantly lower only after consuming barley kernels in the evening compared with evening meals with white wheat bread (P = 0.019) or spaghetti with wheat bran (P = 0.046). There were no significant differences in insulin concentrations at breakfast. Breath hydrogen excretion at breakfast was significantly higher after the evening meal with barley kernels compared with white wheat bread, wheat kernels, and spaghetti (P = 0.026, 0.026, and 0.015, respectively), suggesting the involvement of colonic fermentation of R.S. and D.F. The plasma concentration of propionate at breakfast was significantly higher following the evening meal with barley kernels compared with white wheat bread (P = 0.041), and increased levels of propionate in the blood has been shown to affect hepatic carbohydrate metabolism (Venter et al. 1990). In addition, free fatty acid concentrations were significantly lower after barley kernels compared with white wheat bread (P = 0.042) or spaghetti (P = 0.019).

Day-long Glycemia

In fact, the properties of the breakfast meal may affect day-long glycemic excursions in healthy subjects. In a recent study (Nilsson et al. unpublished observation), glycemic excursion after different whole grain cereal test breakfasts were measured with respect to breakfast to subsequent standardized lunch and dinner meals. In addition to boiled kernels from wheat, rye, oats, and barley, flour-based barley porridge also was included. After breakfast the barley and rye kernels produced a 50% to 55% lower glucose I.A.U.C. than the white wheat bread (P < 0.05). The wheat and oat kernels, as well as the flour-based barley porridge, however, did not differ significantly from the white wheat bread.

At the standardized lunch meal the glycemic areas were significantly smaller (30% to 44%) following test breakfasts with cereal kernels. The glycemic area at lunch after the barley kernel breakfast was lowered substantially (44%). In contrast, the barley-flour porridge breakfast with a G.I. similar to white wheat bread did not improve glucose tolerance at lunch. Therefore, it seems as if low-G.I. cereal foods in general improve four-hour, second meal glucose tolerance, irrespective of D.F. content or other food features. Consequently, all kernel-based products induced significantly lower (30% to 50%) cumulative glucose I.A.U.C.s after breakfast plus lunch.

In addition, the barley kernel breakfasts tended to maintain a lower glycemia at the third standardized meal ingested 9.5 hours after the test breakfasts. In ten out of twelve test subjects, glycemic excursions were lower at the standardized dinner after the barley-kernel breakfast compared with white wheat bread. Consequently, the barley kernel breakfast induced a significantly lower incremental blood glucose area over the course of the entire day.

This indicates that certain low-G.I. foods are more effective in modulating glycemia at subsequent meals, and it could be speculated that low-G.I. barley products of this type could be particularly efficient in reducing metabolic risk factors in a longer-term perspective. The mechanism for the lowering of glycemia over the course of the day in the case of the barley kernels may be related to colonic fermentation, and breath hydrogen excretion was significantly higher when beginning the dinner after the barley kernel test breakfast compared with white wheat bread.

Interestingly, a flour-based barley porridge breakfast from the same raw material was much less effective in generating H_2, suggesting that the RS fraction in the barley kernel may contribute to the increased fermentative activity at the time of the late dinner.

The studies above indicate that it may be possible to tailor not only the acute glycemia with whole grain products, but also to lower the glycemic excursions at subsequent meals. Whereas the four-hour second meal benefits appear to be related to the lente features per se, the semi-acute benefits seen overnight or over the course of the entire day possibly also involve a mechanism related to colonic fermentation of indigestible carbohydrates present, e.g. D.F. and R.S. Information of this type may be significant when designing low-G.I. whole grain foods with the potential for reducing glycemia and insulin demand in a time frame extending beyond the acute meal. It also provides an indication of a synergistic interface between the whole grain and the low-G.I. concepts with respect to metabolic benefits in a longer-term perspective.

Metabolic Potential of Whole Grain Bread with Low G.I. in a Mixed Diet

Is it possible to affect metabolic variables in a longer-term perspective by including tailored low-G.I. cereal foods? To answer this question, common high-G.I. bread was exchanged for tailored low-G.I./high fiber bread (14% D.F., dry weight basis) in the diets of seven women with a history of gestational diabetes (Östman et al. 2005a). The G.I.s of the light and dark bread were 46 and 54, respectively, and they were both based on rye and baked using sourdough fermentation. The light bread also was enriched with oat β-glucans.

Insulin responses to an intravenous glucose challenge were measured before and after each intervention period. No significant difference was noted over the intervention period with common high-G.I. bread in the diet. In contrast, all women displayed a decrease in insulin response to the intravenous glucose challenge over the low-G.I. bread period. The mean decrease was substantial, or close to 40%. The results indicate that the mere exchange of common high-G.I. bread for modified low G.I./high-fiber bread improved insulin economy in women at risk of type 2 diabetes. These data encourage the introduction of newly designed low-G.I. whole grain cereal products.

Conclusions

Evidence is accumulating for a protective role of the whole grain and the low-G.I. concepts in relation to diseases linked to insulin resistance. There are several food factors that can be exploited for development of low-G.I. whole grain cereal products. Tools for quality assurance of the glycemic effect are available, and can be used to predict the physiological effect during product optimization and/or quality assurance during production.

References

Augustin, LS, Polesel, J, Bosetti, C, Kendall, CW, La Vecchia, C, Parpinel, M, Conti, E, Montella, M, Franceschi, S, Jenkins, DJ and Dal Maso, L. 2003. Dietary glycemic index, glycemic load and ovarian cancer risk: a case-control study in Italy. *Annals of Oncology* 14, 78–84.

Augustin, LSA, Dal Maso, L, La Vecchia, C, Parpinel, M, Negri, E, Vaccarella, S, Kendall, CWC, Jenkins, DJA and Franceschi, S. 2001. Dietary glycemic index and glycemic load, and breast cancer risk: A case-control study. *Annals of Oncology.* 12, 1533–1538.

Ball, SD, Keller, KR, Moyer-Mileur, LJ, Ding, YW, Donaldson, D & Jackson, WD. 2003. Prolongation of satiety after low versus moderately high glycemic index meals in obese adolescents. *Pediatrics.* 111, 488–494.

Barnard, RJ, Aronson, WJ, Tymchuk, CN and Ngo, TH. 2002. Prostate cancer: another aspect of the insulin-resistance syndrome? *Obesity Reviews.* 3, 303–308.

Biddinger, SB and Ludwig, DS. 2005. The insulin-like growth factor axis: a potential link between glycemic index and cancer. *American Journal of Clinical Nutrition*. 82, 277–278.

Brand-Miller, JC, Liu, V, Petocz, P and Baxter, RC. 2005. The glycemic index of foods influences postprandial insulin-like growth factor-binding protein responses in lean young subjects. *American Journal of Clinical Nutrition*. 82, 350–354.

Ebbeling, CB, Leidig, MM, Sinclair, KB, Hangen, JP and Ludwig, DS. 2003. A reduced-glycemic load diet in the treatment of adolescent obesity. *Archives of Pediatrics and Adolescent Medicine*. 157, 773–779.

Franceschi, S, Dal Maso, L, Augustin, L, Negri, E, Parpinel, M, Boyle, P, Jenkins, DJA and Vecchia, CL. 2001. Dietary glycemic load and colorectal cancer risk. *Annals of Oncology*. 12, 173–178.

Frost, G, Keogh, B, Smith, D, Akinsanya, K and Leeds, A. 1996. The effect of low-glycemic carbohydrate on insulin and glucose response in vivo and in vitro in patients with coronary heart disease. *Metabolism*. 45, 669–672.

Fung, TT, Hu, FB, Pereira, MA, Liu, S, Stampfer, MJ, Colditz, GA and Willett, WC. 2002. Whole-grain intake and the risk of type 2 diabetes: a prospective study in men. *American Journal of Clinical Nutrition*. 76, 535–540.

Granfeldt, Y, Eliasson, A-C and Björck, I. 2000. An examination of the possibility of lowering the glycemic index of oat and barley flakes by minimal processing. *Journal of Nutrition*. 130, 2207–2214.

Higginbotham, S, Zhang, ZF, Lee, IM, Cook, NR, Giovannucci, E, Buring, JE and Liu, S. 2004. Dietary glycemic load and risk of colorectal cancer in the Women's Health Study. *J Natl Cancer Inst*. 96, 229–233.

Jenkins, DJA, Wolever, TMS, Kalmusky, J, Guidici, S, Giordano, C, Patten, R, Wong, GS, Bird, JN, Hall, M, Buckley, G, Csima, A and Little, JA. 1987. Low-glycemic index diet in hyperlipidemia: use of traditional starchy foods. *American Journal of Clinical Nutrition*. 46, 66–71.

Jensen, MK, Koh-Banerjee, P, Hu, FB, Franz, M, Sampson, L, Gronbaek, M and Rimm, EB. 2004. Intakes of whole grains, bran, and germ and the risk of coronary heart disease in men. *American Journal of Clinical Nutrition*. 80, 1492–1499.

Järvi, AE, Karlström, BE, Granfeldt, YE, Björck, IE, Asp, NG and Vessby, BO. 1999. Improved glycemic control and lipid profile and normalized fibrinolytic activity on a low-glycemic index diet in type 2 diabetic patients. *Diabetes Care*. 22, 10–18.

Kushi, LH, Folsom, AR, Prineas, RJ, Mink, PJ, Wu, Y and Bostick, RM. 1996. Dietary Antioxidant Vitamins and Death from Coronary Heart Disease in Postmenopausal Women. *New England Journal of Medicine*. 334, 1156–1162.

Kushi, LH, Meyer, KA and Jacobs, DR, Jr. 1999. Cereals, legumes, and chronic disease risk reduction: evidence from epidemiologic studies. *American Journal of Clinical Nutrition*. 70, 451S–458.

Liljeberg, HGM and Björck, IME. 1998. Delayed gastric emptying rate may explain improved glycaemia in healthy subjects to a starchy meal with added vinegar. *European Journal of Clinical Nutrition*. 52, 368–371.

Liljeberg, HGM and Björck, IME. 2000. Effects of a low-glycaemic index spaghetti meal on glucose tolerance and lipaemia at a subsequent meal in healthy subjects. *European Journal of Clinical Nutrition*. 54, 24–28.

Liljeberg, HGM, Lönner, CH and Björck, IME. 1995. Sourdough fermentation or addition of organic acids or corresponding salts to bread improves nutritional properties of starch in healthy humans. *Journal of Nutrition*. 125, 1503–1511.

Liljeberg, HGM, Åkerberg, AKE and Björck, IME. 1996. Resistant starch formation in bread as influenced by choice of ingredients or baking conditions. *Food Chemistry*. 56, 389–394.

Liu, S, Willett, WC, Stampfer, MJ, Hu, FB, Franz, M, Sampson, L, Hennekens, CH and Manson, JE. 2000. A prospective study of dietary glycemic load, carbohydrate intake, and risk of coronary heart disease in U.S. women. *American Journal of Clinical Nutrition*. 71, 1455–1461.

McKeown, NM, Meigs, JB, Liu, S, Saltzman, E, Wilson, PWF & Jaques, PF. 2004. Carbohydrate nutrition, insulin resistance, and the prevalence of the metabolic syndrome in the Framingham offspring cohort. Diabetes Care. 27, 538–546.

McKeown, NM, Meigs, JB, Liu, S, Wilson, PW and Jacques, PF. 2002. Whole-grain intake is favorably associated with metabolic risk factors for type 2 diabetes and cardiovascular disease in the Framingham Offspring Study. *American Journal of Clinical Nutrition*. 76, 390–398.

Olthof, MR, van Vliet, T, Boelsma, E and Verhoef, P. 2003. Low dose betaine supplementation leads to immediate and long term lowering of plasma homocysteine in healthy men and women. *Journal of Nutrition*. 133, 4135–4138.

Östman, E, Frid, A, Groop, L and Björck, IME. 2005a. A dietary exchange of common bread for tailored bread of low glycaemic index and rich in dietary fiber improved insulin economy in young women with impaired glucose tolerance. *European Journal of Clinical Nutrition*. (in press)

Östman, E, Granfeldt, Y, Persson, L and Björck, I. 2005b. Vinegar supplementation lowers glucose and insulin responses and increases satiety after a bread meal in healthy subjects. *European Journal of Clinical Nutrition*. 59, 983–988.

Östman, E, Rossi, E, Larsson, H, Brighenti, F and Björck, I. 2005c. Glucose and insulin responses in healthy men to barley bread with different levels of beta-glucans; predictions using fluidity measurement of in vitro enzymatic digestas. *Journal of Cereal Science*. (in press)

Östman, EM, Nilsson, M, Liljeberg Elmståhl, HGM, Molin, G and Björck, IME. 2002. On the effect of lactic acid on blood glucose and insulin responses to cereal products: mechanistic studies in healthy subjects and in vitro. *Journal of Cereal Science*. 36, 339–346.

Pawlak, DB, Ebbeling, CB and Ludwig, DS. 2002. Should obese patients be counselled to follow a low-glycaemic index diet? Yes. *Obesity Reviews*. 3, 235–243.

Raben, A. 2002. Should obese patients be counselled to follow a low-glycaemic index diet? No. *Obesity Reviews*. 3, 245–256.

Salmeron, J, Ascherio, A, Rimm, EB, Colditz, GA, Spiegelman, D, Jenkins, DJ, Stampfer, MJ, Wing, AL and Willett, WC. 1997a. Dietary fiber, glycemic load, and risk of NIDDM in men. *Diabetes Care*. 20, 545–550.

Salmeron, J, Manson, JE, Stampfer, MJ, Colditz, GA, Wing, AL and Willett, WC. 1997b. Dietary fiber, glycemic load, and risk of non-insulin-dependent diabetes mellitus in women. *Journal of the American Medical Association*. 277, 472–477.

Slabber, M, Barnard, HC, Kuyl, JM, Dannhauser, A and Schall, R. 1994. Effects of a low-insulin-response, energy-restricted diet on weight loss and plasma insulin concentrations in hyperinsulinemic obese females. *American Journal of Clinical Nutrition*. 60, 48–53.

Song, Y, Manson, JE, Buring, JE and Liu, S. 2004. Dietary magnesium intake in relation to plasma insulin levels and risk of type 2 diabetes in women. *Diabetes Care*. 27, 59–65.

Warren, JM, Henry, CJ and Simonite, V. 2003. Low glycemic index breakfasts and reduced food intake in preadolescent children. *Pediatrics*. 112, e414.

Venter, CS, Vorster, HH and Cummings, JH. 1990. Effects of dietary propionate on carbohydrate and lipid metabolism in healthy volunteers. *American Journal of Gastroenterology*. 85, 549–553.

World Health Organization. 2003. Diet, nutrition and the prevention of chronic diseases. Report of a Joint WHO/FAO Expert Consultation. World Health Organization, Geneva, p 149.

Wolever, TM. 1990. Relationship between dietary fiber content and composition in foods and the glycemic index. *American Journal of Clinical Nutrition*. 51, 72–75.

Wolever, TMS, Bentum-Williams, A and Jenkins, DJA. 1995. Physiological modulation of plasma free fatty acid concentrations by diet. Metabolic implications in nondiabetic subjects. *Diabetes Care*. 18, 962–970.

Würsch, P and Pi-Sunyer, FX. 1997. The role of viscous soluble fiber in the metabolic control of diabetes. A review with special emphasis on cereals rich in beta-glucan. *Diabetes Care*. 20, 1774–1780.

15 Whole Grain Phytochemicals and Antioxidant Activity

Rui Hai Liu and Kafui Kwami Adom

Introduction

Significant scientific evidence indicates that consumption of whole grains and whole grain products reduces the risk for various types of chronic diseases including cardiovascular disease (Thompson 1994, Morris et al. 1977, Jacobs et al. 1998b, Liu et al. 1999, Anderson et al. 2000), some cancers (Jacobs et al. 1995, Kasum et al. 2002, Nicodemus et al. 2001, Smigel 1992, Thompson 1994, Chatenoud et al. 1998, Jacobs et al. 1998), type 2 diabetes (Meyer et al. 2000, Liu et al. 2000), and all-cause mortality (Jacobs et al. 1999, Jacobs et al. 2001). The 2005 Dietary Guidelines for Americans and Healthy People 2010 recommends the consumption of at least three servings of whole grain (equivalent to three ounces) per day (U.S. Department of Agriculture 2005, U.S. Department of Health and Human Services 2000).

Whole grains are rich sources of fiber, vitamins, minerals, and phytochemicals, including phenolics, carotenoids, lignans, β-glucan, inulin, sterols, phytins, and sphingolipids. Plant-based foods, such as fruit, vegetables, and whole grains, which contain significant amounts of bioactive phytochemicals, may provide desirable health benefits beyond basic nutrition to reduce the risk of chronic diseases (Slavin 2000; Liu 2003, 2004). The additive and synergistic effects of these biologically active components may be responsible for the health benefits that reduce disease risk (Liu 2004). The recent evidence suggests that the complex mixture of bioactives in whole foods may be more healthful than individual, isolated components (Liu 2004). The beneficial effects associated with whole grain consumption are in part due to the existence of the unique phytochemicals of whole grains.

Whole Grain Phytochemicals

Wheat, rice, and corn are the major important grains in the human diet. The minor grains include oats, barley, triticale, sorghum, and millet. Wheat and rice account for one-third and one-fourth of the total worldwide grain production, respectively. Whole grains are important components of the human diet, as is evident by their inclusion in the Food Guide Pyramid and U.S. Dietary Guidelines. However, until recently, the attention given to whole grain consumption has been little compared to that for fruits and vegetables, although the previous nutritional guidelines put grains and grain products at the base of the food guide pyramid to emphasize their consumption as part of a normal diet for optimal health (National Research Council 1989, U.S.D.A. 2000).

Whole grains contain unique phytochemicals that complement those in fruits and vegetables when consumed together. For instance, various classes of phenolic compounds in grains include derivatives of benzoic and cinnamic acids, anthocyanidins, quinones, flavonols, chalcones, flavones, flavanones, and amino phenolic compounds (Lloyd et al. 2000, Maillard and Berset 1995, Shahidi and Naczk 1995, Thompson 1994). Some of these phytochemicals, such as ferulic acid, and diferulates are predominantly found in grains but are not present in significant quantities in some fruits and vegetables (Bunzel et al. 2001, Shahidi and Naczk 1995). Grains also contain tocotrienols, tocopherols, and oryzanols (Lloyd et al. 2000, Thompson 1994).

The type of grain and variety influences the concentration of whole grain phytochemicals (Adom et al. 2003). For instance, total phenolic content of selected wheat varieties did not vary much in one study. This contrasted sharply with results obtained for carotenoids, which showed marked variations (three- to twelve-fold) among the wheat varieties tested (Adom et al. 2003). These phytochemicals play important structural and defense roles in the grain. Ferulic acid and other phenolic acids protect wheat kernels by providing both physical and chemical barriers (Arnason et al. 1992, Hahn et al. 1983). The most important groups of phytochemicals found in whole grains can be classified as phenolics, carotenoids, vitamin E compounds, lignans, β-glucan, and inulin.

Phenolics

Phenolic compounds are structurally characterized by an aromatic ring, with one or more hydroxyl groups attached to it. Plant phenolics are by-products of normal metabolism that produce different classes of phenolic compounds based on type of plant, variety, growing conditions, and state of maturity (Duthie and Crozier 2000, Shahidi and Naczk 1995). Plant phenolics can be grouped into different classes. The most important classes are simple phenols, phenolic acids, hydroxycinnamic acids, coumarins, and flavonoids (Figure 15.1). The most common phenolic compounds found in whole grains are phenolic acids and flavonoids. These compounds usually exist as glycosides linked to various sugar moieties or as other complexes linked to organic acids, amines, lipids, and other phenols. The concentration of phenolic compounds in whole grains is influenced by grain type, variety, and part of the grain sampled (Adom and Liu 2002; Adom et al. 2005, 2003).

Phenolic compounds affect plant growth and reproduction and provide plants with chemical defense against pathogens, parasites, and predators (Shahidi and Naczk 1995). For example, ferulic acid and other phenolic acids protect wheat kernels by providing both physical and chemical barriers through cross-linking carbohydrates, antioxidant activities to combat destructive radicals, and astringency that deters consumption by insects and animals (Arnason et al. 1992, Hahn et al. 1983). A higher concentration of ferulic acid in grains increases dimerization, which in turn affects the physical and chemical properties of grain structure. Significant differences in ferulic acid content among wheat cultivars that correspond with resistance to midge infestation have been reported (Abdel-Aal et al. 2001).

Phenolic compounds also perform several important functions in the human body when ingested. Antioxidant activities of phenolic compounds stem from their ability to donate hydrogen atoms to free radicals and in turn form a resonance-stabilized less reactive phenoxy radical. The total phenolic content of whole grains corresponds to their total antioxidant capacities. The order of total antioxidant activity of tested whole grains was corn-wheat-oats-rice, and the antioxidant activity corresponded to their total phenolic content of 265 mg gallic acid equivalent/100 grams, 136 mg gallic acid equivalent/100 grams, 111 mg gallic acid equivalent/100 grams, and 95 mg gallic acid equivalent/100 grams, respectively (Adom and Liu 2002).

Some of the common phenolic acids found in whole grains include ferulic acid, vanillic acid, caffeic acid, syringic acid, and p-coumaric acid (Sosulski et al. 1982). Their structures are shown in Figure 15.2. Compared to others, ferulic acid is the most studied phenolic acid in whole grains and results so far indicate that it is one of the most important beneficial compounds. Ferulic acid (trans-4-Hydroxy-3-methoxycinnamic acid) is the most common

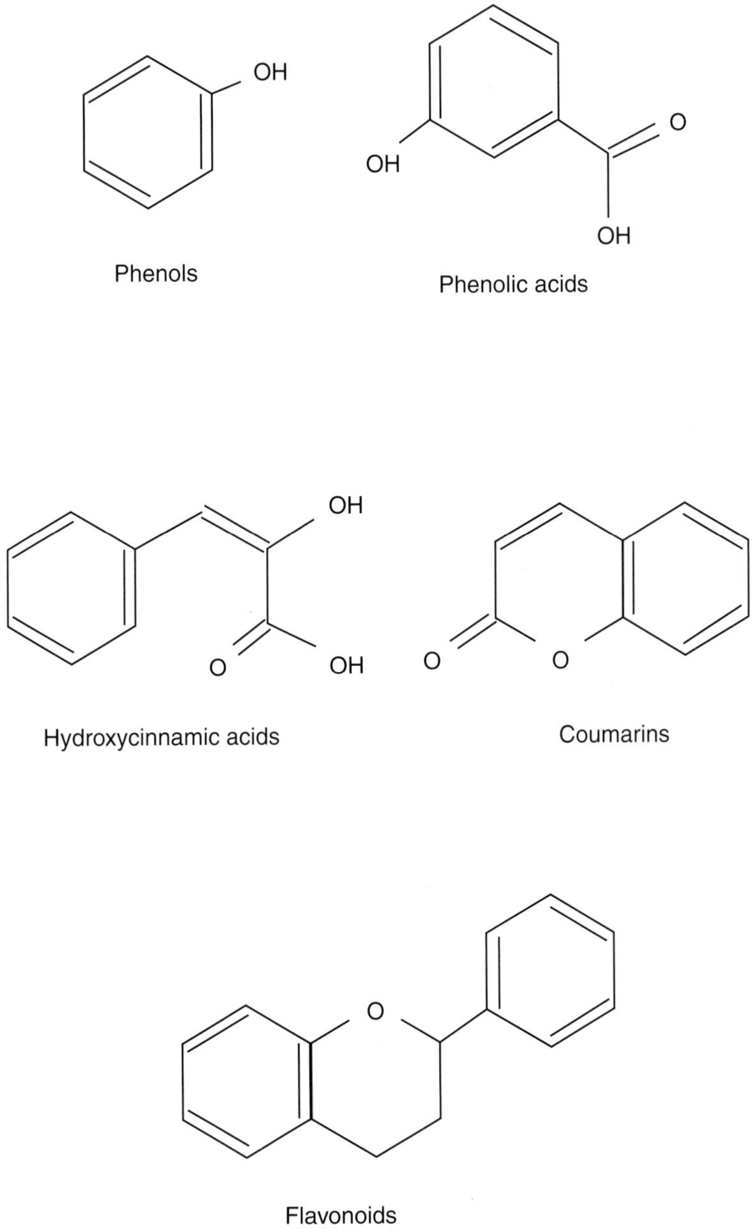

Figure 15.1. Structures of common phenolic compounds.

phenolic acid found in whole grains (Abdel-Aal et al. 2001, Maillard and Berset 1995, Sosulski et al. 1982, Yang et al. 2001). It is abundant in the aleurone, pericarp, and embryo cell walls of various grains, but occurs only in trace amounts in the endosperm (Smith and Hartley 1983). Ferulic acid can exist in the free, soluble-conjugated, and bound forms in whole grains. Bound ferulic acid was significantly higher (more than 93% of total) than free and soluble-conjugated ferulic acid in corn, wheat, oats, and rice (Adom and Liu 2002). For instance, the ratio of free,

(a) Benzoic acid derivatives

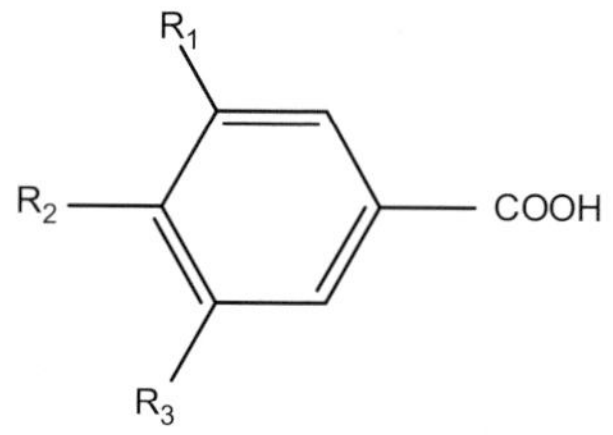

Benzoic acid	Substitutions		
derivatives	R_1	R_2	R_3
Benzoic acid	H	H	H
p-Hydroxybenzoic acid	H	OH	H
Protocatechuic acid	H	OH	OH
Vanillic acid	CH_3O	OH	H
Syringic acid	CH_3O	OH	CH_3O
Gallic acid	OH	OH	OH

(b) Cinnamic acid derivatives

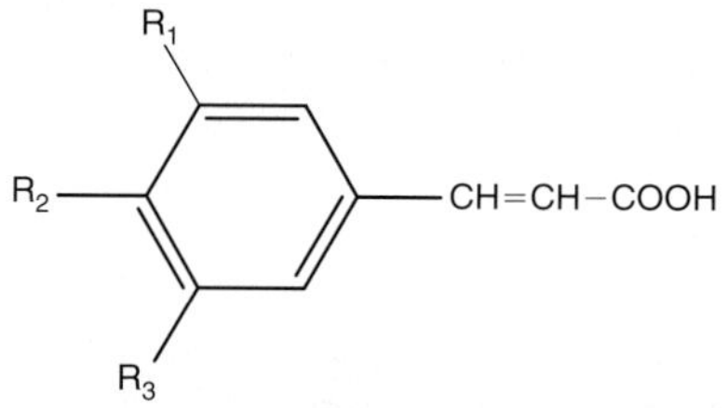

Cinnamic acid	Substitutions		
derivatives	R_1	R_2	R_3
Cinnamic acid	H	H	H
p-Coumaric acid	H	OH	H
Caffeic acid	OH	OH	H
Ferulic acid	CH_3O	OH	H
Sinapic acid	CH_3O	OH	CH_3O

Figure 15.2.   Structures of common phenolic acids: (a) benzoic acid derivatives; (b) cinnamic acid derivatives.

soluble-conjugated, and bound ferulic acid in corn and wheat was 0.1:1:100. The order of total ferulic acid content among the tested grains was corn-wheat-oats-rice (Adom and Liu 2002).

The ferulic acid content of whole grains differs between varieties. Significant differences (up to two-fold) exist among wheat varieties, and ferulic acid also exists mostly in the bound form (more than 97%) in all varieties (Adom et al. 2003). Similarly significant genetic variability in ferulic acid content in durum wheat (three-fold) and common wheat (two-fold) have been reported (Lempereur et al. 1997). Significant differences in ferulic acid content between wheat cultivars that corresponded to levels of enzymes involved in phenolic acid metabolism in wheat plants also have been observed (Rægnier and Macheix 1996). Ferulic acid content was similar during successive phases of grain development, but final concentrations in wheat were different between cultivars. Ferulic acid also varied significantly for some wheat cultivars grown in different environments, with about 13% difference in mean ferulic acid contents (Abdel-Aal et al. 2001).

Ferulic acid and its conjugates have antioxidant properties (Garcia-Conesa et al. 1999). The antioxidant capacity of ferulic acid stems from the free hydroxy group attached to the benzene ring, which can donate a hydrogen atom to quench free radicals. The resulting ferulic acid phenoxy radical is stabilized by resonance delocalization of charges on the benzene ring and the attached carbon-carbon double bond in conjugation with the ring (Garcia-Conesa et al. 1999, Kikuzaki et al. 2002). The electron donating methoxy group increases resonance stability and hence antioxidant activity (Chen and Ho 1997, Graf 1992, Pekkarinen et al. 1999). In addition, the carboxylic acid group adjacent to the carbon-carbon double bond can contribute to resonance stability, as well as provide additional attack sites for free radicals (Graf 1992). Through these mechanisms, ferulic acid can scavenge a whole range of free radicals, including superoxide anions (O^-_2), hydroxyl radicals ($OH^\cdot$), nitrite radical (NO^-), and peroxyl radicals (Kanski et al. 2002, Ogiwaka et al. 2002, Trombino et al. 2004).

The ability of ferulic acid alone and with α-tocopherol, ascorbic acid, and β-carotene to protect against lipid peroxidation induced by A.A.P.H. (peroxyl radical) and tert-B.O.O.H. (alkoxyl radical) was evaluated in rat liver microsomal membranes (Trombino et al. 2004). Ferulic acid inhibited both the initiation and propagation phases of lipid peroxidation and was a stronger antioxidant against tert-B.O.O.H. than A.A.P.H. radicals. In addition, ferulic acid showed a synergistic effect with ascorbic acid, but showed an antagonistic effect with α-tocopherol and β-carotene.

The relative radical scavenging capacity of ferulic acid compared to other compounds depends on a number of factors, including the types of radical, reaction medium, analytical method used, and presence of other antioxidants. For instance, ferulic acid was less potent than α-tocopherol against D.P.P.H. radicals in bulk methyl linoleate, but was as potent as α-tocopherol in ethanol-buffered solution of linoleic acid (Kikuzaki et al. 2002). However, ferulic acid was more potent than α-tocopherol against A.A.P.H. radicals in egg yolk liposomes (Kikuzaki et al. 2002). Ascorbic acid may enhance ferulic acid antioxidant activity by reducing the phenoxy radicals back to initial phenols, as noted by delayed consumption of ferulic acid induced by wheat peroxidase in the presence of ascorbic acid (Garcia et al. 2002). Other phenolic acids found in whole grains include sinapic, vanillic, coumaric, and cinnamic acids (Sosulski et al. 1982). In comparison, ferulic acid with an oxidation potential of 400 mV possessed the greatest antioxidant capacity against the D.P.P.H. radicals (Kanski et al. 2002). Ferulic acid has been used as a food preservative to inhibit auto-oxidation of oils (Dziedzic and Hudson 1984).

The ability of ferulic acid to scavenge free radicals in biological systems can conceivably help modulate the destructive effects of free radicals and thus prevent chronic diseases in humans. Ferulic acid can be effectively absorbed from plant foods into plasma and finally into cells (Bourne and Rice-Evans 1998). The high concentration of ferulic acid in bound fractions of whole grains (Adom and Liu 2002, Adom et al. 2003) is very significant regarding health benefits of whole grain consumption. Bound phytochemicals in grains may resist stomach and small intestinal digestion, and may end up in the colon. Bacterial fermentation processes in the colon may release the high concentration of bound ferulic acid, which in turn may exert health benefits through multi-physiologic mechanisms. Ferulic acid may act in the immediate vicinity of the colon cells or may be absorbed into the plasma (Andreasen et al. 2001, Bourne and Rice-Evans 1998) to exert their health benefits elsewhere.

Epidermiologocal studies have shown that consumption of whole grain products rich in ferulic acid may reduce the risk of chronic diseases (Jacobs et al. 1998b). Ferulic acid effectively prevented the A.A.P.P. radical-induced cell toxicity in cultured hippocampal neuronal cells, as was shown by a reduction in the levels of protein carbonyls, products of oxidative damage to proteins (Kanski et al. 2002). Elevated levels of oxidatively modified proteins have been observed in brains of Alzheimer's patients and in old age (Butterfield and Stadtman 1997, Hensley et al. 1994). Low-density lipoprotein (L.D.L.) oxidation, leading to formation and deposition of foam cells, is one mechanism proposed to explain the link between high plasma L.D.L. levels and the risk of cardiovascular disease (C.V.D.). By this mechanism, protection of L.D.L. is a key to prevent C.V.D. Through its antioxidant activity, ferulic acid has been reported to protect L.D.L. from oxidative damage (Ohta et al. 1997, Schroeter et al. 2000), and could conceivably help prevent C.V.D. The antioxidant activity of ferulic acid in protecting L.D.L. from oxidation in plasma is far greater than that of ascorbic acid (Castelluccio et al. 1996). Lipid peroxidation in cell membranes may follow free radical attack on cell membrane fatty acids. This can lead to membrane disruption and loss of cell integrity. Ferulic acid can inhibit lipid peroxidation and help maintain cell integrity (Trombino et al. 2004, Uchida et al. 1996).

The anti-inflammatory properties of ferulic acid are not clearly understood. In one study, ferulic acid and its esters reduced inflammation in carrageenan-induced rat paw edema (Chawla et al. 1987). Ferulic acid inhibited 1,2-dimethylhydrazine- and 1-methyl-1-nitrosourea induced carcinogenesis and tumor promotion in rats (Imaida et al. 1990). In a similar experiment, curcumin, chlorogenic acid, caffeic acid, and ferulic acid had potent activity inhibiting 12-O-tetradecanoylphorbol-13-acetate induced tumor promotion in mouse skin (Huang et al. 1988).

Carotenoids

Carotenoids are nature's most widespread pigments, with yellow, orange, and red colors. They have received substantial attention because of their provitamin and antioxidant roles. Carotenoids are classified into hydrocarbons (carotenes) and their oxygenated derivatives (xanthophylls). More than 600 different carotenoids have been identified in nature. They occur widely in plants, microorganisms, and animals. Carotenoids have a 40-carbon skeleton of isoprene units (Figure 15.3). The structure may be cyclized at one or both ends, have various hydrogenation levels, or possess oxygen-containing functional groups. Lycopene and β-carotene are examples of acyclized and cyclized carotenoids, respectively. Carotenoid compounds most commonly occur in nature in the all-*trans* form. The most characteristic feature of carotenoids is the long series of conjugated double bonds, forming the central part of the molecule. This gives them their shape, chemical reactivity, and light-absorbing properties.

Lutein, zeaxanthin, β-cryptoxanthin, β-carotene, and α-carotene are some of the carotenoids commonly found in whole grains (Britton, 1995); they are mostly concentrated

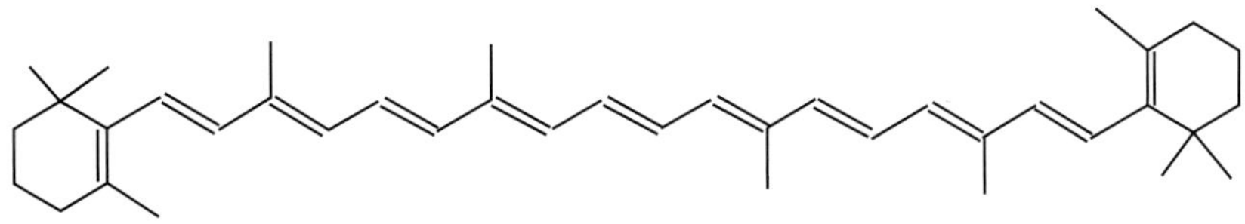

Beta-carotene

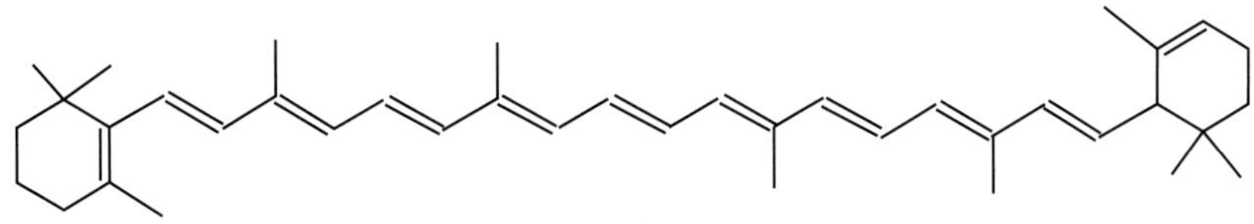

Alpha-carotene

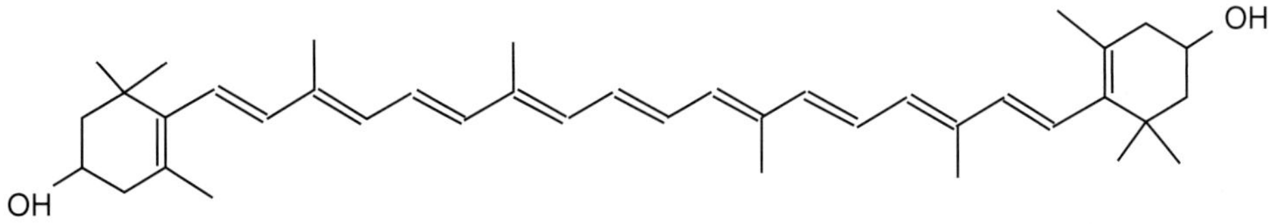

Zeaxanthin

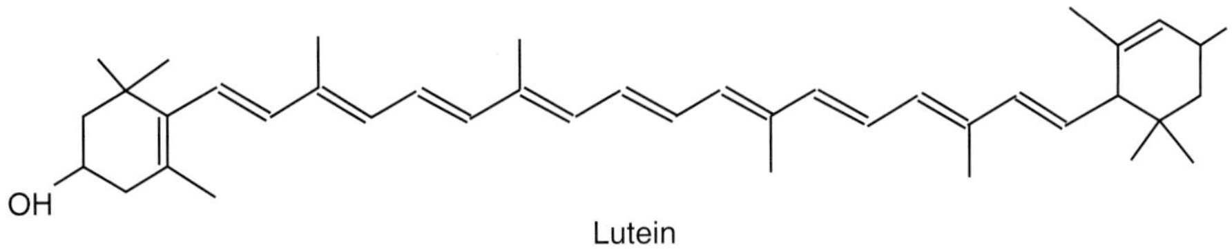

Lutein

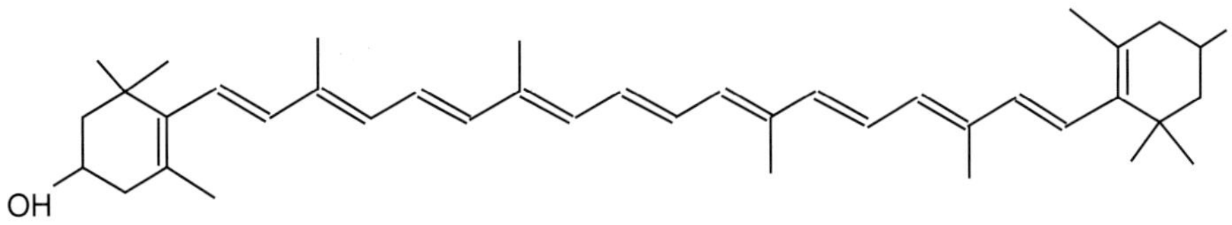

Beta-cryptoxanthin

Figure 15.3. Whole grain carotenoids.

in the bran/germ portion of whole grains (Adom et al. 2005). Carotenoids perform important functions in plants, providing pigmentation essential for photosynthesis, reproduction, and protection. They provide color in whole grain flour.

They also may act as antioxidants in lipid environments of many biological systems through their ability to react with free radicals and form less reactive free radical products. Carotenoid radicals are stabilized by delocalization of unpaired electrons over the conjugated polyene chain of the molecule, allowing the addition of other functional groups to many sites on the radicals (Britton 1995). Carotenoids are especially powerful against singlet oxygen generated from lipid peroxidation, for example. β-carotene, α-carotene, and β-cryptoxanthin have provitamin A activity. Zeaxanthin and lutein are the major carotenoids in the macular region (yellow spot) of the retina in humans.

Vitamin E

Vitamin E is the generic term used to describe a collection of fat-soluble compounds. Their basic structure comprise a six-hydroxychroman group and a phytyl side chain made of isoprenoid units. The chroman group may be methylated at different positions to generate different compounds with vitamin E activity. Vitamin E can exist as two types of structures: the tocopherol and tocotrienol structures (Figure 15.4). Both structures are similar except tocopherols contain saturated phytol side chains, while the tocotrienols have three carbon-carbon double bonds in the phytol side chain.

The eight compounds that exhibit vitamin E activity are α-tocopherol, β-tocopherol, γ-tocopherol, δ-tocopherol, α-tocotrienol, β-tocotrienol, γ-tocotrienol, and δ-tocotrienol. Vitamin E compounds are found in many foods, including whole grains, where they are mostly present in the germ fraction. The concentrations of vitamin E compounds in whole grains are: 75 mg/kg dry weight (D.W.) total tocopherol in soft wheat and barley; 33 mg/kg D.W. to 43 mg/kg D.W. β-tocotrienol in hulled and dehulled wheat; 45 mg/kg D.W. γ-tocopherol in maize; and 56 mg/kg D.W. and 40 mg/kg D.W. α-tocotrienol in oats and barley, respectively (Panfili et al. 2003).

The most important functions of vitamin E in the body are antioxidant activity and maintenance of membrane integrity. The free hydroxyl group on the aromatic ring is responsible for the antioxidant properties. The hydrogen atom from this group can be donated to free radicals, resulting in a resonance-stabilized vitamin E radical. Vitamin E also has been shown to play a role in immune function, D.N.A. repair, and other metabolic processes (Traber 1999).

Other components of whole grains that exert health-beneficial biological activity when ingested include fiber, resistant starch, oligosaccharides, β-glucan, and lignans. Components such as phytates and oxalates may exert negative effects by inhibiting the availability of other beneficial whole grain components.

Lignans

Lignans are one of the important phytochemicals in whole grains. Lignans and neolignans are made up of two coupled C_6C_3 units and are also called secoisolariciresinol diglycoside (S.D.G.) and secoisolariciresinol (Seco) (Figure 15.5). Other examples are isolariciresinol, lariciresinol, matairesinol, pinoresinol, and syringaresinol. They are found in a variety of plants including whole grain corn, oats, wheat, flax seeds, pumpkin seeds, rye, soybeans, broccoli, and some berries (Thompson et al. 1991). The highest concentrations are found in flax (Tham 1998).

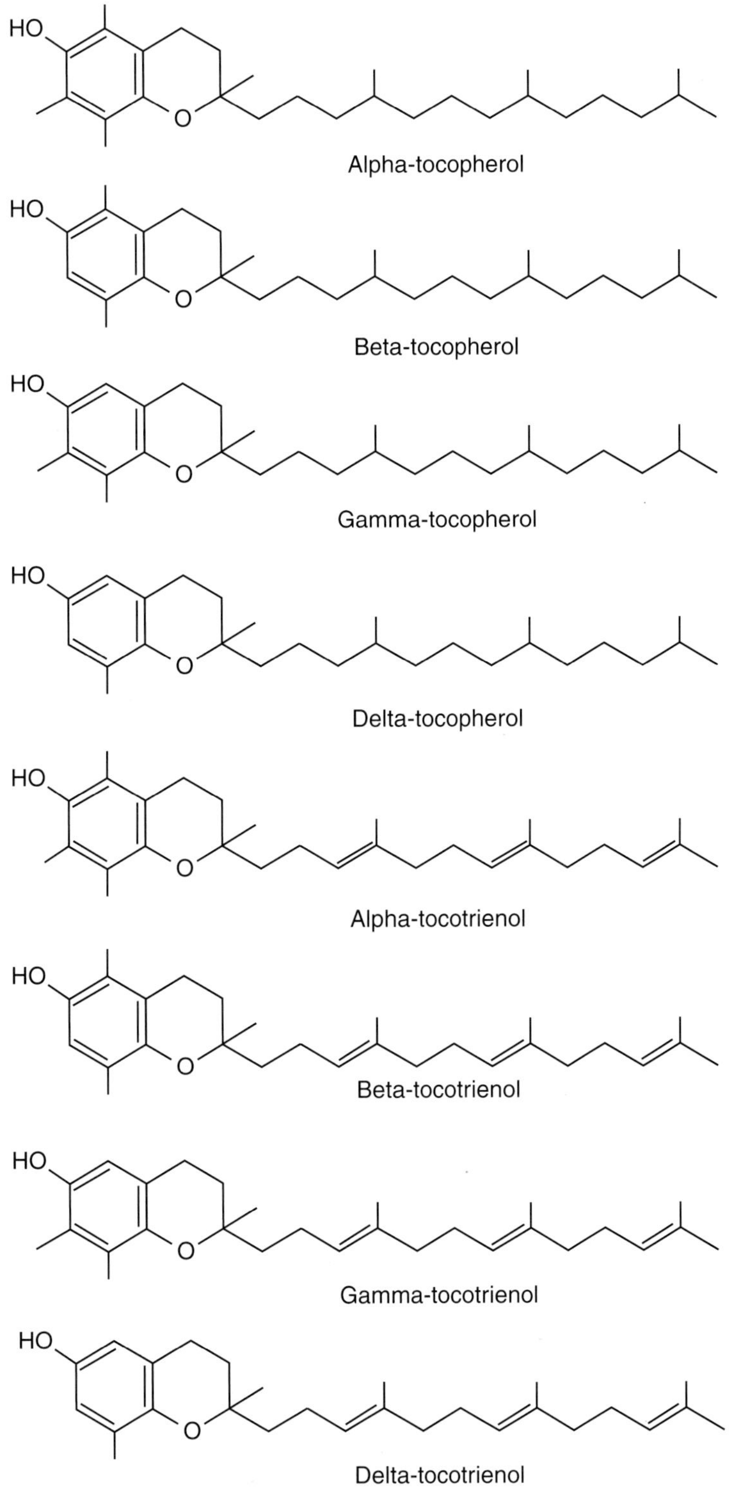

Figure 15.4. Whole grain tocopherols and tocotrienols.

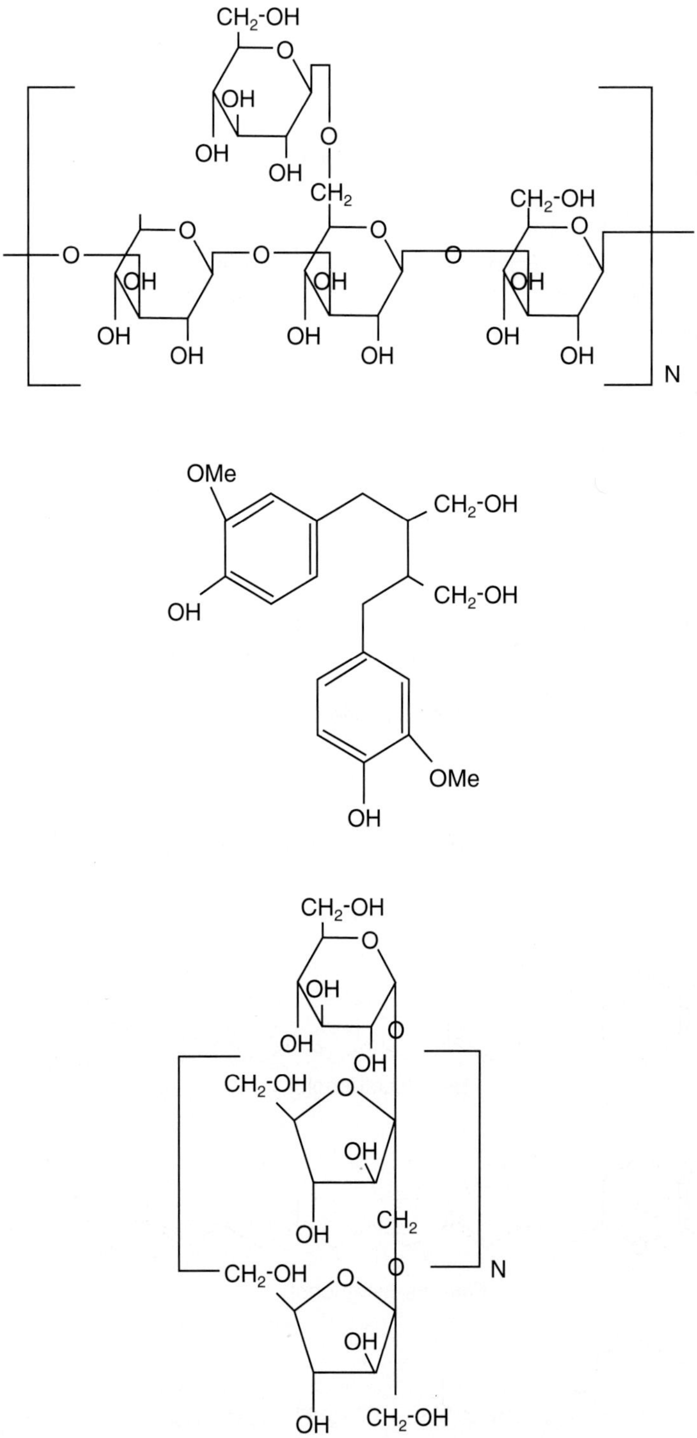

Beta-glucan

Secoisolariciresinol

Inulin

Figure 15.5. Structures of β-glucan, secoisolariciresinol, and inulin.

Lignans have several biological effects that make them unique and very useful in promoting health and combating various diseases. They have strong antioxidant and phytoestrogenic properties that account for their health benefits (Thompson et al. 1991, 1996; Wang et al. 1994). Lignans may prevent diabetes, heart disease, and some hormone-related cancers. Lower cancer rates have been associated with high intakes of lignan (Adlercreutz and Mazur 1997). Intestinal microflora convert ingested plant lignan into mammalian lignans, called enterolactone and enterodiole, that may offer protection against heart disease and hormone-related breast and prostate cancers (Adlercreutz and Mazur 1997, Johnsen et al. 2004). In a Danish study that followed 857 postmenopausal women, women eating the highest amounts of whole grains had significantly higher blood levels of enterolactone (Johnsen et al. 2004). Similarly, in studies involving Finnish men (Vanharanta et al. 2003), blood levels of enterolactone were inversely related to cardiovascular-related deaths, suggesting protective effects of lignans against such conditions.

β-glucan

β-glucan is a soluble fiber made up of complex polysaccharides and commonly found in cell walls of many yeast and cereal fibers such as oats, wheat, and barley. β-glucan consists of a linear polysaccharides chain of linked β-(1-3)- and β-(1-4)-D-glucopyranose units that may contain β-(1-6) branch points (Figure 15.5). Oats and barley contain a mixture of β-1,3-glucan and β-1,4-glucan.

The major biological effects of β-glucan include enhancing the immune system and lowering blood cholesterol levels. In-vivo and in-vitro studies have shown that β-glucan can activate white blood cells, particularly macrophages and neutrophils (Czop 1986, Wakshull et al. 1999). β-glucan-activated macrophages or neutrophils can recognize and kill tumor cells, remove cellular debris resulting from oxidative damage, speed up recovery of damaged tissue, and further activate other components of the immune system (DiRenzo et al. 1991, Ross et al. 1999).

β-glucan is the main component responsible for the cholesterol-lowering effect of oat bran (Bell et al. 1999, Braaten et al. 1994b, Davidson et al. 1991). The cholesterol-lowering effect of β-glucan stems from its ability to bind cholesterol and bile acids and facilitate their elimination from the body (Wood 1990). Results from studies using either oat- or yeast-derived β-glucan show typical reductions of 10% for total cholesterol and 8% for L.D.L. cholesterol after four weeks of use. This was accompanied by up to 16% elevation in H.D.L. cholesterol (Behall et al. 1997, Bell et al. 1999, Uusitupa et al. 1992). Other reports have suggested possible benefits of β-glucan in controlling blood sugar in diabetes subjects. β-glucan was helpful in reducing the elevation in blood sugar levels that normally follow meals (Braaten et al. 1994a, Pick et al. 1996a). β-glucan may cause these effects by delaying gastric emptying, allowing dietary sugar to be absorbed more gradually, and by possibly increasing the tissue sensitivity to insulin (Braaten et al. 1994a, Pick et al. 1996a).

Dietary Fiber, Resistant Starch, and Inulin

Dietary fiber has been identified as an important component of a healthy diet. Whole grains are good sources of dietary fiber. The Association of Official Analytical Chemists (A.O.A.C.) analytically defined dietary fiber as the component of plant cells that resists digestion by the alimentary enzymes of man (Trowel and Burkitt 1986). For whole grains, such components include resistant starch, inulin, lignin, cellulose, hemicellulose, and other constituents distributed in the endosperm and bran parts of the grain. Whole grain dietary fiber performs physiologically important functions in the body and its consumption has been associated with reduced incidence of chronic diseases. In the U.S. Nurses' Study, women with high intakes of cereal fiber showed a 34% lower risk of coronary heart disease events when compared to women with low cereal fiber intake (Wolk et al. 1999). Dietary fiber from fruits and vegetables did not exhibit the same effect in this study.

Results from other studies have demonstrated the protective role of whole grain dietary fiber against myocardial infarction (Rimm et al. 1996), coronary heart disease mortality (Pietinen et al. 1996), some cancers (Kasum et al. 2002), weight gain and diabetes (Koh-Banerjee et al. 2004, Liu et al. 2003, Meyer et al. 2000), and insulin resistance and metabolic syndromes (McKeown et al. 2004). Whole grain dietary fiber may have these effects through multi-physiologic mechanisms that include antioxidant activity, binding and eliminating cholesterol, binding bile acids, modulating hormonal activity, stimulating the immune system, facilitating toxicant transit through the digestive tract, producing short-chain fatty acids in the colon, diluting gut substances, lowering caloric and glycemic index of foods, improving insulin response, and providing bulk in foods. Resistant starch and inulin are some physiologically important and the most studied dietary fiber components of whole grains.

Resistant starch is the portion of starch that can resist upper intestinal digestion and pass into the lower intestine to be fermented by microflora. The three types of resistant starch are physically trapped starch, resistant starch granules, and retrograded starch (Englyst et al. 1993, Muir et al. 1993). Physically trapped starches are trapped within food matrices that severely prevent or delay their interaction with digestive enzymes. They are commonly found in whole or partly ground grains, seeds, cereals, and legumes, and their concentration and distribution is affected by food processing techniques. Resistant starch granules occur in high-amylose maize, potato, and green banana. The granules have crystalline regions that are less susceptible to digestion by acid or α-amylase enzymes. Food processing techniques that gelatinize such starches can aid their digestion. Retrograded starch is formed from gelatinized starch that undergoes the process of retrogradation. High-amylose starch retrogrades faster than high-amylopectin starch. High-amylose starch can be retrograded to a form that resists dispersion in water and digestion by the α-amylase enzyme. Retrograded starch may be generated during food processing (Englyst et al. 1993, Muir et al. 1993).

The physiological functions of resistant starch include improving glycemic response and colon health, providing lower calorie intake, and modulating fat metabolism. Food components that moderate blood sugar levels following food consumption impart important health benefits such as reduced risk of developing diabetes, heart disease, and other major diseases.

Resistant starch is fermented by large intestine microflora to produce short-chain fatty acids butyrate, acetate, and propionate. Butyrate has several physiological effects that promote good colon health (Avivi-Green et al. 2002, Ruemmele et al. 2003). Caloric control is important in combating the obesity epidemic. Resistant starch provides bulk and helps decrease the caloric content of foods. Resistant starch consumption also has been shown to promote lipid oxidation. The relationship between the resistant starch content of a meal and postprandial fat oxidation was investigated in human subjects. The addition of 5.4% resistant starch to the diet significantly increased fat oxidation by 23% compared to a control meal with 0% resistant starch. The results suggested replacing 5.4% of total dietary carbohydrate with resistant starch significantly increased postprandial lipid oxidation and therefore could conceivably decrease fat accumulation in the long-term (Higgins et al. 2004).

Inulin is a natural storage carbohydrate found in several edible plant species, including chicory, artichoke, leek, onion, asparagus, wheat, barley, rye, garlic, and bananas. They belong to a class of carbohydrates known as fructans, which are fructose-containing oligosaccharides. The bond between fructose units in inulin is a β-(2-1) glycosidic linkage (Figure 15.5). Plant inulins contain 2 to 60 fructose units and typically have a terminal glucose unit (Niness 1999). Inulin is sometimes added to food products because of their sweet taste and texture. A U.S.D.A. study showed that American diets typically provide about 2.6 grams of inulin, with wheat (69%) and onions (23%) as the primary sources (Moshfegh et al. 1999).

The major physiological effect of inulin, when ingested, is that it acts as a probiotic to stimulate the growth of friendly and healthy intestinal bacteria that support good colon health. Inulin is a preferred food for lactobacilli in the intestine and can improve the balance of friendly bacteria in the bowel (Gibson et al. 1995, Roberfroid 1993). When subjects in one trial were given 15 grams of inulin a day for fifteen days, the population of *Lactobacillus bifidobacteria* increased by about 10% during that period. At the same time, the population of pathogenic bacteria, such as *Clostridium perfringens* and diarrheogenic strains of *Escherichia coli*, decreased.

Bifidobacteria digest inulin to produce short-chain fatty acids, such as acetic, propionic, and butyric acids. Acetic and propionic acids serve as energy sources for the liver, while butyric acid has cancer-preventing properties in the colon (Reddy et al. 1997, Spiller 1994). Some studies suggest that butyrate may induce differentiation of normal colon cells, but induce growth arrest and upregulate apoptosis in neoplasmic cells (Archer et al. 1998, Avivi-Green et al. 2002, Ruemmele et al. 2003). These three cellular activities are important for anticancer activity. Other health benefits attributed to Bifidobacteria include inhibiting the growth of harmful bacteria, stimulating components of the immune system, aiding the absorption of certain ions, and synthesis of B vitamins. The bifidogenic effect of inulin and oligofructose has been well documented (Bouhnik et al. 1994, Gibson et al. 1995, Gibson and Roberfroid 1995). The effects of inulin and oligofructose in the treatment, prevention or alleviation of symptoms of intestinal diseases have also been reported (Butel et al. 1997).

Inulins also may increase the concentrations of calcium and magnesium in the colon. These cations are important regulators of cellular activity and may help control the rate of cell turnover. High concentrations of calcium also may aid formation of insoluble bile or salts of fatty acids and therefore may reduce the damaging effects of bile or fatty acids on colonocytes (Topping and Clifton 2001). Inulin is sometimes recommended for diabetic patients with low glycemic diet requirements. Inulin does not affect blood sugar levels because it is not absorbed.

Phytates

Phytates are complex esters of phosphorus found in unrefined cereals, legumes, nuts, seeds, and tubers. These negatively charged compounds may combine with positively charged mineral ions of zinc, iron, and calcium, and inhibit their uptake (Harrington et al. 2001, Saha et al. 1994, Zhou and Erdman 1995). This problem may be reduced or overcome using some food processing techniques. Fermentation, for example, may hydrolyze phytates into substances containing fewer phosphate groups. Soaking followed by sprouting tends to reduce phytate content in oats and actually doubles the amount of absorbed zinc in comparison with untreated oats (Sandstrom et al. 1987).

Oxalates

Oxalates are naturally occurring substances found in plants, including whole wheat. High oxalate concentration in the body fluids causes their crystallization and leads to health problems. Oxalates also can combine with divalent cations like Ca^{2+} and inhibit their uptake.

Whole Grains Are Rich in Phytochemicals and High in Antioxidant Activity

Phytochemicals are defined as biologically active compounds of plant origin that, when ingested, provide certain functional benefits beyond basic nutrition (Craig and Beck 1999, Liu 2004). It is estimated that more than 5,000 individual phytochemicals have been identified in fruits, vegetables, and grains. However, a large percentage still remain unknown and need to be identified before we can fully understand the health benefits of phytochemicals in whole foods (Liu 2004). In the meantime, more and more convincing evidence suggests that the benefits of phytochemicals in fruits and vegetables may be even greater than is currently understood because the oxidative stress induced by free radicals is involved in the etiology of a wide range of chronic diseases (Ames and Gold 1991). Because phytochemicals differ widely in composition and ratio from fruit to vegetable to grain, and often have complementary mechanisms to one another, it is suggested that one consume a wide variety of these plant-based foods.

Whole Grain Phytochemicals Were Underestimated

Phytochemicals or antioxidants in grains have not received as much attention as the phytochemicals in fruits and vegetables. Fruits and vegetables are often cited as excellent sources of antioxidants, whereas grains tend not to be mentioned due to relatively low levels of antioxidant activity reported in the literature. Most studies have reported the phenolic levels of grains using various aqueous solutions of methanol, ethanol, and acetone to extract soluble phenolics (Bryngelsson et al. 2002, Dietrych-Szostak and Oleszek 1999, Miller et al. 2000, Velioglu et al. 1998, Zielinski and Kozlowska 2000). These methodologies assumed that long extraction times and/or use of finely powdered samples would ensure maximum extraction of phenolic compounds from grains. These methods at best extracted only the free or loosely attached or readily soluble phenolic compounds in the samples and did not extract phenolic compounds tightly bound to cell wall materials.

Procedures using more exhaustive extraction techniques employ digestion to release bound phytochemicals from whole grains (Adom and Liu 2002; Adom et al. 2003, 2005; Bunzel et al. 2001; Lloyd et al. 2000; Sosulski et al. 1982). These have yielded results that show whole grains contain more phytochemicals than was previously reported. Therefore, the total phenolic contents of whole grains were underestimated in the literature without determining the content of bound phenolics.

Adom and Liu (2002) analyzed and compared the phytochemical profiles of corn, wheat, oats, and rice. The results clearly showed that most grain phenolics were in the bound form. Free phenolics contribution was 15% in corn, 25% in wheat, 25% in oats, and 38% in rice. Bound phenolics contribution was 85% in corn, 76% in wheat, 75% in oats, and 62% in rice. Therefore, it is obvious that without including the bound phenolics, the total phenolic contents of whole grains were previously underestimated in the literature.

A similar observation was made when looking at a specific phenolic compound, ferulic acid. The results showed that bound ferulic acid was significantly higher than free and soluble-conjugate ferulic acid in corn, wheat, oats, and rice. The ratio of free, soluble-conjugated, and bound ferulic acid in corn and wheat was 0.1:1:100 (Adom and Liu 2002). This means the majority of ferulic acid in whole grains is in bound form. Free and soluble-conjugated ferulic acid makes a very small contribution (less than 0.6% and more than 7%, respectively), while bound ferulic acid represents the bulk (more than 93%) of ferulic acid present in the whole grain. These results were consistent with observations by Maillard and Berset (1995), who estimated that free phenolic acids in methanol extracts of barley were 100-fold lower than bound phenolic acids.

We believe that the underestimation of whole grain phytochemicals may have contributed to the little attention previously given to whole grains as a good source of health beneficial phytochemicals when compared to fruits and vegetables. With increasing knowledge of whole grains as a potential source of disease-preventing phytochemicals, whole grains are becoming increasingly more important in the human diet. In fact, current data suggest the concentration of some phytochemicals in whole grains was comparable to that found in some fruits and vegetables (Figure 15.6).

Phenolic compounds in whole grains contribute to antioxidant activity. Some derivatives of phenolic compounds are known to have antioxidant properties. For example, avenanthramides

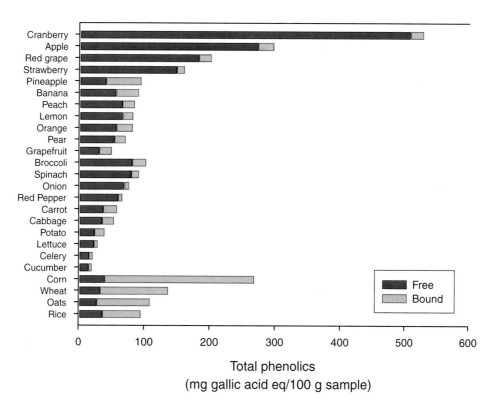

Figure 15.6. Total phenolic content of common fruits, vegetables, and whole grains (adopted from Sun et al. 2002, Chu et al. 2002, and Adom and Liu 2002).

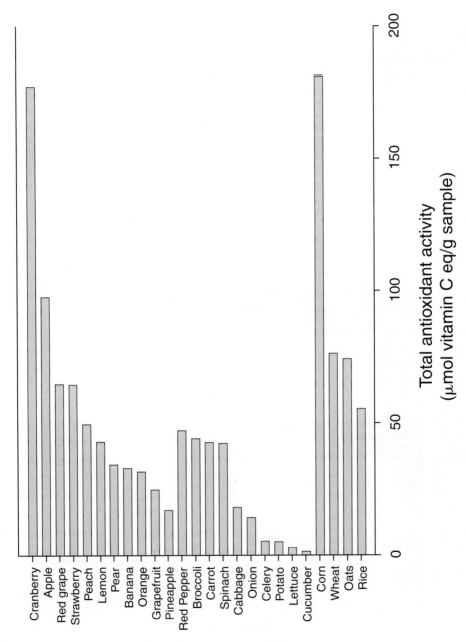

Figure 15.7. Total antioxidant activity of common fruits, vegetables, and whole grains (adopted from Sun et al. 2002, Chu et al. 2002, and Adom and Liu 2002).

are cinnamoyl conjugates that occur in oats and have high antioxidant activity (Bryngels-son et al. 2002, Collins 1989). Long-chain mono- and di-alcohol esters of ferulic and caffeic acids have potent antioxidant activity (Daniels and Martin 1967). The antioxidant activity of 8-8'-diferulic acid compared to antioxidant activities of ferulic acid and other diferulates was reported (Garcia-Conesa et al. 1999). The Trolox equivalent antioxidant capacity (T.E.A.C.) values for various diferulic acid conjugates ranged from 1.49 to 4. Generally, diferulic conjugates were reported to be more potent antioxidants than ferulic acid in both aqueous and lipid phases. Among the diferulates tested, 8-8'-diferulic acid was the most potent antioxidant in the aqueous phase.

In general, high phenolic content strongly correlates with high antioxidant activity (Adom and Liu 2002, Adom et al. 2003, Velioglu et al. 1998, Zielinski and Kozlowska 2000). Results from analyzing different grains showed that total antioxidant activity of corn was 181.42 ± 0.86 μmol/gram grain, and was the highest ($p < 0.01$) compared to wheat, oats, and rice. Total antioxidant activities of wheat (76.70 ± 1.38 μmol/gram grain) and oats (74.67 ± 1.49 μmol/gram grain) were similar ($p > 0.05$), but higher than total antioxidant activity in rice (55.77 ± 1.62 μmol/gram grain) (Adom and Liu 2002). Similarly, when expressed on a per serving basis, the total antioxidant activity of whole grains was comparable to that of some fruits and vegetables (Figure 15.7).

Importance of Bound Phytochemicals—Hypothesis for Colon Cancer Reduction

The health benefits of whole grains have been attributed in part to their phytochemical content. The beneficial phytochemicals of whole grains are uniquely distributed as free, soluble-conjugated, and bound forms. Most of these phytochemicals are in the insoluble bound forms, bound to cell wall materials (Bunzel et al. 2001, Lloyd et al. 2000, Sosulski et al. 1982). Cell wall materials are difficult to digest and may survive upper gastrointestinal digestion to reach the colon. Colonic digestion of such materials would release the bulk of the bound phytochemicals to exert their health benefits locally and beyond upon absorption. For instance, both human and rat gastrointestinal esterase (from intestinal mucosa and microflora) can release ferulic acid and diferulic acids from cereal bran (Andreasen et al. 2001). These compounds have potent antioxidant properties and their absorption into the blood plasma has been reported (Andreasen et al. 2001). This may partly explain the reduced risk of colon cancer associated with increased consumption of whole grains and whole grain products (Jacobs et al. 1995). Thus, the health benefits of whole grain phytochemicals is more site-specific, i.e. they are more effective in the colon (Jacobs et al. 1995, Smigel 1992, Thompson 1994). In contrast, phytochemicals in fruits and vegetables are mainly in free or soluble-conjugate (glycosides) forms that may be more readily available in the upper gastrointestinal tract (Vinson et al. 1998, 2001; Sun et al. 2002; Chu et al. 2002).

Distribution of Phytochemicals in Milled Fractions

The distribution of phytochemicals in the bran, germ, and endosperm parts of the grain is of interest with the recent interest in whole grain. Data on phytochemical profiles and antioxidant activities of milled fractions of different wheat varieties is limited in the literature. Some studies have reported on phytochemical profile and antioxidant activities of whole wheat (Adom and Liu 2002, Adom et al. 2003), while others have focused on the bran fractions (Rondini et al. 2004, Yu et al. 2003, Zhou and Yu 2004) or endosperm fractions alone

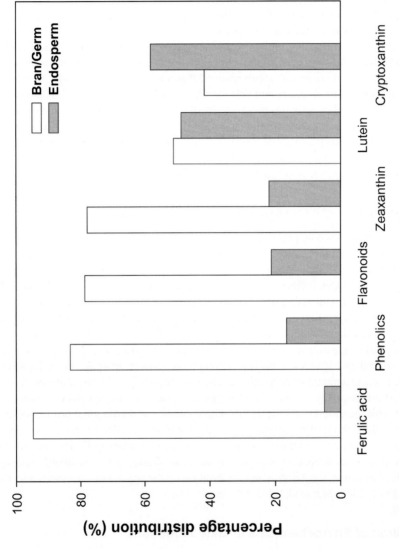

Figure 15.8. Percentage distribution of phytochemicals in milled fractions of whole wheat (adopted from Adom et al. 2005).

(Yu et al. 2004). Reports on the combination of whole wheat grain and milled fractions of wheat only examined a limited number of phytochemicals (Skrabanja et al. 2004, Zhou et al. 2004).

Results reported by Adom et al. (2005) show that the majority of health beneficial phenolic phytochemicals of whole grain wheat are present in the bran/germ fraction (Figure 15.8). For example, phenolic content in the bran/germ fraction was fifteen- to eighteen-fold higher ($p < 0.01$) when compared to the corresponding endosperm samples. The bran/germ parts contribute 83% of the total phenolic content of whole wheat flour (Adom et al. 2005).

Bound wheat phenolics associated with cell walls may survive upper gastrointestinal tract digestion and finally reach the colon, where colonic digestion by intestinal microflora may release the bulk of the bound phenolics. These results suggest the bran/germ fraction would contribute most of the wheat phenolics that may be released in the colon to exert their healthful benefits locally and after absorption (Adom and Liu 2002, Andreasen et al. 2001). This may partly explain the inverse association between increased whole grain consumption and reduced incidence of certain chronic diseases (Jacobs et al. 1999, Kasum et al. 2002, Meyer et al. 2000, Nicodemus et al. 2001, Smigel 1992, Thompson 1994).

The importance of whole wheat flour consumption as compared to refined wheat flour consumption cannot be over emphasized and needs further promotion among consumers. These results would also provide the necessary information for evaluating contributions to health benefits from consumption of whole wheat products. This should help emphasize and further promote whole grain consumption among consumers.

Conclusion

Modifying the diet by increasing the daily consumption of a wide variety of fruit, vegetables, and whole grains is a practical strategy for consumers to optimize their health and reduce the risk of chronic diseases. Use of dietary supplements, nutraceuticals, and functional foods is increasing as industry is responding to consumers' demands. However, more information about the health benefits and possible risks of dietary supplements is needed to ensure their efficacy and safety. The additive and synergistic effects of phytochemicals in fruit, vegetables, and whole grains are responsible for their health benefits. Further research on the health benefits of phytochemicals in whole grains is warranted.

References

Abdel-Aal, E.S.M.; Huci, P.; Sosulski, F.W.; Graf, R.; Gillott, C.; Pietrzak, L. Screening spring wheat for midge resistance in relation to ferulic acid content. *Journal of Agriculture and Food Chemistry.* 2001, 49, 3559–3566.

Adlercreutz, H.; Mazur, W. Phyto-estrogens and Western Diseases. *Annals of Medicine.* 1997, 29, 95–120.

Adom, K.K.; Liu, R.H. Antioxidant activity of grains. *Journal of Agriculture and Food Chemistry.* 2002, 50, 6182–6187.

Adom, K.K.; Sorrells, M.; Liu, R.H. Phytochemicals and antioxidant activity of milled fractions of different wheat varieties. *Journal of Agriculture and Food Chemistry.* 2005, 53, 2297–2306.

Adom, K.K.; Sorrells, M.E.; Liu, R.H. Phytochemical profiles and antioxidant activity of wheat varieties. *Journal of Agriculture and Food Chemistry.* 2003, 51, 7825–7834.

Ames B.N., Gold L.S. (1991) Endogenous mutagens and the causes of aging and cancer. *Mutat Res* 250:3–16.

Anderson, J.W.; Hanna, T.J.; Peng, X.; Kryscio, R.J. Whole grain foods and heart disease risk. *Journal of American College of Nutrition.* 2000, 19, 291S–299S.

Andreasen, M.F.; Kroon, P.A.; Williamson, G.; Garcia-Conesa, M.T. Intestinal release and uptake of phenolic antioxidant diferilic acids. *Free Radical Biology and Medicine.* 2001, 31, 304–314.

Archer, S.Y.; Meng, S.; Shei, A.; Hodin, R.A. p21WAF1 is required for butyrate-mediated growth inhibition of human colon cancer cells. *Proceedings of the National Academy of Sciences. USA*. 1998, 95, 6791–6796.

Arnason, J.T.; Gale, J.; Conilh de Beyssac, B.; Sen, A.; Miller, S.S.; Philogene, B.J.R.; Lambert, J.D.H.; Fulcher, R.G.; Serratos, A.; Mihm, J. Role of phenolics in resistance of maize grain to stored grain insects, Prostphanus truncatus (Horn) and Sitophilus zeamais (Motsch). *Journal of Stored Products and Research*. 1992, 28, 119–126.

Avivi-Green, C.; Polak-Charcon, S.; Madar, Z.; Schwartz, B. Different molecular events account for butyrate-induced apoptosis in two human colon cancer cell lines. *Journal of Nutrition*. 2002, 132, 1812–1818.

Behall, K.M.; Scholfield, D.J.; Hallfrisch, J. Effect of beta-glucan level in oat fiber extracts on blood lipids in men and women. *Journal of American College of Nutrition*. 1997, 16, 46–51.

Bell, S.; Goldman, V.M.; Bistrian, B.R. Effect of beta-glucan from oats and yeast on serum lipids. *Critical Reviews in Food Science and Nutrition*. 1999, 39, 189–202.

Bouhnik, Y.; Flourié, B.; Ouarne, F.; Riottot, M.; Bisetti, N.; Bornet, F.; Rambaud, J. Effects of prolonged ingestion of fructo-oligosaccharides on colonic bifidobacteria, fecal enzymes and bile acids in humans. *Gastroenterology*. 1994, 106, A598–A604.

Bourne, L.C.; Rice-Evans, C. Bioavailability of ferulic acid. *Biochemical and Biophysical Research Communication*. 1998, 253, 222–227.

Braaten, J.T.; Scott, F.W.; Wood, P.J. High beta-glucan oat bran and oat gum reduce postprandial blood glucose and insulin in subjects with and without type 2 diabetes. *Diabetic Medicine: A Journal of the British Diabetic Association*. 1994a, 11, 312–318.

Braaten, J.T.; Wood, P.J.; Scott, F.W. Oat beta-glucan reduces blood cholesterol concentration in hypercholesterolemic subjects. *European Journal of Clinical Nutrition*. 1994b, 48, 465–474.

Britton, G. Structure and properties of carotenoids in relation to function. *FASEB Journal*. 1995, 9, 1551–1558.

Bryngelsson, S.; Dimberg, L.H.; Kamal-Eldin, A. Effects of commercial processing on levels of antioxidants in oats (*Avena sativa L.*). *Journal of Agriculture and Food Chemistry*. 2002, 50, 1890–1896.

Bunzel, M.; Ralph, J.; Martia, J.M.; Hatfield, R.D.; Steinhart, H. Diferulates as structural components in soluble and insoluble cereal dietary fibre. *Journal of the Science of Food and Agriculture*. 2001, 81, 653–660.

Butel, M.J.; Roland, N.; Hibert, A.; Popot, F.; Favre, A.; Tessedre, A.C.; Bensaada, M.; Rimbault, A.; Szylit, O. Clostridial pathogenicity in experimental necrotising enterocolitis in gnotobiotic quails and protective role of bifidobacteria. *Journal of Medical Microbiology*. 1997, 47, 391–399.

Butterfield, D.A.; Stadtman, E.R. Protein oxidation processes in aging brain. *Advance Cell Aging and Gerontology*. 1997, 2, 161–191.

Castelluccio, C.; Bolwell, G.P.; Gerrish, C.; Rice-Evans, C. Differential distribution of ferulic acid to the major plasma constituents in relation to its potential as an antioxidant. *Biochemical Journal*. 1996, 316, 691–694.

Chatenoud, L.; Tavani, A.; La-Vecchia, C.; Jacobs, D.R.J.; Negri, E.; Levi, F.; Franceschi, S. Whole grain food intake and cancer risk. *International Journal of Cancer*. 1998, 77, 24–28.

Chawla, A.S.; Singh, M.; Murthy, M.S.; Gupta, M.P.; Singh, H. Anti-inflammatory action of ferulic acid and its esters in carrageenan-induced rat paw edema model. *Indian Journal of Experimental Biology*. 1987, 25, 187–189.

Chen, J.H.; Ho, C.T. Antioxidant activities of caffeic acid and its related hydroxycinnamic acid compounds. *Journal of Agriculture and Food Chemistry*. 1997, 45, 2374–2378.

Chu, Y.F.; Sun, J.; Wu, X.; Liu, R.H. Antioxidant and antiproliferative activities of common vegetables. *Journal of Agriculture and Food Chemistry*. 2002, 50, 6910–6916.

Collins, F.W. Oats Phenolics: Avenanthramides, Novel Substituted N-Cinnamoylanthranilate Alkaloids from Oats Groats and Hull. *Journal of Agriculture and Food Chemistry*. 1989, 37, 60–66.

Craig, W.; Beck, L. Phytochemicals: health and protective effects. *Canadian Journal of Dietetic Practice and Research*. 1999, 60, 78–84.

Czop, J.K. The role of beta-glucan receptors on blood and tissue leukocytes in phagocytosis and metabolic activation. *Pathology and Immunopathology Research*. 1986, 5, 286–296.

Daniels, D.G.H.; Martin, H.F. Antioxidant in Oats: Mono-esters of caffeic and ferulic acids. *Journal of the Science of Food and Agriculture*. 1967, 18, 589–595.

Davidson, M.H.; Dugan, L.D.; Burns, J.H. The hypocholesterolemic effects of beta-glucan in oatmeal and oat bran. A dose-controlled study. *Journal of the American Medical Association*. 1991, 265, 1833–1839.

Dietrych-Szostak, D.; Oleszek, W. Effect of processing on the flavonoid content in buckwheat (Fagopyrum esculentum Moench) grain. *Journal of Agriculture and Food Chemistry*. 1999, 47, 4384–4387.

DiRenzo, L.; Yefenof, E.; Klein, E. The function of human NK cells is enhanced by beta-glucan, a ligand of CR3 (CD11b/CD18). *European Journal of Immunology*. 1991, 21, 1755–1758.

Duthie, G.; Crozier, A. Plant-derived phenolic antioxidants. *Current Opinion in Lipidology*. 2000, 11, 43–47.

Dziedzic, S.C.; Hudson, B.J.F. Phenolic acids and related compounds as antioxidants for edible oils. *Food Chemistry*. 1984, 14, 45–51.

Englyst, H.N.; Kingman, S.M.; Cummings, J.H. Resistant starch: measurement in foods and physiological role in man. In: *Plant polymeric carbohydrates*, Meuser, F., Manners, D.J., and Seibel, W., eds., p. 137.The Royal Society of Chemistry, Cambridge, U.K. 1993.

Garcia, R.; Rakotozafy, L.; Telef, N.; Potus, J.; Nicolas, J. Oxidation of ferulic acid or arabinose-esterified ferulic acid by wheat germ peroxidase. *Journal of Agriculture and Food Chemistry*. 2002, 50, 3290–3298.

Garcia-Conesa, M.T.; Wilson, P.D.; Plumb, G.W.; Ralph, J.; Williams, G. Antioxidant properties of 4,4′-dihydroxy-3,3′-dimethoxy- b,b′-bicinnamic acid (8-8-diferulic acid, non-cyclic form). *Journal of the Science of Food and Agriculture*. 1999, 79, 379–384.

Gibson, G.R.; Beatty, E.R.; Wang, X.; Cummings, J.H. Selective stimulation of bifidobacteria in the human colon by oligofructose and inulin. *Gastroenterology*. 1995, 108, 975–982.

Gibson, G.R.; Roberfroid, M.B. Dietary modulation of the human colonic microbiota—introducing the concept of prebiotics. *Journal of Nutrition*. 1995, 125.

Graf, E. Antioxidant potential of ferulic acid. *Free Radical Biology and Medicine*. 1992, 13, 435–448.

Hahn, D.H.; Faubion, J.M.; Rooney, L.W. Sorghum phenolic acids, their high performance liquid chromatography separation and their relation to fungal resistance. *Cereal Chemistry*. 1983, 60, 255–259.

Harrington, M.E.; Flynn, A.; Cashman, K.D. Effects of dietary fibre extracts on calcium absorption in rat. *Food Chemistry*. 2001, 73, 263–269.

Hensley, K.; Hall, N.; Subramaniam, R.; Cole, P.; Harris, M.; Aksenov, M.; Aksenova, M.; Gabbita, S.P.; Wu, J.F.; Carney, J.M. Brain regional correspondence between Alzheimer's disease histopathology and biomarkers of protein oxidation. *Journal of Neurochemistry*. 1994, 65, 2146–2156.

Higgins, J.A.; Higbee, D.R.; Donahoo, W.T.; Brown, I.L.; Bell, M.L.; Bessesen, D.H. Resistant starch consumption promotes lipid oxidation. *Nutrition and Metabolism*. 2004, 1, 8–19.

Huang, M.T.; Smart, R.C.; Wong, C.Q.; Conney, A.H. Inhibitory effect of curcumin, chlorogenic acid, caffeic acid, and ferulic acid on tumor promotion in mouse skin by 12-O-tetradecanoylphorbol-13-acetate. *Cancer Research*. 1988, 48, 5941–5946.

Imaida, K.; Hirose, M.; Yamaguchi, S.; Takahashi, S.; Ito, N. Effects of naturally occurring antioxidants on combined 1,2-dimethylhydrazine- and 1-methyl-1-nitrosourea-initiated carcinogenesis in F344 male rats. *Cancer Letters*. 1990, 55, 53–59.

Jacobs, D.R.; Meyer, H.E.; Solvoll, K. Reduced mortality among whole grain bread eaters in men and women in the Norwegian County Study. *The European Journal of Clinical Nutrition*. 2001, 55, 137–143.

Jacobs, D.R.; Meyer, K.A.; Kushi, L.H.; Folsom, A.R. Whole grain intake may reduce risk of coronary heart disease death in postmenopausal women: The Iowa Women's Health Study. *American Journal Clinical Nutrition*. 1998b, 68, 248–257.

Jacobs, D.R.; Slavin, J.; Marquart, L. Whole grain intake and cancer: A review of literature. *Nutrition and Cancer*. 1995, 22, 221–229.

Jacobs, D.R.J.; Meyer, K.A.; Kushi, L.H.; Folsom, A.R. Is whole grain intake associated with reduced total and cause-specific death rates in older women: The Iowa Women's Health Study. *American Journal of Public Health*. 1999, 89, 322–329.

Johnsen, N.F.; Hausner, H.; Olsen, A.; Tetens, I.; Christensen, J.; Knudsen, K.E.; Overvad, K.; Tjonneland, A. Intake of whole grains and vegetables determines the plasma enterolactone concentration of Danish women. *Journal of Nutrition*. 2004, 134, 2691–2697.

Kanski, J.; Aksenova, M.; Stoyanova, A.; Butterfield, D.A. Ferulic acid antioxidant protection against hydroxyl and peroxyl radical oxidation in synaptosomal and neuronal cell culture systems in vitro: structure-activity studies. *Journal of Nutritional Biochemistry*. 2002, 13, 273–281.

Kasum, C.M.; Jacobs, D.R. J.; Nicodemus, K.; Folsom, A.R. Dietary risk factors for upper aerodigestive tract cancers. *International Journal of Cancer*. 2002, 99, 267–272.

Kikuzaki, H.; Hisamoto, M.; Hirose, K.; Akiyama, K.; Taniguchi, H. Antioxidant Properties of ferulic acid and its related compounds. *Journal of Agriculture and Food Chemistry*. 2002, 50, 2161-2168.

Koh-Banerjee, P.; Franz, M.; Sampson, L.; Liu, S.; Jacobs, D. R.; Spiegelman, D.; Willett, W.; Rimm, E. Changes in whole-grain, bran, and cereal fibre consumption in relation to 8-y weight gain among men. *American Journal of Clinical Nutrition*. 2004, 80, 1237–1245.

Lempereur, I.; Rouau, X.; Abecassis, J. Genetic and agronomic variation in arabinoxylan and ferulic acid contents of durum wheat (*Triticum durum L.*) grain and its milling fractions. *Journal of Cereal Science*. 1997, 25, 103–110.

Liu, R.H. Health benefits of fruits and vegetables are from additive and synergistic combination of phytochemicals. Am J Clin Nutr 2003, 78:517S–520S.

Liu, R.H. Potential synergy of phytochemicals in cancer prevention: mechanism of action. *J. Nutr.* 2004, 134: 3479S–3485S.

Liu, S.; Stampfer, M.J.; Hu, F.B.; Giovanucci, E.; Rimm, E.; Manson, J.E.; Hennekens, C.H.; Willett, W.C. Whole grain consumption and risk of coronary heart disease: results from the Nurses' Health study. *American Journal Clinical Nutrition.* 1999, 70, 412–419.

Liu, S.; Willett, W.C.; Manson, J.E.; Hu, F.B.; Rosner, B.; Colditz, G. Relation between changes in intakes of dietary fiber and grain products and changes in weight and development of obesity among middle-aged women. *American Journal of Clinical Nutrition.* 2003, 78, 920–927.

Lloyd, B.J.; Siebenmorgen, T.J.; Beers, K.W. Effect of commercial processing on antioxidants in rice bran. *Cereal Chemistry.* 2000, 77, 551–555.

Lupton, J.R.; Meacher, M.M. Radiographic analysis of the effect of dietary fibers on rat colonic transit time. *American Journal of Physiology.* 1988, 255, G633–639.

Maillard, M.N.; Berset, C. Evolution of antioxidant activity during kilning: Role of insoluble bound phenolic acids of barley and malt. *Journal of Agriculture and Food Chemistry.* 1995, 43, 1789–1793.

McKeown, N.M.; Meigs, J.B.; Liu, S.; Saltzman, E.; Wilson, P.W.; Jacques, P.F. Carbohydrate nutrition, insulin resistance, and the prevalence of the metabolic syndrome in the Framingham Offspring Cohort. *Diabetes Care.* 2004, 27, 538–546.

Meyer, K.A.; Kushi, L.H.; Jacob, D.R.J.; Slavin, J.; Sellers, T.A.; Folsom, A.R. Carbohydrates, dietary fiber, incident type 2 diabetes mellitus in older women. *American Journal Clinical Nutrition.* 2000, 71, 921–930.

Miller, H.E.; Rigelhof, F.; Marquart, L.; Prakash, A.; Kanter, M. Antioxidant content of whole grain breakfast cereals, fruits and vegetables. *Journal of American College of Nutrition.* 2000, 19, 312S–319S.

Morris, J.N.; Marr, J.W.; Clayton, D.G. Diet and heart: A post-script. *British Medical Journal.* 1977, 2, 1307–1314.

Moshfegh, A.J.; Friday, J.E.; Goldman, J.P.; Ahuja, J.K.C. Presence of inulin and oligofructose in the diets of Americans. *Journal of Nutrition.* 1999, 129, 14075–14115.

Muir, J.G.; Young, G.P.; O'Dea, K.; Cameron-Smith, D.; Brown, I.E.; Collier, G.R. Resistant starch—the neglected 'dietary fiber'? Implications for health. *Dietary Fiber Bibliography and Reviews.* 1993, 1, 33–40.

National Research Council. Food and Nutrition Board, *Recommended Dietary Allowance*, 10th ed. National Academy Press, Washington D.C. 1989.

Nicodemus, K.K.; Jacobs, D.R.J.; Folsom, A.R. Whole and refined grain intake and risk of incident postmenopausal breast cancer. *Cancer Causes and Control.* 2001, 12, 917–925.

Niness, K.R. Inulin and Oligofructose: What Are They? *Journal of Nutrition.* 1999, 129, 1402S–1406S.

Ogiwaka, T.; Satoh, K.; Kadoma, Y.; Murakami, Y.; Unten, S.; Atsumi, T.; Sakagami, H.; Fujisawa, S. Radical scavenging activity and cytotoxicity of ferulic acid. *Anticancer Research.* 2002, 22, 2711–2717.

Ohta, T.; Nakano, T.; Egashira, Y.; Sanada, H. Antioxidant activity of ferulic acid beta-glucuronide in the LDL oxidation system. *Bioscience, Biotechnology, and Biochemistry.* 1997, 61, 1942–1943.

Panfili, G.; Fratianni, A.; Irano, M. Normal phase high-performance liquid chromatography method for the determination of tocopherols and tocotrienols in cereals. *Journal of Agriculture and Food Chemistry.* 2003, 51, 3940–3944.

Pekkarinen, S.S.; Stockmann, H.; Schwarz, K.; Heinonen, M.; Hopia, A.I. Antioxidant activity and partitioning of phenolic acids in bulk and emulsified methyl linoleate. *Journal of Agriculture and Food Chemistry.* 1999, 47, 3036–3043.

Pick, M.E.; Hawrysh, Z.J.; Gee, M.I. Oat bran concentrate bread products improve long-term control of diabetes: a pilot study. *Journal of American Dieticians Association.* 1996a, 96, 1254–1261.

Pietinen, P.; Rimm, E.B.; Korhonen, P.; Hartman, A.M.; Willett, W.C.; Albanes, D.; Virtamo, J. Intake of dietary fiber and risk of coronary heart disease in a cohort of Finnish men: the Alpha-Tocopherol, Beta Carotene Cancer Prevention Study. *Circulation.* 1996, 94, 2720 -2727.

Reddy, B.S.; Hamid, R.; Rao, C.V. Effect of dietary oligofructose and inulin on colonic preneoplastic aberrant crypt foci inhibition. *Carcinogenesis.* 1997, 18, 1371–1374.

Rægnier, T.; Macheix, J.-J. Changes in wall-bound phenolic acids, phenylalanine and tyrosine ammonia-lyases, and peroxidases in developing durum wheat grains (Triticum turgidum L. Var. Durum). *Journal of Agriculture and Food Chemistry.* 1996, 44, 1727–1730.

Rimm, E.B.; Ascherio, A.; Giovanucci, E.; Spiegelman, D.; Stampfer, M.J.; Willett, W.C. Vegetable, fruit and cereal fiber intake and risk of coronary heart disease among men. *Journal of the American Medical Association.* 1996, 275, 447–541.

Roberfroid, M. Dietary fiber, inulin, and oligofructose: a review comparing their physiological effects. *Critical Reviews in Food Science and Nutrition.* 1993, 33, 103–148.

Rondini, L.; Peyrat-Maillard, M.N.; Marsset-Baglieri, A.; Fromentin, G.; Durand, P.; Tome, D.; Prost, M.; Berset, C. Bound ferulic acid from bran is more bioavailable than the free compound in rat. *Journal of Agriculture and Food Chemistry*. 2004, 52, 4338–4343.

Ross, G.D.; Vetvicka, V.; Yan, J. Therapeutic intervention with complement and beta-glucan in cancer. *Immunopharmacology*. 1999, 42, 61–74.

Ruemmele, F.M.; Schwartz, S.; Seidman, E.G.; Dionne, S.; Levy, E.; Lentze, M.J. Butyrate induced Caco-2 cell apoptosis is mediated via the mitochondrial pathway. *Gut*. 2003, 52, 94–100.

Saha, P.R.; Weaver, C.M.; Mason, A.C. Mineral bioavailability in rats from intrinsically labelled whole wheat flour of various phytate levels. *Journal of Agriculture and Food Chemistry*. 1994, 42, 2531–2535.

Sandstrom, B.; Almgren, A.; Kivisto, B.; Cederblad, A. Zinc absorption in humans from meals based on rye, barley, oatmeal, triticale, and whole wheat. *Journal of Nutrition*. 1987, 117, 1898–1902.

Schroeter, H.; Williams, R.J.; Matin, R.; Iversen, L.; Rice-Evans, C.A. Phenolic antioxidants attenuate neuronal cell death following uptake of oxidized low-density lipoprotein. *Free Radical Biology and Medicine*. 2000, 29, 1222–1233.

Shahidi, F.; Naczk, M. *Food Phenolics: Sources, Chemistry, Effects, Applications*. Technomic Publishing Company Inc. USA. 1995.

Skrabanja, V.; Kreft, I.; Golob, T.; Modic, M.; Ikeda, S.; Ikeda, K.; Kreft, S.; Bonafaccia, G.; Knapp, M.; Kosmelj, K. Nutrient content in buckwheat milling fractions. *Cereal Chemistry*. 2004, 81, 173–176.

Slavin, J.L. Mechanisms for the impact of whole grain foods on cancer risk. *Journal of the American College of Nutrition*. 2000, 19, 300S–307S.

Smigel, K. Fewer colon polyps found in men with high-fiber, low fat diets. *Journal of the National Cancer Institute*. 1992, 84, 80–81.

Smith, M.M.; Hartley, R.D. Occurrence and nature of ferulic acid substitution of cell wall polysaccharides in gramineous plants. *Carbohydrate Research*. 1983, 118, 65–80.

Sosulski, F.; Krygier, K.; Hogge, L. Free, esterified, and insoluble-bound phenolic acids. 3. Composition of phenolic acids in cereal and potato flours. *Journal of Agriculture and Food Chemistry*. 1982, 30, 337–340.

Spiller, G.A. *Dietary Fiber in Health and Nutrition*. Boca Raton, Florida: C.R.C. Press. 1994.

Sun, J.; Chu, Y.F.; Wu, X.; Liu, R.H. Antioxidant and antiproliferative activities of common fruits. *Journal of Agriculture and Food Chemistry*. 2002, 50, 7449–7454.

Tham, D.M. Potential health benefits of dietary phytoestrogens: A review of the clinical, epidemiological, and mechanistic evidence. *The Journal of Clinical Endocrinology and Metabolism*. 1998, 83, 2223–2235.

Thompson, L.U. Antioxidant and hormone-mediated health benefits of whole grains. *Critical Reviews in Food Science and Nutrition*. 1994, 34, 473–497.

Thompson, L.U.; Robb, P.; Serraino, M.; Cheung, F. Mammalian lignan production from various foods. *Nutrition Cancer*. 1991, 16, 43–52.

Thompson, L.U.; Seidl, M.M.; Rickard, S.E.; Orcheson, L.J.; Fong, H.H. Antitumorigenic effect of a mammalian lignan precursor from flaxseed. *Nutrition and Cancer*. 1996, 26, 159–165.

Topping, D.L.; Clifton, P.M. Short-chain fatty acids and human colonic function: roles of resistant starch and nonstarch polysaccharides. *Physiological Reviews*. 2001, 81, 1031–1064.

Traber, M.G. Vitamin E. In: Shils, M. E.; Olson, J. A.; Shike, M.; Ross, A. C., ed. *Modern Nutrition in Health and Disease*. 10th ed. Baltimore: Williams & Wilkins. 1999, 347–362.

Trombino, S.; Serini, S.; Nicuolo, F.D.; Celleno, L.; Andoa, S.; Picci, N.; Calviello, G.; Palozza, P. Antioxidant effect of ferulic acid in isolated membranes and intact cells: synergistic interactions with alpha-tocopherol, beta-carotene, and ascorbic acid. *Journal of Agriculture and Food Chemistry*. 2004, 52, 2411–2420.

Trowel, H.; Burkitt, D. Physiological role of dietary fiber: a ten year review. *Journal of Dentistry for Children* (Chicago, Illinois.). 1986, 53, 444–447.

Uchida, M.; Nakajin, S.; Toyoshima, S.; Shinoda, M. Antioxidative effect of sesamol and related compounds on lipid peroxididation. *Biological and Pharmacological Bulletin*. 1996, 19, 623–626.

U.S. Department of Agriculture, Department of Health and Human Services. Dietary Guidelines for Americans. Washington, DC: U.S. Government Printing Office. 2000.

U.S.D.A.. Department of Health and Human Services. 2005. Nutrition and Your Health: Dietary Guidelines for Americans. What Are the Relationships between Whole Grain Intake and Health? Washington, D.C http://www.health.gov/dietaryguidelines/dga2005/report/HTML/D6_SelectedFood.htm accessed on 9/16/05.

U.S.D.A., U.S. Department of Health and Human Services, Public Health Service. Office of Disease Prevention and Health Promotion. Healthy People 2010: Volumes I and II. 2000. Washington, D.C: U.S. Government Printing Office.

Uusitupa, M. I; Ruuskanen, E.; Makinen, E. A controlled study on the effect of beta-glucan-rich oat bran on serum lipids in hypercholesterolemic subjects: relation to apolipoprotein E phenotype. *Journal of American College of Nutrition*. 1992, 11, 651–659.

Vanharanta, M.; Voutilainen, S.; Rissanen, T.H.; Adlercreutz, H.; Salonen, J.T. Risk of cardiovascular disease-related and all-cause death according to serum concentrations of enterolactone: Kuopio Ischaemic Heart Disease Risk Factor Study. *Archives of Internal Medicine*. 2003, 163, 1099–1104.

Velioglu, Y.S.; Mazza, G.; Gao, L.; Oomah, B.D. Antioxidants activity and total phenolics in selected fruits, vegetables, and grain products. *Journal of Agriculture and Food Chemistry*. 1998, 46, 4113–4117.

Vinson, J.A.; Hao, Y.; Su, X.; Zubik, L. Phenol antioxidant quantity and quality in foods: Fruits. *Journal of Agriculture and Food Chemistry*. 2001, 49, 5315–5321.

Vinson, J.A.; Hao, Y.; Su, X.; Zubik, L. Phenol antioxidant quantity and quality in foods: vegetables. *Journal of Agriculture and Food Chemistry*. 1998, 46, 3630–3634.

Wakshull, E.; Brunke-Reese, D.; Lindermuth, J. PGG-glucan, a soluble beta-(1,3)-glucan, enhances the oxidative burst response, microbicidal activity, and activates an NF-kappa B-like factor in human PMN: evidence for a glycosphingolipid beta-(1,3)-glucan receptor. *Immunopharmacology*. 1999, 41, 89–107.

Wang, C.; Makela, T.; Hase, T.; Adlercreutz, H.; Kurzer, M.S. Lignans and flavonoids inhibit aromatase enzyme in human preadipocytes. *Journal of Steroid Biochemistry and Molecular Biology*. 1994, 50, 205–212.

Wolk, A.; Manson, J.E.; Stampfer, M.J.; Colditz, G.A.; Hu, F.B.; Speizer, F.E.; Hennekens, C.H.; Willett, W.C. Long-term intake of dietary fiber and decreased risk of coronary heart disease among women. *Journal of the American Medical Association*. 1999, 281, 1998–2004.

Wood, P.J. Physicochemical properties and physiological effects of the (1–3)(1–4)-beta-D-glucan from oats. *Advances in Experimental Medicine and Biology*. 1990, 270, 119–127.

Yang, F.; Basu, T.K.; Ooraikul, B. Studies on germination conditions and antioxidant content of wheat grain. *International Journal of Food Science and Nutrition*. 2001, 52, 319–330.

Yu, L.; Haley, S.; Perret, J.; Harris, M. Comparison of wheat flours grown at different locations for their antioxidant properties. *Food Chemistry*. 2004, 86, 11–16.

Yu, L.; Perret, J.; Harris, M.; Wilson, J.; Haley, S. Antioxidant properties of bran extracts from "Akron" wheat grown at different locations. *Journal of Agriculture and Food Chemistry*. 2003, 51, 1566–1570.

Zhou, J.R.; Erdman, J.W. Phytic acid in health and disease. *Critical Reviews in Food Science and Nutrition*. 1995, 35, 495–508.

Zhou, K.; Laux, J.J.; Yu, L. Comparison of Swiss red wheat grain and fractions for their antioxidant properties. *Journal of Agriculture and Food Chemistry*. 2004, 52, 1118–1123.

Zhou, K.; Yu, L. Antioxidant properties of bran extracts from trego wheat grown at different locations. *Journal of Agriculture and Food Chemistry*. 2004, 52, 1112–1117.

Zielinski, H.; Kozlowska, H. Antioxidant activity and total phenolics in selected cereal grains and their different morphological fractions. *Journal of Agriculture and Food Chemistry*. 2000, 48, 2008–2016.

16 Alkylresorcinols as a Potential Biomarker for Whole Grain Wheat and Rye

Per Åman, Alastair B. Ross, Rikard Landberg, and Afaf Kamal-Eldin

Introduction

Cereal products account for a large portion of the energy and protein intake in the human diet. Most of the grain used for human consumption in the Western world is refined. During processing, the nutritionally important germ and bran are often removed from the white or refined flour (starchy endosperm), thereby depleting many vitamins, minerals and other biologically active constituents (Kris-Etherton et al. 2002). Whole grain products (including the starchy endosperm, germ, and bran), with either intact or milled grains, may lower the risk of chronic diseases (Liu et al. 1999, Hallfrisch and Behall 2000, Murtaugh et al. 2003).

Epidemiological studies strongly suggest a link between consumption of whole grain cereals and decreased risk of heart disease, diabetes, overweight, and certain cancers. However, the mechanisms behind the suggested health benefits are not well established. This is due to the multifactorial nature of diet-related diseases, and relatively low incidences of certain diseases that make it hard to get statistically significant results. This is further compounded by the difficulty that consumers have in identifying whole grain products (Lang and Jebb 2003) and inherent weaknesses of food frequency questionnaires in the estimation of food intake (Kaaks et al. 2002, Bingham et al. 2003)

One of the major obstacles for current epidemiological research on the link between diet and disease is the lack of reliable biomarkers for the intake of specific foods (Asp and Contor 2003). A biomarker of intake can help to overcome some of the problems outlined in the previous paragraph. Dietary biomarkers are compounds that can be measured in a biological sample (e.g. adipose tissue, plasma, or urine) and can be non-subjectively related to the intake of a specific food/food group, which may be linked to a biological activity and/or decreased risk of disease. The use of food intake biomarkers can improve the estimation of food intake because they are independent of errors associated with food frequency questionnaires (Kaaks et al. 2002) which can in turn improve links between diet and disease.

The mammalian lignan enterolactone has been previously proposed to serve as a marker for the intake of plant lignans, including those from whole grain (Johnsen et al. 2004, Bach Kristensen et al. 2005). However, enterolactone lacks specificity because it is produced in the colon from plant lignans present in most non-refined foods, and because it varies in individuals due to their intestinal microflora (Mazur and Adlercreutz 1998). Therefore, there is a need to find new biomarker(s) for the intake of whole grain cereals to link their intake to health effects.

Moreover, there is a great need to select common criteria for how markers should be identified, validated, and used in well-designed studies to explore the links between diet and health. In the past few years, we have started research on alkylresorcinols (A.R.s) and whether they can be used as biomarkers for whole grain wheat and rye. In this chapter we will discuss their structure and occurrence in food; their effect of food processing, intake, absorption and metabolism; and their possible use as a biomarker for whole grain wheat and rye intake.

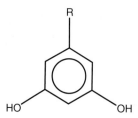

Figure 16.1. Structures and properties of alkylresorcinols (A.R.s) commonly found in cereals.

The Structure of Alkylresorcinols

The structural diversity of alkylresorcinols has recently been reviewed (Kozubek and Tyman 1999). Alkylresorcinols are phenolic lipids with a polar head with two hydroxyl groups and a non-polar hydrocarbon tail. The amphiphilic nature is an important aspect with regard to their analysis, absorption, metabolism, and potential bioactivity. The length of the alkyl tail of A.R.s in cereal grains varies from 15 to 25 carbon atoms (Figure 16.1), but longer side chains also have been suggested (Kozubek and Tyman 1999, Francisco et al. 2005). Normally, the chain is saturated, but unsaturated and oxygenated chain analogues also have been identified. Only about 5% of the A.R.s in wheat have modified alkyl chains, while up to 20% of rye A.R.s are present as unsaturated and/or oxygenated derivatives (Ross et al. 2003a, 2004a). Different A.R. homologues are named according to their chain-length in a similar manner to fatty acids. Therefore, an A.R. with a saturated alkyl chain 17 carbons long is "C17:0."

Concentrations of Alkylresorcinols in Cereals and Cereal Fractions

Quantitative methods for the analysis of A.R.s in cereals include fluorescence measurements, thin layer chromatography, high performance liquid chromatography, gas chromatography, and gas chromatography-mass spectrometry (Gohil et al. 1988). Methods for A.R. analysis have recently been reviewed (Ross et al. 2004b).

A.R.s have been reported to be present exclusively in the outer cuticle of testa in wheat and rye kernels (Tluscik 1978). No A.R.s were found in the pericarp, germ, or starchy endosperm. We recently optimized a gas chromatography method in which A.R.s were extracted with ethyl acetate from intact kernels or milled samples and analyzed by gas chromatography without derivatization with methyl behenate as an internal standard (Ross et al. 2001). A large variation in content (200 μg/gram to 1400 μg/gram) and homologue distribution of A.R.s was found in different *Triticum* species (Table 16.1) (Ross et al. 2003a). *T. compactum* had the highest proportion of shorter chain A.R.s (C15:0 and C17:0) and *T. durum* the highest proportion of longer chains (C23:0 and C25:0). Milling experiments showed that A.R.s were present in the bran and shorts but not in the white flour, providing further evidence that A.R.s are only present in the outer parts of wheat and rye kernels.

The variations in A.R. contents in samples of Swedish wheat (Chen et al. 2004) and rye (Ross et al. 2001) were determined (Figure 16.2). A wide variation in total A.R. content was found for both wheat (230–640 μg/g) and rye (570–1020 μg/g), but the variation in the relative distribution of A.R. homologues was small for both wheat and rye. The dominant A.R.

Table 16.1. Alkylresorcinol homologue composition (relative percentage) and total content (μg/g of D.M.) of *Triticum* species. (Data from Ross et al. 2003a.)

Species	C17:0	C19:0	C21:0	C23:0	C25:0	Total A.R.
T. timophevi	6	28	36	19	11	1480
T. compactum	7	35	42	12	5	1090
T. ispahanicum	N.D.[a]	13	52	23	12	982
T. polonicum	N.D.	9	55	26	10	951
T. paleocolchicum	N.D.	19	53	21	7	916
T. aestivum	6	30	41	19	5	909
T. carthlicum	N.D.	10	55	25	10	876
T. spaerococcum	6	28	50	11	5	862
T. spelta	6	28	43	15	8	819
T. dicoccum	N.D.	20	54	19	8	819
T. dicoccoides	N.D.	13	58	23	6	787
T. orientale	N.D.	9	59	24	8	691
T. durum	N.D.	9	51	27	13	687
T. araraticum	N.D.	11	55	27	8	599
T. turanicum	N.D.	N.D.	74	25	1	200

[a]Not detected (detection limit 5 μg/g)

homologues are C19:0 and C21:0 in wheat and C17:0, C19:0 and C21:0 in rye. In general, it is possible to distinguish between wheat and rye on the basis of the ratio of C17:0 to C21:0, about 0.1 in wheat and about 1.0 in rye. This ratio may be a useful tool to distinguish between the two cereals in cereal foods and maybe biological samples such as plasma as will be discussed below.

Alkylresorcinols as Markers of Whole Grain Wheat and Rye in Cereal Foods

Among plant foods, A.R.s are only found in wheat and rye kernels (Gohil et al. 1988), and in very low levels in barley (Ross et al. 2003a). Mean A.R. content and the ratio of the A.R. homologues C17:0 to C21:0 was analyzed in common Swedish cereal food ingredients (Table 16.2) (Chen et al. 2004). During baking, A.R.s appear to combine with starch, preventing complete extraction by simple methods (Ross et al. 2003a). In cereal products, they can be completely extracted by hot 1-propanol. The A.R. content and C17:0/C21:0 ratio were analyzed in forty-five wheat- and rye-containing food products. The content was well correlated with that calculated from the average content in the cereal ingredients ($R^2 = 0.91$) (Figure 16.3). The ratio of the two A.R. homologues was found to serve as a marker to differentiate wheat food products (ratio approximately = 0.1) from rye food products (ratio ≈ 1.0). Oxidation experiments suggest A.R.s to be stable and resistant to oxidation (Kamal-Eldin et al. 2000). A.R.s also are stable during processing such as cooking and baking (Chen et al. 2004, Ross et al. 2004a, Landberg et al. unpublished results). These results clearly show that A.R.s can be used as markers of whole grain and bran in foods containing wheat and rye and that the C17:0/C21:0 homologue ratio can be used to differentiate between these two cereals in food products.

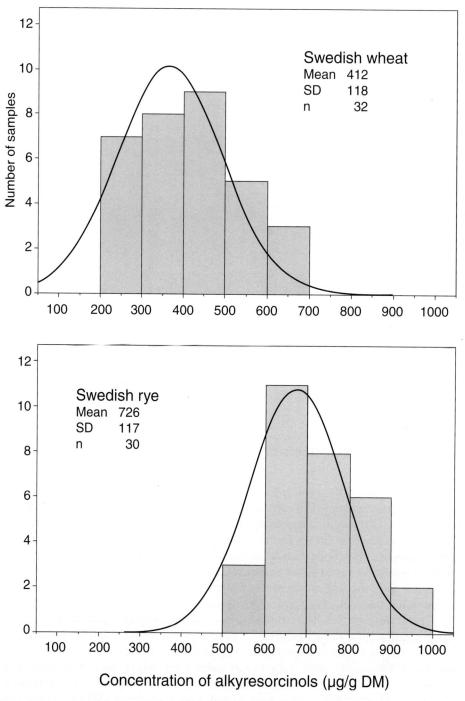

Figure 16.2. Distribution of total alkylresorcinol content in Swedish wheat and rye grain samples. Reproduced from Chen et al. (2004).

Table 16.2. Total alkylresorcinol content (μg/g of D.M.) and ratio of C17:0 to C21:0 alkylresorcinol homologues in Swedish cereal ingredients. (Data from Chen et al. 2004.)

Raw material	n	Total A.R. Mean $\pm$ S.D.	Ratio C17:0/C21:0
Whole grain wheat	32	412 $\pm$ 118	0.1
Whole grain rye	30	726 $\pm$ 117	0.9
Whole grain barley	6	8 $\pm$ 10	0.4
Wheat bran	6	2211 $\pm$ 605	0.1
Rye bran	6	2758 $\pm$ 728	0.9
White wheat flour	6	N.D.[b]	—
Sifted rye flour (100%)	6	99 $\pm$ 35	0.9
Sifted rye flour (40%)[a]	6	37 $\pm$ 15	0.5

[a]Containing sifted wheat flour of higher extraction rate
[b]Not detected (detection limit 5 μg/g)

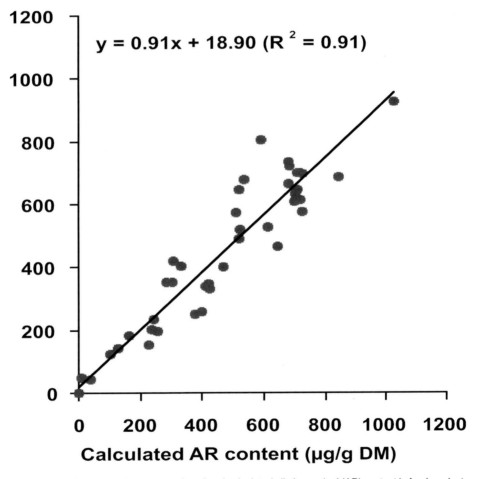

Figure 16.3. Correlation between analyzed and calculated alkylresorcinol (AR) content in food products of Swedish wheat and rye. Reproduced from Chen et al. (2004) with permission from the American Chemical Society.

Absorption and Metabolism of Alkylresorcinols

Absorption and metabolism of A.R.s in humans and animals has been studied. About 60% of the ingested A.R. disappeared from the small intestine of ileostomy-operated humans (Ross et al. 2003b) and 60% to 80% in cannulated pigs (Ross et al. 2003c), indicating that they are readily absorbed. A rat experiment using a radiolabelled A.R. (C21:0) showed that 45% to 55% of the radioactivity was recovered in feces and about 30% in urine in the form of metabolite(s) (Ross et al. 2003c). Small amounts of intact A.R.s (100nmol/L to 300 nmol/L) also have been detected in the plasma of people who eat whole grain rye (Linko et al. 2002). A.R.s, especially the long-chain ones, are present in erythrocyte membranes of humans (Linko and Adlercreutz 2005) and have been detected in the adipose tissues of rats that ate A.R.s (Ross et al. 2004c). The kinetics of A.R.s in the plasma of pigs have been followed (Linko et al. in press). After a single rye-based meal, plasma A.R. concentrations reach a maximum at three hours to four hours, and remain elevated after twelve hours. In the rats fed radiolabelled

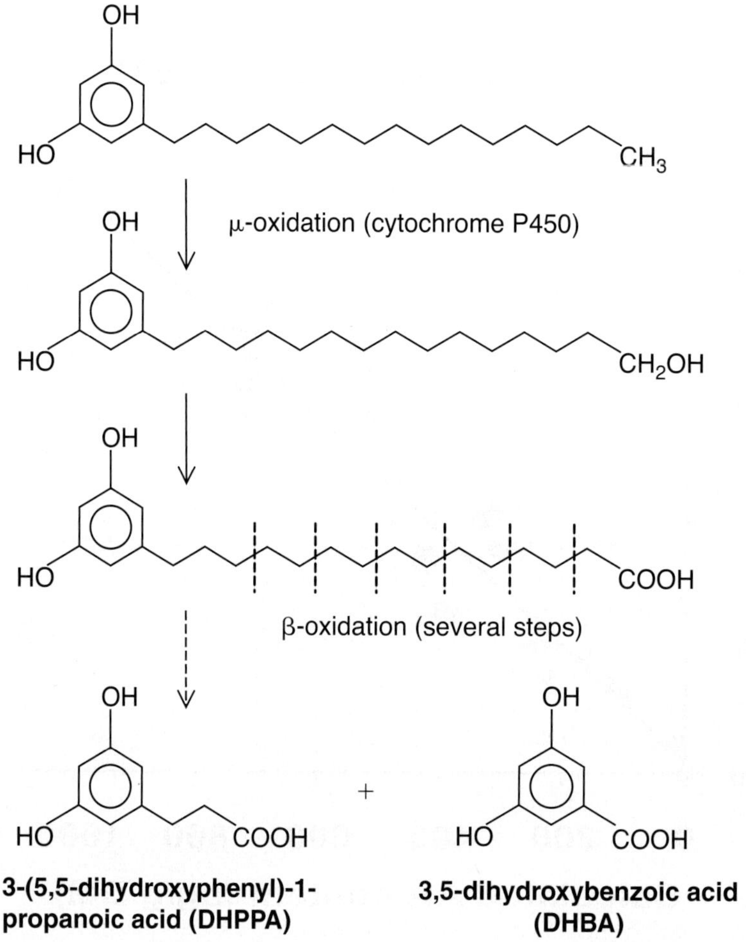

Figure 16.4. Proposed mechanism for the metabolism of alkylresorcinols (Ross et al. 2004a,d). DHBA and DHPPA have been identified in human urine after a wheat bran diet.

C21:0, radioactivity peaked between seven and twelve hours and was mostly cleared from the rats by sixty hours (Ross et al. 2003c).

Two probable urinary metabolites of A.R.s, 3-(3,5-dihydroxyphenyl)-1-propanoic acid (D.H.P.P.A.) and 1,3-dihydroxybenzoic acid (D.H.B.A.) were detected in human urine after consumption of wheat bran (Ross et al. 2004d). The metabolism of A.R.s probably occurs by shortening of the side chain by β-oxidation after ω-hydroxylation in a similar way to tocopherols (McClanahan and Robertson 1984, Birringer et al. 2001) (Figure 16.4). This is backed up by the research showing that rats that ate a diet high in alkylresorcinols had elevated liver and lung γ-tocopherol concentrations, and that rye A.R.s inhibited γ-tocopherol metabolism *in vitro* (Ross et al. 2004c). The resorcinol part of the molecule is presumably not affected by phase 1 enzymes but is converted to glucuronide and sulphate conjugates for excretion in urine (Kim and Matthews 1987, Freudenthal et al. 2000). Future studies using labeled compounds are needed to confirm that these metabolites exclusively come from A.R.s.

Alkylresorcinols as a Potential Biomarker for Whole Grain Wheat and Rye Intake

The important criteria for a useful dietary biomarker include: specificity for the food, presence in the food in amounts and forms that can be easily analyzed, consumption of these foods at levels that allow reasonable intake of the biomarker, reasonable absorption into the body, metabolism to one or a few major metabolites that can easily be analyzed in serum and/or urine, stability of the biomarker during storage of blood and/or urine samples, a plausible dose-response relationship, and a consistent response across studies, etc. (Crews et al. 2001, Weber 2001, Wild et al. 2001). As discussed above, A.R.s are present in food almost exclusively in whole grain wheat and rye and in the bran of these cereals, and methods are available for analyzing A.R.s in cereal fractions and foods.

For a biomarker to be useful it must be consumed in reasonable amounts and be bioavailable to allow quantification in bodily fluids/tissues. The daily intake of A.R.s in the United Kingdom and Sweden was estimated with two different methods (food supply data and food consumption data) and was found in the U.K. to be 12 mg/person/day with both methods, and in Sweden 18 mg/person/day using food supply data and 23 mg/person/day using food consumption data (Ross et al. 2005). Ninety-six percent of all Swedes consumed some A.R.s, compared with only 50% in the U.K. The results show that the intake of A.R.s varies widely both within and between countries and indicate that they may be good markers of diets rich or poor in whole grain wheat and rye products.

Methods for the analysis of intact A.R.s in plasma and erythrocytes by gas chromatography-mass spectrometry are available (Linko et al. 2002, Linko and Adlercreutz 2005) and recently plasma A.R. concentrations were correlated with whole grain bread intake in Finnish women (Linko et al. 2005). However, further studies are needed to develop reliable and simple quantitative methods and to strengthen the possible relationship between intake and concentration in biological samples and to allow rapid analysis of large numbers of samples from clinical and epidemiological studies. A method for the extraction and analysis of the A.R. metabolites, D.H.P.P.A. and D.H.B.A., in blood and/or urine from humans needs to be developed and possible relationships between intake of A.R.s and concentration of metabolites in biological samples from humans need to be established. Possibilities are discussed in the review by Ross et al. (2004b).

Mainly epidemiological studies suggest that whole grains are a major part of a potential dietary prevention of many diet-related diseases, but stronger evidence is needed. A dietary biomarker for whole grain cereals also is needed for investigating the relationship between whole grain cereal intake and health and disease. Due to their stability and specificity for cereal brans, A.R.s are potential biomarkers for whole grain wheat and rye. If this is proven correct, it will open up new possibilities for studying the link between a diet high in whole grains and health. After establishing the methods described above and testing their applicability, human studies will be performed to evaluate the relationship between whole grain rye and wheat intake and levels of A.R.s and their metabolites in blood and/or urine. Blood banks with large numbers of samples can be used to retrospectively establish relationships between the concentration of A.R.s in blood, whole grain intake, and certain diseases. These would provide a powerful tool to help link whole grain wheat and rye intake to proposed health benefits.

References

Asp N-G, and Contor L (2003) Process for the assessment of scientific support for claims on foods (PASSCLAIM): overall introduction. *European Journal of Nutrition.* 42(Supl 1):3–5.

Bingham SA, Luben R, Welch A, Wareham N, Khaw K-T, and Day N (2003) Are imprecise methods obscuring a relation between fat and breast cancer? *Lancet* 362:212–214.

Birringer M, Dragon D, and Brigelius-Floche R (2001) Tocopherols are metabolized in HepG2 cells by side chain Ω-oxidation and consecutive β-oxidation. *Free Radical Biology and Medicine.* 31:226–32.

Chen Y, Ross AB, Åman P, Kamal-Eldin A (2004) Alkylresorcinols as markers of whole grain wheat and rye in cereal products. *Journal of Agricultural and Food Chemistry.* 52:8242–8246.

Crews H, Alink G, Anersen R, Braesco V, Holst B, Maiani G, Oversen L, Scotter M, Solfrizzo M, van den Berg R, Verhagen H and Williamson G (2001) A critical assessment of some biomarker approaches linked with dietary intake. *British Journal of Nutrition.* 86:S5–S35.

Francisco JDC, Danielsson B, Kozubek A and Dey ES. (2005) Extraction of rye bran by supercritical carbon dioxide: influence of temperature CO_2, and cosolvent flow rate. *Journal of Agricultural and Food Chemistry.* In press.

Freudenthal RI, McDonald LJ, Johnson JV, McCormick DL, and Henrich RT (2000) Comparative metabolism and toxicokinetics of ^{14}C-resorcinol bis-diphenylphosphate (RDP) in the rat, mouse and monkey. *International Journal of Toxicology.* 19:233–242.

Gohil S, Pettersson D, Salomonsson A-C, and Åman P (1988) Analysis of alkyl- and alkenylresorcinols in triticale, wheat and rye. *Journal of Agricultural and Food Chemistry.* 45:43–52.

Hallfrisch J, and Behall KM (2000) Mechanisms of the effects of grains on insulin and glucose responses. *Journal of the American College of Nutrition* 19:S320–S325.

Johnsen N, Hauser H, Olsen A, Tetens I, Christensen J, Bach Knudsen KE, Overvad K, and Tjønneland A. (2004) Intake of whole grains and vegetables determines the plasma enterolactone concentration of Danish women. *Journal of Nutrition.* 134:2691–2697.

Kaaks R, Ferrari P, Ciampi A, Plummer M, and Riboli E (2002) Advances in the statistical evaluations and interpretations of dietary data: Uses and limitations of statistical accounting for random error correlations in the validation of dietary questionnaire assessment. *Public Health Nutrition.* 5:969–976.

Kamal-Eldin A, Pouru A, Eliasson C, and Åman P (2000) Alkylresorcinols as antioxidants: hydrogen-donation and peroxyl radical scavenging effects. *Journl of the Science of Food and Agriculture.* 81:353–356.

Kim, YC, and Matthews HB (1987) Comparative metabolism and excretion of resorcinol in male and female F344 rats. *Fundamental and Applied Toxicology.* 9:409–414.

Kozubek A, and Tyman JHP (1999) Resorcinolic lipids, the natural amphiphiles and their biological activity. *Chemical Reviews.* 99:1–26.

Kris-Etherton PM, Hecker KD, Bonanome A, Coval SM, Binkoski AE, Hilpert KF, Griel AE, and Erherton TD. (2002) Bioactive compounds in foods: Their role in prevention of cardiovascular disease and cancer. *American Journal of Medicine.* 113(Suppl. 2):71–88.

Bach Kristensen M, Hels O, and Tetens I. (2005) No change in serum enterolactone levels after eight weeks' intake of rye-bran products in healthy young men. *Scandinavian Journal of Nutrition.* 49:62–67.

Lang R, and Jebb SA (2003) Who consumes whole grains, and how much? *Proceedings of the Nutrition Society.* 62:123–127.

Linko A-M, and Adlercreutz H (2005) Whole grain rye and wheat alkylresorcinols are incorporated into human erythrocyte membranes. *British Journal of Nutrition*. 93:11–13.

Linko A-M, Juntunen KS, Mykkänen HM, and Adlercreutz H (2005) Whole-grain rye bread consumption by women correlates with plasma alkylresorcinols and increases their concentration compared with low-fiber wheat bread. *Journal of Nutrition*. 135:580–583.

Linko A-M, Parikka K, Wähälä K, and Adlercruetz H (2002) Gas chromatographic-mass spectrometric method for the determination of alkylresorcinols in human plasma. *Analytical Biochemistry*. 308:307–313.

Linko A-M, Ross AB, Kamal-Eldin A, Serena A, Bjørnbak Kjær AK, Jørgensen H, Penalvo JL, Adlercreutz H, Åman P, and Bach Knudsen KE. Kinetics of the appearance of cereal alkylresorcinols in pig plasma. *British Journal of Nutrition*. In press.

Liu S, Stampfer MJ, Hu FB, Giovannucci E, Rimm E, Manson JE, Hennekens CH, and Willett WC (1999) Whole-grain consumption and risk of coronary heart disease: results from the Nurses' Health Study. *American Journal of Clinical Nutrition*. 70:412–419.

Mazur W, and Adlercreutz H (1998) Natural and anthropogenic environmental oestrogens: the scientific basis for risk assessment: naturally occurring oestrogens in food. *Pure and Applied Chemistry*. 70:1759–1776.

McClanahan RH, and Robertson, LW (1984) Biotransformation of Olivetol by *Syncephalastrum racemosum*. *Journal of Natural Products* 47:828–834.

Murtaugh MA, Jacobs DR, Jacob B, Steffen L, and Marquart L. (2003) Epidemiological support for the protection of whole grains against diabetes. *Proceedings of the Nutrition Society*. 62:143–149.

Ross AB, Kamal-Eldin A, Jung C, Shepherd MJ, and Åman P (2001) Gas chromatographic analysis of alkylresorcinols in rye (*Secale cereale* L.) grains. *Journal of the Science of Food and Agriculture*. 81:1405–1411.

Ross AB, Shepherd MJ, Schüpphaus M, Sinclair V, Alfaro B, Kamal-Eldin A, and Åman P (2003a) Alkylresorcinols in cereals and cereal products. *Journal of Agricultural and Food Chemistry*. 51:4111–4118.

Ross AB, Kamal-Eldin A, Lundin E, Zhang J-X, Hallmans G, Åman P (2003b) Cereal alkylresorcinols are absorbed by humans. *Journal of Nutrition*. 133:2222–2224.

Ross AB, Shepherd MJ, Bach Knudsen K-E, Glisø LV, Bowey E, Phillips J, Rowland I, Guo Z-X, Massy DJR, Åman P, and Kamal-Eldin A (2003c) Absorption of dietary alkylresorcinols in ileal cannulated pigs and rats. *British Journal of Nutrition*. 90:787–794.

Ross AB, Kamal-Eldin A, and Åman P (2004a) Dietary alkylresorcinols: absorption, bioactivities, and possible use as biomarkers of whole grain wheat and rye rich foods. *Nutrition Reviews*. 62:81–95.

Ross AB, Åman P, Andersson R, and Kamal-Eldin A (2004b) Chromatographic analysis of alkylresorcinols and their metabolites—a review. *J. Chromatography A*. 1054:157–164.

Ross AB, Chen Y, Frank J, Swanson JE, Parker RS, Kozubec A, Lundh T, Vessby B, Åman P, and Kamal-Eldin A (2004c) Cereal alkylresorcinols elevate γ-tocopherols levels in rats and inhibit γ-tocopherol metabolism in vitro. *Journal of Nutrition*. 134:506–510.

Ross AB, Åman P, and Kamal-Eldin A (2004d) Identification of cereal alkylresorcinol metabolites in human urine—potential biomarkers of whole grain wheat and rye intake. *Journal of Chromatography B*. 809:125–130.

Ross AB, Becker W, Chen Y, Kamal-Eldin A and Åman, P. (2005) Intake of alkylresorcinols from wheat and rye in the United Kingdom and Sweden. *British Journal of Nutrition*. In press.

Tluscik F. (1978) Localization of alkylresorcinols in rye and wheat caryopses. *Acta Societatis Botanicorum Poloniae*. 47:211–218.

Weber P (2001) Role of biomarkers in nutritional science and industry—a comment. *British Journal of Nutrition*. 86:S93–S95.

Wild CP, Andersson C, O'Brien NM, Wilson L, and Woods JA (2001) A critical evaluation of the application of biomarkers in epidemiological studies on diet and health. *British Journal of Nutrition*. 86:S37–S53.

17 Resistant Starch as a Contributor to the Health Benefits of Whole Grains

David Topping, Anthony Bird, Shusuke Toden, Michael Conlon, Manny Noakes, Roger King, Gulay Mann, Zhong Yi Li, and Matthew Morell

Introduction

Morbidity and mortality from non-infectious diseases are significant problems in affluent, developed economies, and they include cardiovascular disease (C.V.D.), type 2 diabetes, and colo-rectal cancer (Jemal et al. 2005). Diet and lifestyle are modifiable risk factors for these conditions and prevention is the optimal strategy for lowering their socio-economic impact. The risk of these illnesses is exacerbated by obesity, and there is evidence that they are emerging as serious issues in developing countries through greater affluence with industrialization (Mascie-Taylor and Karim 2003).

Whole grain foods have a great potential to contribute to both the prevention and management of diet-related diseases and obesity. A number of prospective population studies have shown that consumption of whole grain products is associated with lowered risk of C.V.D., colo-rectal cancer, and diabetes (Hill 1999, Jacobs and Gallaher 2004, Truswell 2002). Greater intake of whole grain foods also is associated with lesser obesity (Koh-Banerjee et al. 2004).

This protection is apparently strong and dose-dependent, and the effect remains after correction for potentially confounding lifestyle factors. However, the specific agency in whole grains which mediates the benefits has not been identified. Dietary non-starch polysaccharides (N.S.P.), major components of dietary fiber, are potential contributors; these are generally present at higher levels in whole grain foods compared with refined products. There is good evidence that soluble N.S.P. are effective in lowering plasma cholesterol, an established risk factor for C.V.D. (Lupton and Turner 2003).

However, soluble fiber is found at high concentrations in only a few cereals, notably oats and barley, while others (e.g. wheat and rye) are low in these N.S.P. Further, the range of conditions for which whole grain foods lower risk is very broad, which leads to two plausible hypotheses to account for the observational data. The first is that compared to refined cereal foods, whole grains contain such a complete portfolio of protective agents (phytochemicals, micronutrients, fats, fiber, etc.) that they can protect against diverse targets. This is the "whole grain package" model (Jacobs and Gallaher, 2004). The other hypothesis is that whole grains possess a general characteristic (and not specific components) that offers comprehensive protection.

Both suggestions have merit, but the latter has yet to be examined in detail. We propose that the limited small intestinal digestibility of whole grains (compared with highly refined foods) is the unifying factor. Specifically, we suggest that the lower digestibility of starch in whole grains leads to lowered glycemic responses (G.R.) and greater resistant starch (R.S.).

This combination leads to slower and less small intestinal glucose absorption and the passage of more starch into the large bowel, where it is fermented by the resident bacteria with the production of substantial quantities of metabolites (short-chain fatty acids, S.C.F.A.) with specific health-promoting attributes. Our proposal is supported by a body of human and animal experimental and population data and also by the fact that dietary fiber does not seem to be responsible for the inverse relationship between whole grain consumption and overweight (Koh-Banerjee et al. 2004).

Historical Perspective

Significant community interest in the preventive potential of whole grain cereal foods can be said to have started with the observational studies of Burkitt and colleagues (1973) in East Africa. They noted that the native Africans consumed a diet high in unrefined cereals (principally maize) and were at a much lower risk of the diseases of affluence which affected Europeans living in the same environment but who ate highly refined foods. Although the initial focus was on the diet as a whole, attention became directed specifically on its fiber content, which was assumed to be high relative to that of Europeans.

Without entering into a detailed description of the limitations of the then-current analytical methodology for dietary fiber, it appears likely there were serious underestimates of the fiber content of human foods (Topping and Clifton 2001). The development of improved methodologies with greater specificity and their application to staple African and European foods showed that although the native Africans ate unrefined products, their fiber intakes were actually lower than those of the high-risk Europeans (O'Keefe et al. 1999).

This apparent paradox can be reconciled by two substantial differences between the two populations. The first was that the Africans ate considerably more unrefined starch than the Europeans. The second was that their cooking practices were rather different, especially their habit of eating unrefined starchy foods which had been cooked in water and then cooled and stored for some time. The starch in cooked whole grain foods appears to be digested more slowly (i.e. lower glycemic response or G.R.) and less completely (i.e. higher R.S.) than in comparable refined food (Jenkins et al. 1988). Similarly, starch in whole grain foods has a higher R.S. content than refined foods, as measured by excretion in ileostomists (Livesey et al. 1995). While cooking increases the digestibility of starch and other nutrients, cooling and storage leads to retrogradation of starch and the formation of resistant starch (R.S.). There is good evidence from human studies that this is the case (Ahmed et al. 2000). Thus, it seems possible that this combination (i.e. unrefined and retrograded starch), rather than fiber alone, could contribute to the altered risk profile of this ethnic group through slowing starch digestion.

R.S., Lowered Small Intestinal Starch Digestibility, and Human Health

Humans possess only one intestinal polysaccharidase, α-amylase, which can hydrolyze a single dietary polysaccharide—starch. This enzyme, plus the complement of human small intestinal saccharidases, can degrade starch to glucose, a conversion which can go to completion (at least theoretically). All other food polysaccharides (i.e. N.S.P.) resist small intestinal digestion completely and pass into the large bowel. This resistance helps to explain their fecal bulking capacity and effectiveness as laxating agents. Indeed, there is evidence that fecal bulking per se is an important contributor to the laxative properties of N.S.P. as plastic "bran" flakes (which are quite inert) are as effective as wheat bran in improving laxation (Lewis and Heaton 1997).

The potential for complete hydrolysis of starch to glucose in the small intestine, coupled with the absence of starch in normal human feces, led to the widespread perception that no starch escaped past the ileo-caecal valve into the large bowel. This is despite indirect evidence obtained from breath H_2 evolution patterns of incomplete small intestinal starch digestion in normal humans (Anderson et al. 1981). In fact, it is quite clear that a fraction of starch escapes from the small intestine into the human large bowel. This is R.S., defined as all starch and starch degradation products which resist small intestinal digestion and enter the large bowel in normal humans (Asp 1992).

R.S. is a physiological quantity which occurs for a variety of reasons. These include the rates of transit, particle size of the food, degree of gelatinization and retrogradation, and the presence of other food components (such as N.S.P.). This is reflected in the four main classifications (Brown et al. 1995). $R.S._1$ occurs through the physical inaccessibility of the starch to digestive enzymes, either through partial milling of the grain or the presence N.S.P. in intact cell walls. $R.S._2$ is a result of the ingestion of granular (raw) starches. $R.S._3$ is formed through retrogradation of cooked (i.e. gelatinized) starches on cool storage. The $R.S._4$ classification encompasses the range of chemically modified starches used industrially in processed food manufacture.

Starches acylated with S.C.F.A. recently have found potential use as vehicles to deliver those S.C.F.A. to the large bowel. This approach offers the opportunity to deliver specific S.C.F.A. (plus undigested starch) to the large bowel (Annison et al. 2003).

In terms of modern convenience foods, it seems that processing conditions favor more rapid and complete small intestinal starch digestibility, i.e. high G.R. and low R.S. An in vitro assay for R.S. under development at C.S.I.R.O. Human Nutrition has shown that the R.S. content of processed foods such as French fries, cookies, and white bread is very low indeed (Figure 17.1).

A few processed foods, such as beans, are relatively high in R.S. (Topping et al. 1993), but these seem to be the exception. The reasons for the generally high digestibility of modern foods seem to lie in the use of highly refined starches for product formulation coupled with the extensive degree of starch gelatinization and the absence of retrogradation in modern processing. These data strongly suggest that R.S. intakes in affluent industrialized countries are low and could contribute to their disease risk profile. However, the lack of data on the R.S. content of the full range of R.S. in processed food consumed by low- and high-risk populations is a serious impediment in establishing the true potential contribution of R.S. to health outcomes (Topping and Clifton 2001). Wider application of the validated methodology should help fill this critical gap in knowledge.

One of the more poorly understood relationships in starch digestion is that of R.S. to G.R. R.S. reflects the sum total of starch which escapes small intestinal digestion, while G.R. is a measure of the rate of small intestinal starch hydrolysis. Conventionally, G.R. is expressed as either glycemic index (G.I.) or glycemic load (G.L.). G.I. is the integrated excursion in blood glucose after a test meal against a standard (such as glucose) containing a similar amount of available carbohydrate. The glycemic load concept is being used increasingly as a measure of the impact of any given amount of carbohydrate on blood glucose levels.

However, it must be recognized that G.R. also may have a specific meaning in that it is a measure of the rise in blood glucose after consumption of a particular portion of a given food. This is an attempt to relate actual food consumption to glycemia. Controversy remains as to which index is optimal for dietary management of diabetes (Barclay et al. 2005).

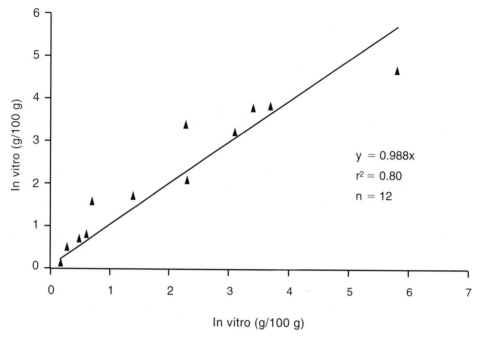

Figure 17.1. The relationship between resistant starch content of a range of convenience foods (including breads, beans, cookies, and cold breakfast cereals) determined *in vivo* in humans with ileostomy and *in vitro*.

There is ambiguity about the relationship between R.S. and G.R. because they both reflect the susceptibility of starch to human small intestinal digestion. However, G.R. is a measure of the rate of glucose release, while R.S. is an index of ileal starch digestibility, i.e. the fraction of starch which remains undigested at the terminal small intestine. Given that a wide range of factors (such as transit) affect R.S., one can postulate that it is possible to have high G.R. (through rapid hydrolysis) and high R.S. (through rapid transit). This point has been made very effectively by Truswell (1992). Nevertheless, it is still true that foods with low G.R. and high R.S. are optimal because they seem to offer the greatest health benefits. Evidence is accumulating from population studies that have shown that diets with low G.R. (expressed as G.L.) are associated with a lower risk of the serious non-infectious diseases found in affluent industrialized societies (Brand-Miller 2003).

N.S.P., R.S., Large Bowel Fermentation, and Human Health

N.S.P. resist human small intestinal digestion completely, but not all N.S.P. are excreted quantitatively in feces (Stephen and Cummings 1980). A fraction, which varies by N.S.P. type, is degraded by the large bowel microflora of normal humans. This breakdown is small for some N.S.P. (such as cellulose) and nearly complete for others (especially water-soluble carbohydrates such as pectin). Large bowel carbohydrate fermentation is affected by a very complex bacterial ecosystem which is numerically large and comprised of several hundred species (or more) (Eckburg et al. 2005). The process is anaerobic and resembles that in the rumen of obligate herbivores and has similar end products. i.e. S.C.F.A., gases (CH_4, H_2 and CO_2), some heat, and more bacteria (Topping and Clifton 2001). The process consumes nitrogen (largely as urea or ammonia) for bacterial protein and nucleotide synthesis. It also provides energy for the host, because more than 90% of S.C.F.A. are absorbed and metabolized by the viscera (McNeil et al. 1978).

The three principal S.C.F.A. (acetate, propionate, and butyrate) have a number of general effects in the colonic lumen. For example, their production lowers digesta pH through their intrinsic acidity and also the consumption of NH_4^+. This is thought to control the overgrowth of potentially pathogenic bacteria and lower the risk of infectious diarrhea. S.C.F.A. absorption is coupled to water and cation absorption, which leads to their salvage. Formerly it was thought the effect was limited to Na^+ and K^+, but it is becoming apparent that there is substantial absorption of Ca^{2+} and Mg^{2+}.

It is thought that one of the S.C.F.A., butyrate, has more specific actions (Brouns et al. 2002, Topping and Clifton 2001). It is believed to be the principal metabolic substrate for normal colonocytes, especially in the distal colon—the site of most organic colonic disease, including cancer. Butyrate is thought to modulate colonic muscular activity with relaxation at lower concentrations and contraction at higher levels. Butyrate also promotes large bowel blood flow through relaxing resistance vessels, improving tissue perfusion. However, it is the potential of butyrate to maintain a normal cell phenotype in colonocytes which has attracted the most interest.

A wealth of experimental data in vitro shows that butyrate inhibits the growth of cancer cells, especially through the induction of apoptosis. Butyrate also stimulates the growth of normal cells and promotes D.N.A. in damaged cells. These actions of butyrate are achieved at concentrations which occur in the colon and there is evidence from animal studies that suggests the acid can promote a normal colonocyte population. However, it must be recognized that demonstration of a direct inhibitory effect of higher butyrate concentrations on human colon carcinogenesis is yet to be obtained. Propionate seems to have many of the beneficial effects of butyrate but at much higher concentrations.

While N.S.P. contribute to fermentation, it appears that these polysaccharides are insufficient to maintain the bacterial microflora and to account for the quantities of S.C.F.A. that they produce. This is the "carbohydrate gap" and it is thought that R.S. fills the deficit (Stephen 1991). As noted above, there is evidence that the native African population studied by Burkitt and colleagues consumed relatively little fiber compared to high-risk Europeans living in the same region. However, the Africans did eat much more starch (as maize corn) and their cooking practices seem to encourage the formation of R.S. in the finished product. Briefly, they cook milled corn in water and then let the porridge cool over a period of time, which would allow retrogradation to occur.

There is evidence that fecal S.C.F.A. were substantially higher in Africans consuming their traditional diet than in whites (Segal et al. 1995). Direct proof that consumption of staled maize porridge raises large bowel S.C.F.A. (including butyrate) comes from a study in which volunteers with a transverse colostomy consumed fresh and stale maize porridge. Excretion of total S.C.F.A. and butyrate were substantially higher when the latter was consumed, compared with the fresh maize (Ahmed et al. 2000). This is a potentially important finding and adds weight to the proposal that R.S. is an important contributor to the health effects of this traditional diet. It also has implications for the relative roles of N.S.P and R.S. in health promotion and suggests that excessive attention may have been given to the former at the expense of R.S.

Whole Grain Starch Digestibility, S.C.F.A., and Energy

There is considerable evidence that the ileal digestibility of whole grains is less than that of refined cereals. Studies in humans with ileostomy have shown greater excretion of starch and other nutrients when whole grains were consumed, compared with refined cereals (Livesey et al. 1995). This lesser digestibility could come from the limited access of starch to amylase through the presence of cell wall material (i.e. $R.S._1$). Jenkins et al. (1988) showed that the G.I. of whole cracked maize and barley was significantly lower than that of milled whole grain; the difference persisted (but was less) when whole grains were milled to a flour.

While there is no direct link between G.I. and R.S., these data support the suggestion of lower starch digestibility in whole grains compared with refined foods. They also suggest that physical accessibility is critical to the lowered starch digestibility of whole grain foods. If this is the case it means that the properties of whole grain foods could be affected by the physical state of the grain and that the presence of whole grain is not necessarily the sole predictor of the health benefits of a food.

Evidence of greater R.S. in whole grain foods comes from animal and human experimentation. Studies in rats fed whole grain wheat flour have shown greater large bowel digesta and S.C.F.A., compared with animals fed refined flour made from the same wheat (Choct et al. 1998). That this difference was not due to gross differences in dietary fiber has been shown in animals fed whole grain barley where large-bowel S.C.F.A. were substantially higher than in those fed fiber (as wheat bran) plus refined starch at equivalent fiber intakes (Bird et al. 2004). Studies with intact humans have shown increased fecal output and S.C.F.A. with whole grain foods compared with refined products (McIntosh et al. 2003).

Some of this increase may be ascribed to the fiber component but fecal butyrate was significantly higher when whole grain rye was consumed, compared with whole grain wheat (Gråsten et al. 2000). R.S. fermentation is thought to favor butyrate production (Weaver et al. 1992), which is consistent with these observations.

The contribution of fiber in determining the digestibility of whole grains has been shown in studies with wheats of different apparent metabolizable energy (A.M.E.). Broiler chickens are reared intensively and the apparent metabolizable energy of the feed is critical to growth performance. Wheats of apparently similar fiber content can have A.M.E. values which differ by 20% to 30% as measured by weight accretion. The discrepancy seems to reside in relatively small differences in the soluble N.S.P. content of the endosperm (Annison 1991).

When rats were fed diets containing whole grain wheats of low- and high-metabolizable energy (as determined in broilers), large bowel digesta and S.C.F.A. were higher with the low A.M.E. wheat (at roughly equivalent N.S.P. intakes). The difference between the two wheats persisted when refined flours were fed to rats. While the absolute digesta mass and cecal S.C.F.A. levels were lower than when whole wheat flours were fed, the values were still significantly higher when rats consumed the flour made from low A.M.E. wheat.

Similar data were obtained with a novel barley cultivar with a single gene modification in one enzyme in the amylopectin synthesis pathway leading to a relatively greater proportion of amylose plus a higher content of N.S.P. Feeding trials with this cultivar have shown relatively higher R.S. and large bowel S.C.F.A. (Bird et al. 2003), indicating that N.S.P. and the altered starch composition could have influenced starch digestibility.

These data have some implications for whole grains and disease risk. R.S. is believed to protect against colo-rectal cancer through its fermentation products. Similarly, R.S. has an intrinsic lower energy value than readily digested starch (Livesey 1990) and also seems to trigger greater fat oxidation in humans consuming it in relatively small quantities (Higgins et al. 2004). This would contribute to whole grain consumption's apparent protection against obesity. It also would explain the relative lack of importance of dietary fiber in health promotion beyond laxation.

The studies with plastic bran indicate that laxation can be effected by fiber without any apparent change in S.C.F.A. This proposition is supported by the studies with psyllium with and without R.S. Volunteers were asked to consume a low-fiber diet and then take supplements (approximately 10 grams/day) either as a psyllium drink or that drink with R.S. (as a high amylose starch). Large bowel S.C.F.A. were raised above a low fiber control only with the psyllium plus R.S. combination (Clifton and Topping unpublished).

R.S., Dietary Protein, and Colo-Rectal Cancer Risk

One of the most promising prospects for whole grains in improving human health lies in the area of colo-rectal cancer. While interventions examining the effects of dietary fiber have proved inconclusive (Schatzkin et al. 2002), a large prospective study European Prospective Investigation into Cancer (E.P.I.C.) is showing a protective effect of dietary fiber against this malignancy (Bingham et al. 2003). The measure of fiber intake in this study was total dietary fiber (T.D.F.), which includes a fraction of R.S. A meta analysis of a number of population studies indicated a negative relationship between starch and calculated R.S. intakes and colo-rectal cancer (Cassidy et al. 1994). This analysis is weakened by the lack of a robust method giving accurate values (as opposed to estimates) of the R.S. content of foods. However, it (together with the wider body of literature) suggests that R.S. could protect against cancer in this viscus.

Experimental support for this proposition is relatively sparse. While there is abundant evidence of a direct inhibitory effect of butyrate on colo-rectal cancer cell lines *in vitro*, there is no direct evidence *in vivo*. Genomic damage is thought to be one prerequisite for carcinogenesis and recently we have shown that R.S. may have the potential to lower this biomarker (Toden et al. 2005a). When rats were fed a diet high in protein, genetic damage in colonocytes measured by the comet assay was increased by more than 100%. This effect was obtained by raising the casein content of a standard experimental diet from 15% to 25% by weight and did not involve treatment with a carcinogen. The increased comet tail moment occurred in a diet containing fiber (as wheat bran) and a highly digestible starch. When the latter was replaced by R.S. as a high amylose maize starch, the genetic damage was completely reversed. The study has been replicated with casein, soy protein, and whey protein, with damage occurring with the former two protein sources but not with whey (Toden et al. 2005b). Again, the damage was abolished by incorporating R.S. in the diet. Genetic damage is thought to be a prerequisite for carcinogenesis, and these studies show that R.S. has the potential to stabilize the colonocyte genome in the face of genotoxic insult.

Conclusions

Perhaps the greatest significance of whole grains lies in their potential to lower the risk of serious diseases when consumed regularly. This potential has emerged from a number of large prospective population studies, but as yet there has been no randomized controlled trial of the effects of whole grain consumption on disease outcome in the general population. It may be that such a trial is unlikely in the foreseeable future for reasons of expense.

Nevertheless, there is considerable evidence that the prospects for primary disease prevention through consumption of whole grain foods are good. Until now, no single component of whole grains has been identified as the protective agency. The central idea of this chapter is that the digestibility of whole grains and whole grain foods is less than that of refined cereal products and that this leads to lower G.R. and higher R.S., and, so, to health benefits. If this proposition is correct, it offers a scope for the quantification of starch digestibility and its potential relationship to risk modification.

It also follows that if starch digestibility is important in R.S., then it is a component that can be manipulated by cultivar selection and processing. This has implications for the consumer, because not all whole grain foods may be equivalent. Further, the fiber content of whole grain foods is the current indicator of the level of whole grain incorporation. This may not be the most appropriate measure of the health benefits of those foods. A measure of small intestinal whole grain food digestibility may need to be developed to gauge their effectiveness.

References

Ahmed R, Segal I, Hassan H (2000) Fermentation of dietary starch in humans. *Am J Gastroenterol* 95:1017–1020.

Anderson IH, Levine AS, Levitt MD (1981) Incomplete absorption of the carbohydrate in an all purpose wheat flour. *New Eng J Med* 304:891–892, 1981.

Annison G (1991) Relationship between the levels of soluble nonstarch polysaccharides and the apparent metabolizable energy of wheats assayed in broiler-chickens *J Ag Food Chem* 39 (7):1252–1256.

Annison G, Illman RJ, Topping DL (2003) Acetylated, propionylated or butyrylated starches raise large bowel short-chain fatty acids preferentially when fed to rats. *J Nutr* 133:3523–3528.

Asp N-G (1992) Resistant starch. *Eur J Clin Nutr* 46: suppl 2, S1.

Barclay AW, Brand-Miller JC, Wolever TM (2005) Glycemic index, glycemic load, and glycemic response are not the same. *Diabetes Care* 28:1839–1840.

Bingham SA, Day NE, Luben R, Ferrari P, Slimani N, Norat T, Clavel-Chapelon F, Kesse E, Nieters A, Boeing H, Tjonneland A, Overvad K, Martinez C, Dorronsoro M, Gonzalez CA, Key TJ, Trichopoulou A, Naska A, Vineis P, Tumino R, Krogh V, Bueno-de-Mesquita HB, Peeters PH, Berglund G, Hallmans G, Lund E, Skeie G, Kaaks R, Riboli E; (2003) European Prospective Investigation into Cancer and Nutrition Dietary fibre in food and protection against colorectal cancer in the European Prospective Investigation into Cancer and Nutrition (E.P.I.C.): an observational study. *Lancet* 361:1496–1501.

Bird AR, Flory C, Davies DA, Usher S, Topping DL (2004) A novel barley cultivar (*Himalaya 292*) with a specific gene mutation in starch synthase IIa raises large bowel starch and short-chain fatty acids in rats. *J Nutr* 134:831–835.

Brand-Miller JC (2003) Glycemic load and chronic disease. *Nutr Rev* 61:S49–S55.

Brown IL, McNaught KJ, Moloney E (1995) *Hi-maize*[TM]: new directions in starch technology and nutrition. *Food Aust* 47:272–275.

Brouns F, Kettlitz B, Arrigoni E (2002) Resistant starch and "the butyrate revolution." *Trends Food Sci Technol* 13:251–261.

Burkitt DP (1973) Some diseases characteristic of western civilization. *Br Med J* 2:274–263.

Cassidy A, Bingham SA, Cummings JH (1994) Starch intake and colo-rectal cancer risk: an international comparison. *Br J Cancer* 69:937–942.

Choct M, Illman RJ, Biebrick DA, Topping DL (1998) White and wholemeal flours from wheats of low and higher apparent metabolisable energy differ in their nutritional effects in rats. *J Nutr* 128:234–238.

Eckburg PB, Bik EM, Bernstein CN, Purdom E, Dethlefsen L, Sargent M, Gill SR, Nelson KE, Relman DA (2005) Diversity of the human intestinal microbial flora. *Science* 308:1635–1638.

Gråsten SM, Juntunen KS, Poutanen KS, Gylling HK, Miettinen TA, Mykkanen HM (2000) Rye bread improves bowel function and decreases the concentrations of some compounds that are putative colon cancer risk markers in middle-aged women and men. *J Nutr* 130:2215–2221.

Higgins JA, Higbee DR, Donahoo WT, Brown IL, Bell ML, Bessesen DH (2004) Resistant starch consumption promotes lipid oxidation. *Nutr Metab* 6:8.

Hill MJ (1999) Mechanisms of diet and colon carcinogenesis. *Eur J Cancer Prev* 8 (suppl 1):S95–S98.

Jacobs DR Jr, Gallaher, DD (2004) Whole grain intake and cardiovascular disease: a review. *Curr Atheroscler* Rep 6:415–423.

Jemal A, Ward E, Hao Y, Thun M (2005) Trends in the leading causes of death in the United States, 1970–2002. *JAMA* 294, 1255–1259.

Jenkins DJA, Jenkins AL, Klamusky J, Giudici S, Wesson V (1988) Wholemeal versus wholegrain breads: proportion of whole or cracked grain and glycaemic response. *Br Med J* 297:958–960.

Koh-Banerjee P, Franz M, Sampson L, Liu S, Jacobs DR jr, Spiegelman D, Willett W, Rimm E (2004) Changes in whole-grain, bran and cereal fiber consumption in relation to 8-y weight gain among men. *Am J Clin Nutr* 80:1237–1245.

Lewis SJ, Heaton KW (1997) The intestinal effects of bran-like plastic particles: is the concept of 'roughage' valid after all? *Eur J Gastroenterol Hepatol* 9:553–557.

Livesey G, Wilkinson JA, Roe M, Faulks R, Clark S, Brown JC, Kennedy H, Elia M (1995) Influence of the physical form of barley grain on the digestion of its starch in the human small intestine and implications for health. *Am J Clin Nutr* 61:75–81.

Lupton JR, Turner ND (2003) Dietary fiber and coronary disease: does the evidence support an association. *Curr Atheroscler Rep* 5:500–505.

Mascie-Taylor CG, Karim E (2003) The burden of chronic disease. *Science* 302:1921–1922.

McIntosh GH, Noakes M, Royle PJ, Foster PR (2003) Whole-grain rye and wheat foods and markers of bowel health in overweight middle-aged men. *Am J Clin Nutr* 77:967–974.

McNeil NI, Cummings JH, James WPT (1978) Short chain fatty acid absorption by the human large intestine. *Gut* 19:819–822.

O'Keefe SJ, Espitalier-Noel G, Owira P (1999) Rarity of colon cancer in Africans is associated with low animal product consumption, not fiber. *Am J Gastroenterol* 94:1373–1380.

Schatzkin A, Lanza E, Corle D, Lance P, Iber F, Caan B, Shike M, Weissfeld J, Burt R, Cooper MR, Kikendall JW, Cahill J (2000) Lack of effect of a low-fat, high-fiber diet on the recurrence of colorectal adenomas. Polyp Prevention Trial Study Group. *N Engl J Med* 342:1149–1155.

Segal I, Hassan H, Walker ARP, Becker P, Braganza J (1995) Fecal short chain fatty acids in South African urban Africans and Whites. *Dis Colon Rectum* 38:732–734.

Stephen AM (1991) Starch and dietary fibre: their physiological and epidemiological interrelationship. *Can J Physiol Pharmacol* 69:116–120.

Stephen AM, Cummings JH (1980) Mechanism of action of dietary fibre in the human colon. *Nature* 284:283–284, 1980.

Toden S, Bird AR, Topping DL, Conlon MA (2005a) Resistant starch attenuates colonic DNA damage induced by high dietary protein in rats. *Nutr Cancer* 51:45–51.

Toden S, Bird AR, Topping DL, Conlon MA (2005b) Differential effects of dietary whey and casein on colonic DNA damage in rats. *Aust J Dairy Technol* 60:146–148.

Topping DL, Clifton PM (2001) Short chain fatty acids and human colonic function—roles of resistant starch and non-starch polysaccharides. *Physiol Rev* 81:1031–1064.

Topping DL, Illman, RJ, Clarke JM, Trimble RP, Jackson KA, Marsono Y (1993) Dietary fat and fiber alter large bowel and portal venous volatile fatty acids and plasma cholesterol but not biliary steroids in pigs. *J Nutr* 123:133–143.

Truswell AS (1992) Glycaemic index of foods. *Eur J Clin Nutr* 46 (suppl 2):S91–S101.

Truswell, AS (2002) Cereal grains and coronary heart disease. *Eur J Clin Nutr*.56:1–14.

Weaver GA, Krause JA, Miller TL, Wolin MJ (1992) Cornstarch fermentation by the colonic microbial community yields more butyrate than does cabbage fermentation; cornstarch fermentation rates correlate negatively with methanogenesis. *Am J Clin Nutr* 55:70–77.

18 Influence of Germination Conditions on the Bioactivity of Rye

Kirsi-Helena Liukkonen, Kati Katina, Anu Kaukovirta-Norja, Anna-Maija Lampi, Susanna Kariluoto, Vieno Piironen, Satu-Maarit Heinonen, Herman Adlercreutz, Anna Nurmi, Juha-Matti Pihlava, and Kaisa Poutanen

Introduction

Whole grains are high in useful macronutrients and dietary fiber as well as vitamins, especially B vitamins, and they are good sources of minerals, particularly the trace minerals (Liukkonen et al. 2005, Lampi et al. 2002). Whole grains are also the source of many phytochemicals, such as phytoestrogens, phenolic compounds, antioxidative compounds, phytic acid, enzyme inhibitors and sterols (Liukkonen et al. 2005, Piironen et al. 2002, Ross et al. 2003). The bioactive compounds of whole grains, as well as those of fruits and berries, are being intensively studied for their protective role in prevention of cardiovascular disease, diabetes, and cancer. These compounds vary widely in chemical structure and function, and therefore many possible mechanisms have been postulated (Willcox et al. 2004; Kris-Etherton et al. 2002; Slavin et al. 1999, 2001).

Rye is an important source of whole grains in Northern and Eastern European diets. The bioactive compounds are concentrated in the germ and the outer layers of the kernel; the outer parts are also the richest in dietary fiber (Lampi et al. 2004, Liukkonen et al. 2003, Piironen et al. 2002, Glitsø and Bach Knudsen 1999, Nilsson et al. 1997).

Phenolic acids and alkylrecorcinols are major phenolic compounds in rye (Liukkonen et al. 2005). Ferulic acid is the most abundant phenolic acid in rye (approximately equal to 85%, Andreasen et al. 2000a,b), and it can covalently link to cell wall polysaccharides and lignin (Faulds and Williamson 1999). A portion of ferulic acid in the cell wall is present as dehydrodimers (Faulds and Williamson 1999). Rye alk(en)ylresorcinols occur as the three major homologs: C17:0 ($\approx$ 24%), C19:0 (approximately equal to 32%), and C21:0 (approximately equal to 24%) (Ross et al. 2003). Matairesinol and secoisolariciresinol were long assumed to be the main plant lignans in rye. Lately, new lignans, pinoresinol, syringaresinol, lariciresinol, and isolariciresinol, have been found, comprising more than 80% of the total lignan content of rye (Heinonen et al. 2001).

Sitosterol is the main sterol in rye (approximately equal to 50%). The other sterols, in decreasing order, are campesterol (15% to 18%), sitostanol (12% to 15%), campestanol (8% to 10%), and sigmasterol (2% to 4%) (Piironen et al. 2002). Rye folates occur as six vitamers formylfolates (5-HCO-H4-folate, 10-HCO-H2-folate, and 10-HCO-folic acid) and 5-CH3H4-folate are the most abundant vitamers. Folic acid and H4-folate are present only in minor amounts (Vahteristo et al. 1999). α- and β-tocopherols and tocotrienols are the major vitamers of vitamin E in rye (Bramley et al. 2000). A less known group of bioactive compounds in rye is benzoxazinoids, which are cyclic hydroxyamine acids.

Malting is a controlled germination process mainly known for barley. However, it also is an interesting way of changing whole grain properties. During germination the biosynthetic potential of grains is taken into use and a number of hydrolytic enzymes are synthesized. They degrade storage macromolecules and allow mobilization of the nutrients in the grains. Moisture, temperature and germination time are the major variables in germination, which is terminated by a drying process. The reactions in germinating grain lead to structural modification (Autio et al. 1998) and development of new compounds, many of which have high bioactivity and can increase the nutritional value and stability of the grains (Kaukovirta-Norja et al. 2004). For example, germinating rye grains for six days at 15°C to 25°C has been shown to lead to two- to 3.5-fold increase in the contents of folates and methanol soluble phenolic compounds (Liukkonen et al. 2003).

The aim of this work was to study the effect of germination temperature, germination time, and drying temperature on the amounts of total phenolics, phenolic acids, alkylresorcinols, lignans, folates, sterols, and benzoxazinoids of rye by using a statistical experimental design and response surface modeling.

Materials and Methods

Large-grained rye Amilo, harvested in summer 2000 in Finland, was used in this study.

Germination

The germination experiments were performed in commercial malting equipment (Joe White Malting Systems, Melbourne, Australia) in darkness at 8°C, 15°C, or 22°C. The grains were steeped for eight hours followed by an air rest of sixteen hours, and a second steep of eight hours (at 8°C), six hours (at 15°C) or four hours (at 22°C). The samples were then germinated at a grain moisture content of approximately 42% to 46%. The total germination time (including steeping) depended on the temperature: seven days at 8°C, five days at 15°C, and three days at 22°C. The samples were dried to a final temperature of 50°C, 75°C or 100°C or freeze-dried. The loosened rootlets were separated from the respective grains and the rootlets and the grains were analyzed separately for the amounts of bioactive compounds.

Analysis of Bioactive Compounds

Sterols were analyzed after acid and alkaline hydrolysis by gas chromatography (GC) (Piironen et al. 2002). Folates were analyzed by a microbiological assay method, including extraction and trienzyme treatment, as described by Kariluoto et al. (2001). Tocopherols and tocotrienols were analyzed after saponification by high-performance liquid chromatography (HPLC) (Ryynänen et al. 2004). Alkylresorcinols (ARs) were analyzed after methanol extraction by HPLC (Mattila, Pihlava, Helström 2005). Benzoxazinoids (Bxs) were analyzed by the same HPLC run as ARs.

Primary identification of the four (and in rootless six) Bxs was done by lc-dad-ms. In the routine work the identification of Bxs were based on their characteristic UV-spectra. Quantitation of Bxs was done at 370 nm with DIMBOA as the reference compound (a gift from Lars P. Christensen, Danish Institute of Agricultural Sciences, Tjele, Denmark). Because the analyzed Bxs UV-absorption maximas differ from that of DIMBOA, the amounts of Bxs is to be considered only as indicative. Phenolic acids were analyzed as free, esterified, glycosylated

Table 18.1. Values of germination condition factors used in experiments of central composite design.

Experiment	Germination time (days)	Germination temperature (°C)	Drying temperature (°C)
1	3	8	50
2	7	8	50
3	3	22	50
4	7	22	50
5	3	8	100
6	7	8	100
7	3	22	100
8	7	22	100
9	3	15	75
10	7	15	75
11	5	8	75
12	5	22	75
13	5	15	50
14	5	15	100
15	5	15	75
16	5	15	75
17	5	15	75
18	5	15	75

and insoluble-bound fractions by HPLC (a modified method based on Hatcher and Kruger 1997, Hertog et al. 1992). In the results, phenolic acids are presented as a sum of free, esterified, glycosylated and bound phenolic acids. Lignans were analyzed with GC-MS. Samples were pretreated by using a modification of the original lignan method earlier published by Mazur et al. (1996). Total phenolics: Methanolic extracts of freeze-dried and ground rye samples were obtained by an ultrasonication-assisted extraction procedure. The residue was further extracted at alkaline conditions. The content of total phenolic compounds (gallic acid equivalents) in methanolic and alkaline extracts was determined using the Folin-Ciocalteu procedure (Singleton and Rossi 1965).

Experimental Design and Statistical Methods

To study the effect of germination conditions on the amount of bioactive compounds in rye, the parameters selected as independent variables were germination time (three to seven days), germination temperature (8°C to 22°C) and final drying temperature (50°C to 100°C). A central composite design was used to arrange the experiments, and four replicates were made at the center point of the design to allow estimation of the pure error at the sum of the square. The experimental design is presented in Table 18.1. Levels of variables were selected on the basis of commonly used ones in real germinations.

The results were analyzed by multiple regression methods (multiple linear regression or partial least squares), which describes the effects of variables in the second-order polynomial models. For each response (amounts of bioactive compounds) a quadratic model was used:

$$Y = \beta_0 + \beta_1 GerTi + \beta_2 GerTe + \beta_3 DryTe + + \beta_{11} GerTi^2 + \beta_{22} GerTe^2 + \beta_{33} DryTe^2$$
$$+ \beta_{12} GerTi*GerTe + \beta_{13} GerTi*DryTe + \beta_{23} GerTe*DryTe + \epsilon$$

This model considered the effects of the variables alone (e.g. germination time), the effects of the interactions between two variables (e.g. germination time $\times$ germination temperature) and quadratic effects of the variables alone (germination time^2). Regression analysis was calculated and the response surfaces were plotted with the Modde 4.0 (Umetrics AB, Umeå, Sweden). The fit of model to the experimental data was given by the coefficient of determination, R^2, which explains the extent of the variance in a modeled variable that can be explained with the model. Each model was validated by calculating predictive power of the model, Q^2, which is a measure of how well the model will predict the responses for a new experimental condition. Large Q^2 indicates that the model has good predictive ability and will have small prediction errors. Q^2 should be greater than 0.5 if conclusions are to be drawn from the model.

Results and Discussion

The rye grains germinated well; after three days, the proportion of germinated grains was 95% to 98% independent of germination temperature. The rootlets comprised 5% to 10% of the total weight of the grains, depending on the germination time. The rootlets were separated from the respective grains for analyses of bioactive compounds.

Bioactivity of Rootlets

In the case of rootlets, the levels of bioactive compounds were analyzed only in selected germination conditions and therefore, response surfaces are not presented for the rootlets. Table 18.2 shows the levels of folates, benzoxazinoids, sterols, tocopherols, and -trienols and alkylresorsinols in rootlets and in respective germinated grains after germination (at 15°C) and subsequent freeze-drying. In rootlets, the level of folates was ten- and nineteen-fold compared to that of respective germinated and ungerminated grains, respectively. The level of benzoxazinoids was twenty-five and forty-two times higher in rootlets than in germinated and ungerminated grains, respectively. The levels of sterols and tocols were 1.5 to four times

Table 18.2. Effect of germination at 15°C on the distribution of folates, benzoxazinoids, sterols, tocopherols and -trienols and alkylresorsinols between the rootlet and the respective grain. (The samples were freeze-dried after germination at 15°C. The loosened germs were separated from the respective grains and analyzed separately for the amounts of bioactive compounds.)

Germination time (d)	Folates μg/100g	Bendoxazinoids mg/100g	Sterols mg/100g	Tocophenols and -trienols mg/100g	Alkylresorcinols mg/100g
Grains					
0	65	6	91	5	109
3	122		92	5	
5	130	10	98	5	57
7	122		102	5	
Rootlets					
3	1255	255	313	12	5
5	1183		257	7	58
7	1239		263	8	

higher in the rootlets than in the grains and there were practically no differences in the levels between germinated and ungerminated grains. Among the studied bioactive compounds, alkylresorcinols were an exception because their concentration decreased during the germination and the concentration was the same in the rootlets and in the grains.

The results show that a remarkable increase in the levels of most bioactive compounds occurs in the rootlets during germination, and therefore, the use of rootlets is highly recommended. On the other hand, high concentrations of phytochemicals in rootlets can cause off-flavors such as bitterness. Therefore, it is important to understand the role of phytochemicals both as bioactive health-related compounds and as flavor-active compounds. Yang et al. (2001) have shown that sprouts formed during germination of wheat grains are very rich in vitamin C, β-carotene, vitamin E, and phenolic acids. They also showed that both high bioactivity and sensory acceptability of rootlets can be obtained by optimization.

Bioactivity of Germinated Grains

Eighteen experiments were performed according to an experimental design. For each response group a quadratic equation was formed with relevant terms ($p < 0.05$) to obtain as high R^2 and Q^2 values as possible. Table 18.3 shows the coefficients of particular models and R^2 and Q^2 values obtained. Based on these equations, the behavior of responses could be predicted within an experimental area and is presented as response surfaces (Figures 18.1-4).

Table 18.3. Effects of factors with significant coefficients in models for amounts of bioactive conditions during germination[a].

Bioactive compound	Regression equations	Effectiveness of fit and predictive power
Total phenolics *Free (after MeOH extraction)	$110.2 + 9.69GerTi + 17.9GerTe$	$R^2 = 0.75$, $Q^2 = 0.56$
*Bound (after alkaline extraction)	$248.5 - 20.18DryTe - 42.80GerTe^2 - 15.47GerTi \times DryTe$	$R^2 = 0.73$, $Q^2 = 0.52$
*Free + Bound	$358.9 + 19.02GerTi + 15.27GerTe - 16.37DryTe - 47.19GerTe^2 - 14.64GerTi*DryTe$	$R^2 = 0.82$, $Q^2 = 0.65$
Phenolic acids	$129.9 + 6.14GerTi + 10.64GerTe - 7.40GerTi^2$	$R^2 = 0.85$, $Q^2 = 0.73$
Lignans	$3.50 + 0.34GerTi + 0.41GerTe$	$R^2 = 0.72$, $Q^2 = 0.57$
Alkylresorcinols	$68.23 - 5.85GerTi - 8.01GerTe + 11.76GerTe^2$	$R^2 = 0.79$, $Q^2 = 0.68$
Folates	$143.7 + 8.06GerTi + 11.00GerTe - 6.36DryTe - 20.68GerTe^2$	$R^2 = 0.87$, $Q^2 = 0.73$
Benzoxazinoids	$18.52 + 1.09GerTi + 2.29GerTe$	$R^2 = 0.71$, $Q^2 = 0.59$
Sterols	$100.7 + 2.15GerTi + 4.67GerTe$	$R^2 = 0.82$, $Q^2 = 0.66$

[a]Only values of significant coefficients are presented (95% confidence level), GerTi = germination time, GerTe = germination temperature, DryTe = drying temperature, GerTi × DryTe = germination time-drying temperature interaction, $GerTe^2$ = quadratic effect of germination temperature, R^2 = measure of fit of the model, Q^2 = predictive power of the model.

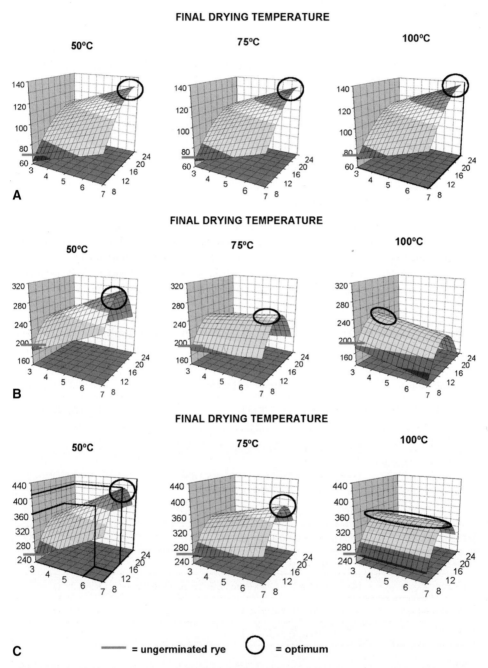

Figure 18.1. Effect of germination conditions on the amount of total phenolics: A. free (free + glyco-sidic + esterified), B. bound, and C. free + bound.

Total Phenolics

In native, ungerminated rye grains, 28% of total phenolics was methanol extractable (free) and the rest (72%) alkaline extractable (bound). Figure 18.1a shows that the level of free phenolics (= methanol extractable fraction) increased linearly as a function of germination time and germination temperature. This could reflect to increased synthesis of phenolics but also to the liberation of bound phenolic compounds from polymeric rye grain structure as a result of germination-induced biochemical reactions. This part of germination remains to be studied.

The germination temperature expressed a quadratic effect on the level of bound phenolics (= alkaline extractable fraction after methanol extraction, Figure 18.1b), which means that the level of bound phenolic compounds was at its highest at a narrow germination temperature area (14°C to 16°C), which was independent of the germination time. Instead, interaction was seen between germination time and final drying temperature, indicating that influence of time was dependent on final drying temperature (Table 18.3; equation for bound phenolics). When the lowest drying temperature (50°C) was used, increasing germination time increased the level of bound phenolics, probably due to their increased extractability in analyses (Figure 18.1b). When the final drying temperature was increased to 75°C or to 100°C, the level of bound phenolics decreased and became practically independent of the germination time, indicating that at higher drying temperatures part of the bound phenolic compounds were destroyed or converted to compounds which could not be detected by the used Folic C method.

For the highest possible level of free phenolics, germination at 22°C for seven days seemed the most optimal (Figure 18.1a). The highest level of total phenolics (free + bound) could be obtained by the seventh day of germination at 14°C to 16°C and subsequent drying to the final temperature of 50°C (Figure 18.1c). In a previous study on another rye variety, Akusti (Liukkonen et al. 2003), we showed a 2.7- and 1.6-fold increase in the relative amounts of free and bound total phenolic of rye, respectively, during germination at 25°C for six days, which is consistent with the current study. In studies with sorghum, both several-fold increase and decrease of total phenolic compounds upon germination has been observed (Dicko et al. 2005, Nwanguma et al. 1996). It is obvious that analysis of total phenolics by the Folic C method is a very crude method, which also may partly explain the different results. The changes of phenolic compounds during grain processing deserve more attention at the level of individual compounds.

Phenolic Acids, Lignans, and Alkylresorcinols

Figure 18.2 shows the effect of the germination conditions on the levels of total phenolic acids, lignans and alkylresorcinols. As the effect of the drying temperature on levels of these phenolic groups was minor (Table 18.3), the response surface plots are only presented for the experiments in which the middle drying temperature of 75°C was used.

The level of phenolic acids increased linearly as a function of increasing germination time and germination temperature until 18°C. At higher germination temperatures (over 18°C), the germination time seemed to have a negatively quadratic effect on the amount of phenolic acids (Figure 18.2).

The level of lignans decreased from that of ungerminated grains when low germination temperature (5°C to 15°C) and short germination time (three to five days) was used, reaching

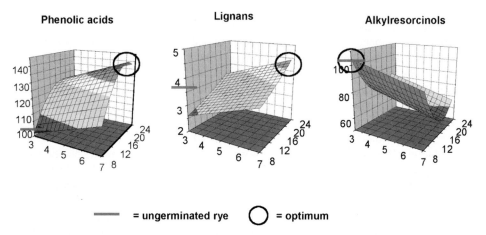

Figure 18.2. Effect of germination conditions on the amount of phenolic acids, lignans, and alkylresorcinols.

the level of ungerminated grains after five days of germination at 15°C. This suggests that lignans are probably converted into other phenolic compounds at low germination temperatures. Above 15°C, the level of lignans increased linearly as a function of germination temperature and time. The highest level of phenolic acids was obtained by six to seven days germination at 18°C, and the highest level of lignans by the seventh day of germination at 22°C.

The levels of alkylresorcinols decreased rapidly during germination. Germination temperature had a quadratic effect on the level of alkylresorcinols so that the loss of alkyresorcinols was at its highest at a temperature range of 14°C to 16°C. The results show that low germination temperature and short germination time are needed to prevent the loss of alkylresorcinols.

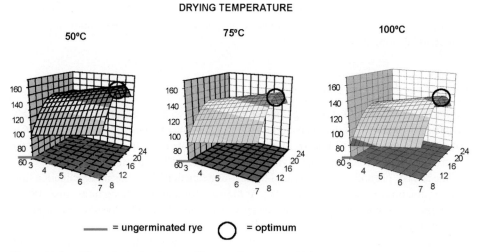

Figure 18.3. Effect of germination conditions on the amount of folates.

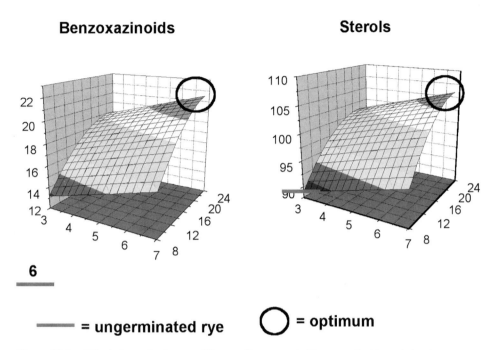

Figure 18.4.   Effect of germination conditions on the amount of benzoxazinoids and sterols.

Folates, Benzoxazinoids and Sterols

Figure 18.3 shows that the germination temperature expressed a strong quadratic effect on the level of folates. The highest concentration of folates was obtained by germinating grains at 14°C to 16°C. Most of the increase in the level of folates took place during the first three days. The same rapid increase of folate level also was recently observed in barley (Jägerstad et al. 2005). As compared to the level of folates in native, ungerminated rye grains, a 2.5-fold increase could be obtained by the germination process. Jägerstad et al. (2005) measured folate contents of industrially malted rye grains and had a range of 140 μg/100 grams to 330 μg/100 grams fresh weight, which is at the same level as in the current study where the highest folate level was about 160 μg/100 grams dry matter.

The amounts of benzoxazinoids and sterols increased linearly as a function of optimum germination time (seven days) and germination temperature (22°C) (Figure 18.4). The highest increase in the level of benzoxazinoids took place during the first three days.

Conclusions

With the exception of alkylresorcinols, the levels of bioactive compounds of rye increased in germination (up to four-fold). Synthesis of folates and benzoxazinoids was induced in rootlets. Germination temperature expressed a quadratic effect on levels of folates and total phenolics, which means that their formation had a clear optimum temperature area (14°C to 16°C), which was independent of the germination time. Increasing the drying temperature from 50°C to 100°C was accompanied by a gradual reduction in the levels of folates and total phenolics.

It was clearly demonstrated that processing cannot only decrease but also increase the levels of the grain constituents that have been suggested to contribute to the health benefits of whole grains. The malting process can be regarded as a pre-treatment of raw cereal material with the aims of modifying the structure, composition, and flavor of the kernel for further processing. A desired combination of valuable properties may be obtained in malted grains by using statistical modeling in the process design. Therefore, malting offers new possibilities for incorporating whole grains into foods such as breads, breakfast cereals, biscuits, and snacks. Furthermore, various malts are used more and more in baking nowadays.

Acknowledgments

The Ministry of Agriculture and Forestry of Finland, the National Technology Agency of Finland (Tekes), Fazer Bakeries Ltd., Vaasan & Vaasan Oy, Raisio Group plc, and Laihian Mallas Oy are gratefully acknowledged for financial support. The research was done as part of the VTT research program "Tailored Technologies for Future Foods."

References

Andreasen MF, Christensen LP, Meyer AS, Hansen Å. 2000a. Ferulic acid dehydrodimers in rye (*Secale cereale L.*). *Journal of Cereal Science* 31:303-307.

Andreasen MF, Christensen LP, Meyer AS, Hansen Å. 2000b. Content of phenolic acids and ferulic acid dehydrodimers in 17 rye (*Secale cereale L.*) varieties. *Journal of Agricultural and Food Chemistry* 48:2837–2842.

Autio K, Fabritius M, Kinnunen A. 1998. Effect of germination and water content on the microstructure and rheological properties of two rye doughs. *Cereal Chemistry* 75:10–14.

Bramley PM, Elmadfa I, Kafatos A, Kelly FJ, Manios Y, Roxborough HE, Schuch W, Sheehy PJA, Wagner KH. 2000. Review Vitamin E. *Journal of the Science of Food and Agriculture* 80:913–938.

Dicko MH, Gruppen H, Traore AS, van Berkel WJH, Voragen AGJ. 2005. Evaluation of the effect of germination on phenolic compounds and antioxidant activities in sorghum varieties. *Journal of Agricultural and Food Chemistry* 53:2581–2588.

Faulds CB, Williamson G. 1999. The role of hydroxycinnamates in the plant cell wall. *Journal of the Science of Food and Agriculture* 79:393–395.

Glitsø LV, Bach Knudsen KE. 1999. Milling of whole grain rye to obtain fractions with different dietary fibre characteristics. *Journal of Cereal Science* 29:89–97.

Hatcher DW, Kruger JE. 1997. Simple phenolic acids in flours prepared from Canadian wheat: Relationship to ash content, colos, and polyphenolic oxidase activity. *Cereal Chemistry* 74:337–343

Heinonen S, Nurmi T, Liukkonen K-H, Poutanen K, Wähälä K, Deyama T, Nishibe S, Adlercreutz H. 2001. *In Vitro* Metabolism of Plant Lignans: New Precursors of Mammalian Lignans Enterolactone and Enterodiol. *Journal of Agricultural and Food Chemistry* 49:3178–3186.

Hertog M, Hollman P, Venema D. 1992. Optimization of quantitative HPLC determination of potentially anticarcinogenic flavonoids in vegetables and fruits. *Journal of Agricultural and Food Chemistry* 40:1591–1598

Jägerstad M, Piironen V, Walker C, Ros G, Carnovale E, Holasova M, Nau H. 2005. Increasing natural folates through bioprocessing and biotechnology. *Trends in Food Science and Technology* 16:298–306.

Kariluoto SM, Vahteristo LT, Piironen VI. 2001. Applicability of microbiological assay and affinity chromatography purification followed by high-performance liquid chromatography (HPLC) in studying folate contents in rye. *Journal of the Science of Food and Agriculture* 81:938–942.

Kaukovirta-Norja A, Wilhelmson A, Poutanen K. 2004. Germination: a means to improve the functionality of oat. *Scandinavian Journal of Agricultural and Food Science* 13:100–112.

Kris-Etherton PM, Hecker KD, Bonanome A, Coval SM, Binkonski AE, Hilpert KF, Griel AM, Etherton TD. 2002. Bioactive compounds in foods: their role in the prevention of cardiovascular disease and cancer. *The American Journal of Medicine* 113:71S–88S.

Lampi AM, Moreau RA, Piironen V, Hicks KB. 2004. Pearling barley and rye to produce phytosterol-rich fractions. *Lipids* 39:783–787.

Lampi AM, Kamal-Eldin A, Piironen V. 2002. Tocopherols and tocotrienols from oil and cereal grains. In: *Functional Foods, Biochemical and Processing Aspects, vol. 2, edited by* J Shi, G Mazza, and M Le Maguer (Eds). pp.1–38. CRC Press LLC. Boca Raton, FL.

Liukkonen KH, Heiniö RL, Salmenkallio M, Autio K, Katina K, Poutanen K. Rye. In *Bakery Products: Science and Technology*, Chapter 5, edited by YH Hui, H Corke, I de Leyn, WK Nip, N. Cross (In press).

Liukkonen KH, Katina K, Wilhelmson A, Myllymäki O, Lampi AM, Kariluoto S, Piironen V, Heinonen SM, Nurmi T, Adlercreutz H, Peltoketo A, Pihlava JM, Hietaniemi V, Poutanen K. 2003. Process-induced changes on bioactive compounds in whole grain rye. *Proceedings of Nutrition* 62:117–122.

Mattila, P., Pihlava, J.-M., Hellström, J. 2005. Contents of phenolic acids, alk(en)ylresorcinols and avenanthramides in commercial grain products. *Journal of Agricultural and Food Chemistry*, In press.

Mazur W, Fotsis T, Wähälä K, Ojala S, Salakka A, Adlercreutz, H. 1996. Isotope dilution gas chromatographic-mass spectrometric method for the determination of isoflavonoids, coumesterol, and lignans in food samples. *Analytical Biochemistry* 233, 169–180.

Nwanguma BC, Eze MO. 1996. Changes in concentration of the phenolic constituents of sorghum during malting and mashing. *Journal of Agricultural and Food Chemistry* 70:162–166.

Nilsson M, Åman P, Härkönen H, Bach Knudsen KE, Mazur W, Adlercreutz H. 1997. Content of nutrients and lignans in roller milled fractions of rye. *Journal of the Science of Food and Agriculture* 73:143–148.

Piironen V, Toivo J, Lampi AM. 2002. Plant sterols in cereals and cereal products. *Cereal Chemistry* 79:148–154.

Poutanen K. 2000. Effect of processing on the properties of dietary fibre. In *Advanced Dietary Fibres,* B, edited by B McCleary, pp. 262–267. London: Blackwell Science.

Ross A, Shepherd MJ, Schupphaus M, Sinclair V, Alfaro B, Kamal-Eldin A, Åman P. 2003. Alkylresorcinols in cereals and cereal products. *Journal of Agricultural and Food Chemistry* 51:4111–4118.

Ryynänen M, Lampi AM, Salo-Väänänen P, Ollilainen V, Piironen V. 2004. A small-scale preparation method with HPLC analysis for determination of tocopherols and tocotrienols in cereals. *Journal of Food Composition Analysis* 17:749–765.

Singleton VL, Rossi JA. 1965. Colorimetry of total phenolics with phosphomolybdic-phosphotungstic acid reagents. *Am J Enol Vitic* 16:144–158.

Slavin JL, Jacobs D, Marquart L, Wiemer K. 2001. The role of whole grains in disease prevention. *Journal of the American Dietetic Association* 101:780–785.

Slavin JL, Martini MC, Jacobs DR, Marquart L. 1999. Plausible mechanisms for the protectiveness of whole grains. *American Journal of Clinical Nutrition* 70:459S–63S.

Vahteristo L, Kariluoto S, Finglas PM. 1999. High folate content in rye and rye products brings additional value to rye as a healthy dietary choice. In *Functional foods—a new challenge for the food chemist. Proc. Euro Food Chem X,* edited by Lasztity R, Pfannhauser W, Simon-Sarkadi L, Tömösközi S, pp. 603–606, Hungary.

Willcox JK, Ash SL, Catignani GL. 2004. Antioxidants and prevention of chronic disease. *Critical Reviews in Food Science and Nutrition* 44:275–295.

Yang F, Basu TK, Ooraikul B. 2001. Studies on germination conditions and antioxidant contents of wheat grain. *International Journal of Food Sciences and Nutrition* 52:319–330.

Part IV

Whole Grains and Consumer and Regulatory Issues

19 Barriers to the Consumption of Whole Grain Foods

Chris J. Seal and Angela R. Jones

Current Whole Grain Consumption Patterns in the U.K.

Data collected from questionnaires which were not specifically designed to quantify whole grain intakes are the basis of causal relationships that have been established between whole grain consumption and a reduced risk of certain diseases. Thus, questionnaires used a limited range of whole grain foods with varying descriptions of those foods. As a result, they may have led to an underestimation and inaccurate measure of whole grain intake.

For example, the use of "dark" bread may not have been interpreted as whole meal bread. Often, reported intakes are based on eating occasions or portions in which estimates of portion size and detail of the whole grain content have been less than ideal.

Despite these limitations, the data universally show that whole grain intakes are extremely low both in the U.S. and the U.K. (Adams and Engstrom 2000, Cleveland et al. 2000, Lang et al. 2003, Jensen et al. 2004). More detailed dietary estimates such at those provided by the National Diet and Nutrition Surveys (N.D.N.S.) in the U.K. give good information on food consumption but still require additional re-analysis to give a more accurate measure of whole grain intake.

We have recently undertaken such analyses which included identifying whole grain foods containing more than 10% whole grain and calculating whole grain content using manufacturer's data and standard recipes. Again, these analyses clearly show that whole grain intakes, at least in the U.K., are not only extremely low but have declined in recent years (Thane et al. 2005a,b). In the most recent N.D.N.S. of British people aged 19 to 64 years (Henderson et al. 2005), 93% of men and 89% of women consumed white bread, whereas only 33% of men and 39% of women consumed whole meal bread. Only 48% of the population surveyed consumed whole grain and high fiber breakfast cereals.

Separately, within the North East of England, data from 827 individuals show that the median intake of whole grains was only 12.3 grams per day; 37% of those studied consumed no whole grains at all; and less than 10% achieved the equivalent of three servings of whole grain per day (Figure 19.1).

Before we can increase consumption of whole grain foods, we must understand why current consumption patterns are so low. This information can then be used to formulate strategies to more effectively communicate the appropriate health messages associated with whole grains.

Methods to Assess Consumer Knowledge about Whole Grains

Investigating the acceptability of and barriers to whole grain foods requires a range of methodologies which can be applied in different groups of individuals. These include people with different demographic variables such as age, gender, and socio-economic background,

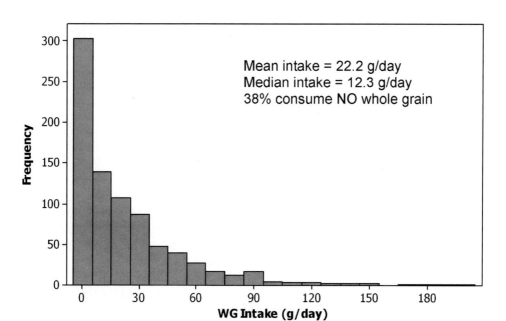

Figure 19.1. Frequency distribution of whole grain (WG) intake in 827 subjects from the North East region of England.

as well as groups with different exposures to whole grain foods. We have adopted a range of techniques based on small focus groups and questionnaires administered within a closed environment and on a wider population-based level.

The level of exposure to whole grain foods is an important factor in the application of these methods. Table 19.1 demonstrates the intimate relationship between these different levels of exposure. It also shows the heterogeneity in potential study groups within the "study" population and underlines that information from all of these groups is essential to develop public health policy.

Table 19.2 shows a number of additional factors, both positive and negative, which the participants may have experienced that would increase whole grain food consumption and further influence the results obtained from these studies. Consideration of these factors suggests that no one single method should be taken in isolation, since each may unwittingly contribute bias to the interpretation of the results.

Table 19.1.   Ranges of exposure to whole grain (WG) foods. Advantages and disadvantages in their use in evaluating acceptability of and barriers to consumption of whole grain foods.

Study group	Advantages to researcher	Disadvantages to researcher
Individuals randomly selected from general population—no specific exposure to whole grain foods prior to subject evaluation/interview	Representative of the 'general population' Will include WG consumers and non-consumers Easy to repeat at different time points and in different geographical locations Can be applied across a range of different research methods, e.g. focus group discussions, large-scale questionnaire use, nutrition studies	Depending on numbers surveyed may not represent all sectors of the population equally, e.g. consumers and non-consumers, demographic variables Requires skilled researcher to facilitate focus group discussions Participants may be biased due to prior interest and knowledge about nutrition and healthy eating
Individuals given advice about healthfulness of whole grain foods, target consumption levels, etc., but not provided with foods	May be representative of the 'general population' Reflects the effect of a 'real' public health strategy to promote whole grain consumption Can be used to test the effectiveness of the public health strategy(ies)	Population may be biased if self selecting for involvement Time scale may be difficult to determine Compliance will be varied, and some marker of intake may be required to characterize the individual May be affected by other external factors, e.g. promotional campaigns
Individuals given a test meal containing whole grain foods on single or multiple occasions	Can investigate the effects of a single meal on hedonic, satiety, nutritional, and wider attitudinal factors Easier to identify likes/dislikes associated with a single meal Possible to control eating environment, portion size, etc.	Possible issues of repeatability and reliability of data Single meal effects may be influenced by previous meal factors which are uncontrolled Artificial environment outside the home may affect results
Individuals provided with test whole grain foods given information on healthy properties of whole grain foods and asked to adopt whole grain foods as part of their diet without constraint	Foods provided can be well characterized and made readily available to the subjects Provision of foods removes the cost and availability barriers Intake of whole grain foods will be very variable between subjects Measures acceptability of selected whole grain foods and barriers associated with the consumption of the selected foods Information can be gathered during the intervention and at specified time points after the intervention	Provision of foods removes the cost and availability barriers Only tests the effects of the specific foods selected if individuals do not seek out other options Foods consumed may be completely different from those provided Compliance may be affected by likes/dislikes of whole grain foods Need a good measure of whole grain intake, preferably with a marker of intake to assess compliance

(*continued*)

Table 19.1. Ranges of exposure to whole grain (WG) foods. Advantages and disadvantages in their use in evaluating acceptability of and barriers to consumption of whole grain foods. (*continued*)

Study group	Advantages to researcher	Disadvantages to researcher
Individuals provided with test whole grain foods and asked to adopt the foods as part of their diet at a fixed level of intake without consuming other whole grain foods. No additional information on the healthfulness of whole grain foods given.	Foods can be well characterized and made readily available to the subjects Provision of foods removes the cost and availability barriers If compliance is good, intake of whole grain foods will not vary between subjects Measures acceptability of selected whole grain foods and barriers associated with the consumption of the selected foods Intake level can be controlled, portion sizes regulated and set in line with recommendations Can measure metabolic consequences of consuming well-characterized whole grain foods at fixed intakes Information can be gathered during the intervention and at specified time points after the intervention	Provision of foods removes the cost and availability barriers Only tests the effects of the specific foods selected and individuals must not seek out other options Compliance must be monitored and individuals encouraged not to exceed target intake Only tests the effects of the specific foods selected if individuals do not seek out other options Whole grain foods selected may contain different grains (e.g. oats, wheat, rye, rice) and hence have very different nutrient compositions Need a good measure of whole-grain intake, preferably with a marker of intake to assess compliance

Table 19.2. Positive and negative factors associated with taking part in whole grain interventions reported by participants (Smith 2004).

Category	Facilitating factors	Barrier factors
Participation in intervention	Focus on individual diet—recognition of need for improvement in diet Prompted other healthful practices, e.g. eating a generally healthier diet, increased fruit and vegetable intake, increased physical activity New awareness of the 'whole grain' concept	
Provision of foods	Opportunity to try new foods Overcome negative preconceptions Assisted variety and compliance Reintroduction to previously eaten products	Choice of foods may have been limiting, subjects became bored with foods
Recommendations/meeting target levels of consumption	Easy to follow	Struggle to consume more than 3 portions daily Compromised intakes of other healthful foods Increased boredom at high intakes

(*continued*)

Table 19.2. Positive and negative factors associated with taking part in whole grain interventions reported by participants (Smith 2004). (*continued*)

Category	Facilitating factors	Barrier factors
Food-specific characteristics	Favorable taste evaluations for many products More filling than refined products 'Righteous' snacking	Unfavourable food characteristics, e.g. dry bread, gluey pasta Taste preferences for refined varieties Increased cooking times: decrease in convenience Difficulty in finding suitable accompaniments Reduced variety and availability compared with refined foods
Perceived health benefits of participating in whole grain intervention	Made diet healthier Important for balanced diet Help protect against disease	Other factors may be more influential in determining health. Diet already high in fiber Incompatible dietary patterns (low consumption levels of cereals or bread) High incidence of reported intestinal discomfort Surprise of healthfulness of sweet-tasting products
Social eating contexts		Limited choice of whole grain options Negative choices and attitudes of family members

Knowledge about Whole Grain Foods

Whole grains have not achieved the same profile within the U.K. as they have within the U.S. Industry advertising has dominated the exposure, and it has focused on breakfast cereals, followed by bread. It is not surprising, therefore, that whole grain consumption is dominated by these products. In the younger age groups there is modest consumption of whole grain biscuits. Nevertheless, the level of consumption of all of these products is low, as discussed above (Lang et al. 2003; Thane et al. 2005a,b).

There are no specific recommendations for whole grain consumption in the U.K. as there are in the U.S. That nation has embraced the importance of these foods in the latest U.S. Department of Agriculture (U.S.D.A.) Dietary Guidelines for Americans 2005 and the "My Pyramid" system (U.S.D.A. 2005). The plate model introduced with the U.K. Balance of Good Health in 1995 (Health Education Authority, 1995) gives a pictorial representation of the proportion of the diet (by weight) of five food groups recommended as part of a balanced healthy diet. Grains are contained within the "bread, other cereals, and potatoes" group and are described as foods which should be eaten "most often." The more recent descriptions (see, for example, Food Standards Agency 2005) advise most people to "eat more starchy foods such as rice, bread, pasta (try to choose whole grain varieties when you can) and potatoes." However, this message is not yet widespread.

It is now accepted that education alone may not be enough to influence purchasing behaviors. However, awareness of an issue must be raised before it can be addressed. Information from the Diet and Health Knowledge Survey (D.H.K.S.) suggested that intake of grain servings was significantly greater for adults who knew how many grain servings were recommended than those who did not. This increase included a significantly greater intake of whole grains than non-whole grains (Kantor et al. 2001). In the same survey, only 7% of consumers were aware that they should consume six to eleven servings daily (Kantor et al. 2001).

We assessed knowledge about whole grains in a 2001 postal survey of 507 subjects from the North East of England (Newcastle upon Tyne) and the North West of England (Chester, Cheshire) (Smith et al. 2001, 2003). The results showed that more people agreed than disagreed with the statement "whole grain products may protect against cancer" (average score 2.81 where 1 = agree strongly, 5 = disagree strongly). They were equally divided on the statement "whole grain products may protect against heart disease" (average score 2.54 on the same scale). The majority, however, disagreed with the statement that "white rice contains more nutrients than brown rice" (average score 4.36 on the same scale), perhaps implying that there is apparently good knowledge of the nutritional differences between the two products. Subjects under the age of 25 scored higher on the statements on disease risk and disagreed less with the statement on the nutrient content of white rice, indicating that knowledge is strongly age-dependent.

In open discussions, subjects often were confused about and unable to describe whole grain foods. When asked to name whole grain foods, subjects correctly identified a range of foods and products, but also confused a number of them, especially cereal products (Table 19.3). Even within the scientific community, there is some conflict in the terminology for whole grains. For example, we have not included wild rice as a whole grain because it is not a

Table 19.3. Foods correctly and incorrectly identified as whole grain foods within seven different focus group sessions.

Correct	Incorrect
Breads	Breads
Whole grain bread	Brown bread
Whole meal bread	
Cereals	Cereals
Shredded wheat*	All bran
Shreddies	Bran cereals
Porridge oats	Kellogg's Special K
Muesli (including named brands)	
Weetabix	
Kellogg's Bran Flakes	
Pasta and rice	Pasta and rice
Brown rice	Brown pasta
Wheat meal/whole meal pasta	Wild rice
Others	Others
Whole grain flour	Pearl barley
	Baked beans
	Pulses
	Brown sugar

*One subject stated that Shredded wheat would be a whole grain if the sugar content was reduced.

member of the Graminaea family, although others have included it in their definition (Cleveland et al. 2000). In botanical terms, maize/corn also is not a "grain." It has not been included in our estimates of whole grain intake when reported as "sweet corn" or "corn on the cob" because in the N.D.N.S. these were coded as vegetables rather than grains (Thane et al. 2005b). It is, however, included in U.S. data (Harnack et al. 2003). Corn and corn-based products were not identified among the list of whole grain foods named by subjects in our studies, perhaps reflecting the smaller contribution of corn-based products to the U.K. diet compared with that of the U.S.

When discussing whole grain foods, the concept of "wholeness" is most commonly associated with phrases such as "brown," "whole grain has the husk on," "nothing taken out of it," and "having the seed coat on the outside as well as the inside." For some individuals, nutrition knowledge is related to whole grain and may extend to include "fiber," "carbohydrate," and general references to healthiness, but when probed, this knowledge is often superficial. Identification of whole grain products is generally through the terms "whole grain" or "whole meal" on food packaging and the whole grain logo present on specific cereal products.

Barriers to Consumption of Whole Grain Foods

A number of other factors, apart from the lack of knowledge of whole grain foods described above, have been identified as influencing the consumption of these products, (Figure 19.2). Taste is a critical factor for all food selection, and adverse taste experiences or expectations can deter choice. For many subjects, whole grain foods were given negative descriptions: ". . . just the taste . . . wholegrain rice was just, I don't know, strange . . ." (younger female), "just find (whole meal bread) dry and a bit tasteless" (younger male), and "I've had whole meal spaghetti . . . it's kind of chewier".

Wardle (1993) examined the relationship between health and taste appraisal and food consumption frequency among family members, and showed that taste index was consistently higher than health index. Thus, food choice appears to be determined by considerations of

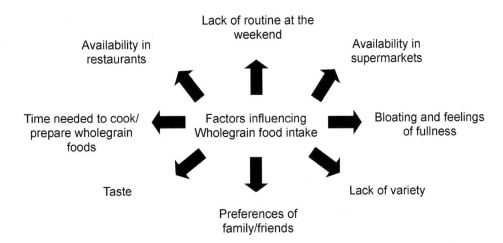

Figure 19.2. Summary of factors identified as affecting consumption of whole grain foods.

taste rather than health, and is a consistent finding in our studies. For whole grain foods, the health message is not yet strong enough to overcome preconceived taste ideals. The food industry must, therefore, develop new products with improved taste, texture, and appearance characteristics to tempt consumers into this market.

Technological improvements for preparing whole grain products also are important. Many consumers found cooking whole grain alternatives more difficult. For instance, "The pasta (shapes)—I didn't like that at all. But I did say to you that I hadn't cooked it very well—it was the only one I had actually microwaved rather than boiled, according to the instructions, but it came out kinda mushy and not very nice. I don't know what it would have been like if I had boiled it."

This also impacts on the time it takes to prepare meals; whole grain alternatives often take longer to cook and require more care in preparation. Some comments: "You gave us two types of rice and one took a lot longer to cook than the other, so if I was going to the supermarket, because I'm pushed for time a lot of the time, I would actually choose based on what's the quickest to cook rather than what's the best." Modern consumers expect products that are quick and easy to prepare, and can be direct substitutions for refined products. Consumers complain that they need to make pasta sauces more flavorful to mask the stronger taste associated with whole grain pasta: "I have no problem with rice, but with whole meal pasta we've yet to find a sauce which makes it tasty. That was one thing where it was a struggle to eat. It was difficult because it definitely tasted different from usual pasta. We tried to cook it for longer and not as long and no matter what you do there was still a texture to it that we couldn't even disguise with a sauce."

Two other principle barriers to consumption of whole grain foods are cost and availability. Almost without exception, whole grain foods are more expensive than the refined grain option in U.K. supermarkets; in some cases there can be a two-fold difference between refined and whole grain versions of a product sitting on the same supermarket shelf. Although this price differential is declining, for many consumers this still represents a considerable barrier to their use. Whole grain products are not displayed prominently on supermarket shelves; brown rice is usually on lower shelves, with less brand choice, and can only be purchased in small bags. This often exaggerates the cost differential against supermarket brands and the much-larger economy bags.

Some consumers take issue with the reduced availability and variety of whole grain products, which compromises the extent to which whole grains can be introduced to the diet without feelings of restriction or monotony. This is often cited as the main reason for poor compliance in the studies in which we asked volunteers to increase their whole grain intake above three portions per day. Availability of whole grain foods outside the home also is an issue. With the possible exception of health-food or vegetarian restaurants, whole grain ingredients are rare on menus, and family and friends may not have embraced their use. For example, "eating out or eating at friends you know most people just wouldn't have brown pasta. So even in a restaurant you'd struggle to find a whole meal—unless it was maybe a very good vegetarian restaurant"; "No chance of getting whole meal rice in a curry house."

The influence of the family and social context of eating also affects food choice (for a British and European perspective, Lennernas et al. 1997; Roos et al. 1998, Stratton and Bromley 1999). The dominant factors affecting food choice at the family level are whether the food is acceptable to other family members (i.e. is it enjoyable and/or will it be eaten): "we don't have a lot of control over everything that we eat because other people have a part to play in what we eat"; "I know for a fact they'll (children) push it (brown rice) away; they won't even try it so if I bought it I think it would be a total waste of money." As a result, nutrition issues generally are a low priority (Lappalainen et al. 1997).

Reasons for Consuming Whole Grain Foods

The reasons for consuming whole grain foods are complex and depend strongly on knowledge of their health benefits. Often these are associated with perceptions of the degree of processing of whole grain foods, even though this may not be true: "It means that the grain has not been heavily processed" (older male); "Fiber . . . very low additives I think . . ." (younger male). When prompted, many individuals suggest that whole grain foods may aid digestion and prevent the development of bowel diseases. This is further related to their higher fiber content and their ability to act as "natural laxatives": "I don't think I was aware of 'whole grain' as a concept, I was aware of fiber."

Very few individuals cite the ability of whole grain foods to reduce heart disease, despite this being the main thrust of some high profile cereal advertisement campaigns. The imagery of these campaigns is often recalled, i.e. the names of the celebrities in advertisements are remembered but the "message" behind the advertisement is often not. One participant, however, did recall, "It's supposed to lower your cholesterol . . . because (names celebrity)'s on the telly doing adverts for it."

Not surprisingly, for the U.K. subjects in our studies, there was no knowledge of any form of dietary recommendations for whole grain foods. When prompted further and asked to comment on the U.S. recommendation to consume "three servings per day" there was confusion about the difference between "servings" and "portions," and how these could be translated into dietary amounts. However, in the context of the interventions, once the concept of the portion and serving were explained and the target level of intake established, most participants were able to embrace the concepts. In our interventions we have stressed the "substitution" of whole grain varieties for refined varieties and this proved a successful strategy: "the nicest bit was that it didn't actually disrupt your normal day's routine and it wasn't a change in lifestyle, really; it was just an adaptation of what you were currently doing."

Eating Whole Grain Foods Can be a Positive Experience

Providing specific foods in intervention studies or taste sessions facilitates the testing of new foods and eliminates personal "risks" to the participants, such as waste associated with purchasing unfamiliar products, and other potential barriers to consumption, such as cost and availability. We also found that it enables participants to overcome negative taste preconceptions and helps them comply with intervention recommendations: "I would have found it much harder because of preconceptions about the foods. So I would have had it in my head, 'oh, my husband hates brown rice, I can't buy that; the kids won't eat brown bread.' But because the things you gave us, we had them, so we tried them and discovered that they would eat them."

Many volunteers taking part in intervention studies continue to consume the whole grain foods after the study has ended and the supply of the sample foods has ceased. Six months post-intervention, the volunteers also recall health-related messages given at the start of the intervention period, as shown in Table 19.4, clearly demonstrating greater awareness of the health benefits of whole grain foods. This suggests that health messages associated with whole grain foods, if delivered effectively, can be effective.

Table 19.4. Various belief and attitude statements on whole grains and their importance in whole grain food selection for males and females (n = 16) six months post-intervention.

Statement My main reasons for eating wholegrain foods are:	Mean score*
I didn't eat enough whole grain foods before	1.8
They are healthier for me/my family	1.2
They taste good	2.2
They are not expensive	2.9
They are convenient	2.9
My partner/family likes them	2.8
Whole grains are important for a balanced diet	1.2
They fill me up better than refined products	1.8
Including whole grains has improved my diet	1.6
I didn't eat enough fiber before	2.4
They are more nutritious than refined products	1.7
They will help protect me from developing heart disease and certain cancers	1.3

*1 = Agree strongly; 2 = agree slightly; 3 = neither agree/disagree; 4 = disagree slightly; 5 = disagree strongly.

Promoting Whole Grain Consumption

It is clear that the message about whole grains' health benefits is not being transmitted to consumers effectively. Communication of many nutrition messages to the public has often been unsuccessful, but recent campaigns such as 'Five-a-day' in the U.K. and U.S. (Department of Health 2005, U.S. Department of Health and Human Services 2005) to promote increased fruit and vegetable consumption have become widely recognized. According to Schwartz (1994), healthy eating messages should have the following attributes to be effective: a positive message, simplicity, practicality, flexibility, and consistency. There is a particular need to standardize terminology for "portions" and "servings" and agreement is necessary on the quantities of whole grain required for beneficial effects. This information, which must be related in a consumer-friendly way, can then be incorporated on food packaging and labels within the legislative framework which currently exists.

For any health promotion strategy to be successful it must also address the needs and aspirations of the target audience; it must reflect their current knowledge, attitudes, and behaviors (Barker et al. 1995). Consumers must be motivated to change; they must perceive personal consequences from undertaking (i.e. reduced risk of disease) or not undertaking (i.e. no improvement in risk) change. Our experience shows that, not surprisingly, these factors vary widely across different population groups, and therefore different approaches will be required if food intakes are to change for the population as a whole.

It is essential that industry be involved in the development of new whole grain products, which meet the criteria for health claims in the U.S. and across Europe, to increase market penetration and awareness. It is important to create an environment in which consumers can implement dietary change which is cost-effective and does not negatively affect time and effort. This could be particularly valuable for products targeted at children, who might then develop lifelong whole grain-eating habits (outside whole grain breakfast cereals).

Adoption of the "whole grain message" by health professionals also is important; Chase et al. (2003) recently reported a surprising lack of knowledge and self efficacy for dietitians in their ability to help clients to consume more whole grains. Although the sample response rate was relatively low in this study (39% of those mailed were returned), and therefore the results may not be representative of the profession as a whole, these results suggest an urgent need for additional training for health care professionals. To our knowledge there are no comparable data for the profession in the U.K., but such information would be useful before initiating new policies.

Promoting whole grain consumption in a positive light represents a change in philosophy from the negative connotations associated with some health promotion strategies aimed at changing diet. For example, the emphasis on *reducing* fat, *reducing* cholesterol, and *avoiding* high fat has negative associations with diet and implications of denial and removal. In contrast, emphasis on *increasing* consumption of whole grain foods, *substituting* for refined products, and *enhancing* health invokes positive associations which may be more successful in the longer term in achieving the required dietary change.

Acknowledgements

The authors acknowledge the funding for this work from the Biotechnology and Biological Sciences Research Council, the Food Standards Agency, Nestlé U.K. Ltd., and Cereal Partners U.K. The views expressed in this article are those of the authors alone.

References

Adams JF and Engstrom A (2000) Dietary intake of whole grain vs. recommendations. *Cereal Foods World* 45, 75–78.

Barker ME, Thompson KA and McClean SI (1995) Attitudinal dimensions of food choice and nutrient intake. *British Journal of Nutrition* 74, 649–659.

Chase K, Reicks M and Jones JM (2003) Applying the theory of planned behavior to promotion of whole-grain foods by dietitians. *Journal of the American Dietetic Association* 103, 1639–1642.

Cleveland LE, Moshfegh AJ, Albertson AM and Goldman JD (2000) Dietary intake of whole grains. *Journal of the American College of Nutrition* 19, 331S–338S.

Department of Health (2005) Just Eat More (fruit and veg). http://www.5aday.nhs.uk/. Date accessed: October, 2005

Food Standards Agency (2005) Eat well, be well. Helping you make healthier choices. http://www.eatwell.gov.uk/. Date accessed: 01.10.05, 2005

Harnack L, Walters SAH and Jacobs DR (2003) Dietary intake and food sources of whole grains among U.S. children and adolescents: Data from the 1994-1996 Continuing Survey of Food Intakes by Individuals. *Journal of the American Dietetic Association* 103, 1015–1019.

Health Education Authority (1995) *Enjoy Healthy Eating, The Balance of Good Health*. London: H.E.A.

Henderson L, Gregory J and Swan G (2005) *The National Diet and Nutrition Survey: Adults Aged 19 to 64 Years. Types and Quantities of Food Consumed*. London: The Stationery Office.

Jensen MK, Koh-Banerjee P, Hu FB, Franz M, Sampson L, Gronbaek M and Rimm EB (2004) Intakes of whole grains, bran, and germ and the risk of coronary heart disease in men. *American Journal of Clinical Nutrition* 80, 1492–1499.

Kantor LS, Variyam JN, Allshouse JE, Putnam JJ and Bing-Hwan L (2001) Choose a variety of grains daily, especially whole grains: A challenge for consumers. *Journal of Nutrition* 131, 473S–486S.

Lang R, Thane CW, Bolton-Smith C and Jebb SA (2003) Consumption of whole grain foods by British adults: findings from further analysis of two national dietary surveys. *Public Health Nutrition* 6, 479–484.

Lappalainen R, Saba A, Holm L, Mykkanen H and Gibney MJ (1997) Difficulties in trying to eat healthier: descriptive analysis of perceived barriers for healthy eating. *European Journal of Clinical Nutrition* 51, S36–S40.

Lennernas M, Fjellstrom C, Becker W, Giachetti I, Schmitt A, deWinter AMR and Kearney M (1997) Influences on food choice perceived to be important by nationally-representative samples of adults in the European Union. *European Journal of Clinical Nutrition* 51, S8–S15.

Roos E, Lahelma E, Virtanen M, Prattala R and Pietinen P (1998) Gender, socioeconomic status and family status as determinants of food behaviour. *Social Science and Medicine* 46, 1519–1529.

Schwartz NE (1994) Narrowing the gap—practical strategies for increasing whole grain consumption. *Critical Reviews in Food Science and Nutrition* 34, 513–516.

Smith A (2004) Sociological and dietary responses to the consumption of low-fat and wholegrain foods. Ph.D., University of Newcastle.

Smith AT, Kuznesof S, Richardson DP and Seal CJ (2003) Behavioural, attitudinal and dietary responses to the consumption of wholegrain foods. *Proceedings of the Nutrition Society* 62, 455–467.

Smith S, Smith A, Richardson DP and Seal CJ (2001) Regional variations in consumer knowledge and purchasing of whole grain foods. *Proceedings of the Nutrition Society* 60, (OCB) 218A.

Stratton P and Bromley K (1999) Families' accounts of the causal processes in food choice. *Appetite* 33, 89-108.

Thane CW, Jones AR, Stephen AM, Seal CJ and Jebb SA (2005a) Secular trends in whole-grain intake and sources of British adults. *Proceedings of the Nutrition Society* 64, In press.

Thane CW, Jones AR, Stephen AM, Seal CJ and Jebb SA (2005b) Whole-grain intake of British young people aged 4-18 years. *British Journal of Nutrition* 94, 825–831.

U.S. Department of Agriculture (2005) My Pyramid. http://www.mypyramid.gov/. Date accessed: August, 2005

U.S. Department of Health and Human Services (2005) Eat 5 to 9 a Day for Better Health. http://www.5aday.gov/. Date accessed: October, 2005

Wardle J (1993) Food choices and health evaluation. *Psychology and Health* 8, 65–75.1

20 Consumer Acceptance of Refined and Whole Wheat Breads

Alyssa Bakke, Zata Vickers, Len Marquart, and Sara Sjoberg

Introduction

The preceding chapters have clearly shown that whole grain consumption and, more specifically, whole grain bread consumption is much less than the consumption of refined breads. Other chapters have examined some of the many factors that may explain the failure of people to eat more bread made from whole grains. The goal of this chapter is to examine in more depth the relative liking of whole wheat bread and refined wheat breads. In other words, do people prefer refined wheat bread to whole wheat bread? We compare liking ratings of whole wheat and white breads from several questionnaire studies and from the very few published taste test studies we could find. Then we present results of three recent taste tests conducted at the University of Minnesota comparing whole wheat and refined wheat breads.

Questionnaire Liking Ratings

Peryam et al. (1960), in their examination of food preferences of men in the United States Armed Forces, showed that white bread was preferred to whole wheat bread with scores of 7.7 and 6.8, respectively on a nine-point hedonic scale (1 = dislike extremely and 9 = like extremely). The survey was repeated eight times between 1950 and 1954, with more than 4,000 men taking the survey at each occasion. Soldiers preferred white bread to 89% of the foods surveyed, while they preferred whole wheat bread to 59% of the other foods surveyed. Taste preferences change over time, so these data may no longer apply to current consumers. The data also are limited to adult males in the U.S. Armed Forces, so they may not be applicable to more diverse populations. However, their more general comment—that the best-liked foods, such as white bread, on average were liked by nearly everyone, whereas everyone did not, on average, dislike the least liked foods—is likely still true today.

Vickers et al. (1981) measured food preferences in a relatively older consumer population of cancer patients and age-matched controls (40 to 75 years). Their 205 subjects (controls) significantly preferred whole wheat bread to white bread (scores of 2.5 for whole wheat and 3 for white bread on a 9 point hedonic scale with 1 = like extremely and 9 = dislike extremely). These data show the opposite trend to that observed by Peryam et al. (1960), and like the Peryam study, may only apply to the relatively specific population included in the study at that time.

In a more recent study with children, Berg et al. (2003) studied bread choices of 181 children. They asked the children to use pictures to construct three breakfasts: their usual breakfast, a tasty breakfast, and a healthy breakfast. The bread pictures, listed in order of increasing fiber content, included: white bread, a combination rye and white bread, rye bread, and crisp bread. Children's tasty breakfasts contained breads with less fiber than their usual breakfasts, which in turn contained breads with less fiber than their healthy breakfasts. Sixty-eight percent of the breads in the tasty breakfasts were white breads. Although this study included rye breads and not whole wheat breads, it supports the hypothesis that refined white breads are preferred by children.

These three studies suggest that younger consumers may generally prefer white breads to whole wheat breads, while the opposite may be true of older consumers. All three population groups had reasonably large percentages of subjects, even if not the majority, that preferred each type of bread. This reinforces the observation of Peryam et al. (1960) that relatively more disliked foods still have reasonably large groups of likers.

Taste Tests—Published Studies

Questionnaire data often does not predict liking ratings of actual food products when they are tasted (Cardello and Maller 1982). So we next searched the literature for taste tests comparing liking of refined and whole wheat breads. We were surprised at the dearth of information available on this topic in contrast to widespread assumptions (perhaps based on well-documented consumption data) that people like whole wheat breads less than white breads.

Mialon et al. (2002) had 79 Chinese Malaysian and 82 Australian consumers (mean ages of the two ethnic groups were 19.3 and 18.5, respectively) rate their expected liking and actual liking of white and whole meal breads. The Australian consumers expected to like and actually did like the white bread better than the whole wheat bread. The Malaysian consumers exhibited the same pattern of liking; actual liking was significantly greater for white breads than the whole wheat breads, but their expected liking was not significantly different.

King et al. (1937) conducted taste tests to determine the influence of flour grade on bread preference. They examined the preferences of 96 adults for bread made from three flours: 85% extraction patent flour, 70% extraction patent flour, and straight grade flour. Their judges ranked bread samples made from the three flours as best, intermediate, or poorest based first on the bread odor, and then again based on the bread taste. Their judges preferred 85% extraction patent flour over both 70% extraction patent flour and straight grade flour on the basis of both taste and odor. That study did not directly address preference between whole wheat bread and refined white bread, but it showed that a higher extraction flour, which would include more of the bran and germ fractions of the grain, was preferred to 70% extraction patent flour and straight grade flours, which would contain less of those fractions and more starchy endosperm.

Ludkow et al. (2004) examined whether children preferred whole wheat bread made from a white wheat variety to whole wheat bread made from a red wheat variety. One hundred thirty children rated both their visual and taste preferences between the two breads. To rate visual preference, children rated their liking on a seven-point facial hedonic scale anchored from "super bad" to "super good." Forty-five percent of the children preferred the appearance of the white whole wheat bread, 17% preferred the appearance of the red whole wheat bread, and 38% of the children had no visual preference. Children then tasted the bread and rated their liking on the same scale. Forty-eight percent of the children preferred the white whole wheat bread, 27% preferred the red whole wheat bread, and 25% had no taste preference.

Taste Tests—Recent University of Minnesota Studies

Because of the lack of information available in the literature, we have conducted a series of three studies examining consumer preferences between refined and whole wheat breads.

Study #1

In this study our objective was to examine liking of breads containing different levels (100%, 50%, 25%, 0%) of whole wheat flour. A local artisan bakery prepared all the breads, including two made with 0% whole wheat flour: one with caramel coloring added to mimic the color of the 100% whole wheat bread ("brown bread") and one without coloring added ("white bread"). We had 103 subjects rate their overall liking, flavor liking, texture liking, and appearance liking of all five breads on nine-point hedonic scales.

We observed a trend of increased liking with increased whole wheat flour content. Judges preferred the 100% whole wheat bread to the white, the brown, and the 25% whole wheat bread (Figure 20.1). Other liking differences were not statistically significant.

In response to an accompanying questionnaire, 23% percent of the consumers in the study classified themselves as white bread likers; the remaining 77% preferred some other listed type of bread (wheat, whole wheat, or cracked wheat). When we separated the judges into two groups, those who preferred white bread and those who preferred any of the other types of breads, we observed no product by preference interaction. The white bread likers also preferred the 100% whole wheat bread to the white bread.

We think the increasing preference for increasing amounts of whole wheat in these breads was due to the increasing amount of honey added as the amount of whole wheat flour increased. Because the amount of honey (and the sweetness, softness, and suppression of bitterness it imparts to bread) was completely confounded with the amount of whole wheat flour, we could not determine if the liking increased due to the whole wheat flour or the honey.

Study #2

In our second study we compared the liking of whole wheat breads made from whole white wheat flour and whole red wheat flour. Four of the breads formed a 2×2 factorial design (two white wheat vs. two red wheat and two laboratory made vs. two commercial). The fifth was a commercial refined flour white bread. The five breads in the study included: a whole white wheat bread and a whole red wheat bread (both made in a laboratory according to American Association of Cereal Chemists (A.A.C.C.) International Approved Method 10-10B Optimized Straight-Dough Bread-Baking Method), commercial samples of a whole white wheat bread (Natural Ovens[TM]), a whole red wheat bread (Cub[TM]), and the refined flour white bread (Cub[TM]).

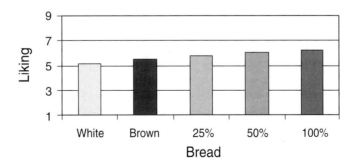

Figure 20.1. Liking ratings from 103 subjects for breads of varying (0%, 25%, 50%, and 100%) whole wheat content. The white bread contained 0% whole wheat flour. The brown bread also contained 0% whole-wheat flour, but it had added caramel coloring.

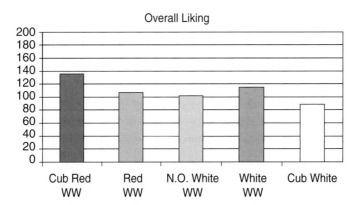

Figure 20.2. Liking ratings from 107 subjects for the five breads in study #2. From left to right the breads are: Cub[TM] red whole wheat, laboratory made red whole wheat, Natural Ovens[TM] white whole wheat, laboratory made white whole wheat, and Cub[TM] refined white bread. Ratings are on a 200-point labeled affective magnitude scale where 200 = greatest like imaginable, 100 = neutral, and 0 = greatest dislike imaginable.

One-hundred-seven subjects rated their overall liking, flavor liking, texture liking, and appearance liking of all five breads on labeled affective magnitude (L.A.M.) scales (Schutz and Cardello 2001). Prior to the test, subjects were given a definition of whole wheat bread and asked to indicate whether they preferred whole wheat bread or white bread. Sixteen subjects preferred white bread; the remaining ninety-one subjects preferred whole wheat bread.

Our subjects gave their highest ratings to the commercial red whole wheat bread, followed by our laboratory white whole wheat bread. Our laboratory red whole wheat bread and the commercial white whole wheat bread were less well liked. The commercial refined white

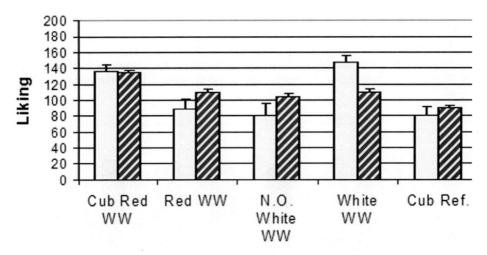

Figure 20.3. Liking scores from study #2 broken down by subjects' preferences for white or 100% whole wheat breads. Plain light bars represent those preferring white bread; striped bars represent those preferring 100% whole wheat bread. From left to right the breads are: Cub[TM] red whole wheat, laboratory made red whole wheat, Natural Ovens[TM] white whole wheat, laboratory made white whole wheat, and Cub[TM] refined white bread. Ratings are on a 200-point labeled affective magnitude scale where 200 = greatest like imaginable, 100 = neutral, and 0 = greatest dislike imaginable.

bread was the least liked product (Figure 20.2). The overall liking pattern between the breads seemed to mirror that of the flavor liking pattern, while the texture liking and appearance liking patterns were quite different, possibly indicating that flavor was the most important factor in overall bread liking.

When we divided the subjects into those who preferred white bread and those who preferred whole wheat bread, and then examined the liking responses of those two groups, the subjects who preferred white bread liked the laboratory samples of whole white wheat breads significantly better and the laboratory samples of whole red wheat breads significantly less than those who preferred whole wheat bread (Figure 20.3). No other differences between the two subject groups were observed.

Study #3

Our third study sought to measure consumer liking for several whole wheat and refined white breads. This study focused on the following four separate comparisons between whole wheat and white breads:

1. Laboratory-prepared loaves of a whole red wheat bread and a refined red wheat bread plus an additional laboratory sample of whole red wheat bread with added sodium stearyl lactylate (S.S.L.). The addition of the S.S.L. produced a whole wheat bread with a loaf volume equal to that of the refined red wheat bread.
2. Laboratory prepared loaves of a whole white wheat bread and a refined white wheat bread
3. The top-selling (according to Nielsen ratings) whole wheat bread and white bread for the Twin Cities area
4. A high-quality whole wheat bread and white bread obtained from a local artisan bakery (Breadsmith^{TM})

The laboratory samples in group 1 and group 2 were prepared using A.A.C.C. International Method 10-10B Optimized Straight-Dough Bread-Baking Method and commercially available flours. We chose breads in groups 3 and 4 to be representative samples of breads available locally to subjects in our study.

Eighty-nine subjects rated their overall liking, flavor liking, texture liking, and appearance liking of all nine breads on L.A.M. scales. After the taste test, we asked subjects if they preferred whole wheat bread or white bread. Twenty-nine percent preferred white bread, 65% preferred whole wheat bread, and 6% provided no response.

Subjects that preferred white bread and those that preferred whole wheat liked the refined breads made in the laboratory (groups 1 and 2) better than the whole wheat breads made in the laboratory (Figure 20.4). The size of this difference in liking was greater for people preferring white bread. We observed no difference in preference for white wheat vs. red wheat for either group of subjects. People who preferred white bread liked the artisan white bread better than the artisan whole wheat bread, and the "best selling" white bread better than the "best selling" whole wheat bread. Conversely, people who preferred whole wheat bread generally liked the artisan whole wheat bread better than the artisan white bread, and showed a trend toward preferring the "best selling" whole wheat bread to the 'best selling' white bread.

We compared the pattern of liking scores for overall liking with the patterns of scores for flavor liking, texture liking, and appearance liking. The pattern for flavor liking was nearly identical with the pattern for overall liking (Figure 20.5). Thus, flavor is likely a very important factor driving the overall liking of these breads.

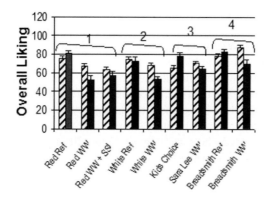

Figure 20.4. Liking ratings of the nine bread samples broken into the four groups described in the text. Solid bars represent subjects who preferred white breads (29% of the 89 subjects); striped bars represent subjects who preferred whole wheat breads (65% of subjects). Error bars represent standard errors. From left to right the breads are: hard red refined, hard red whole wheat, hard red whole wheat plus sodium stearyl lactylate, hard white refined, hard white whole wheat, Kids Choice[TM], the best selling local refined wheat bread, Sara Lee[TM] 100% whole wheat—the best selling local whole wheat bread, Breadsmith[TM] refined, and Breadsmith[TM] 100% whole wheat. Ratings were on a 120-point labeled affective magnitude scale where 120 = greatest like imaginable, 60 = neutral, and 0 = greatest dislike imaginable.

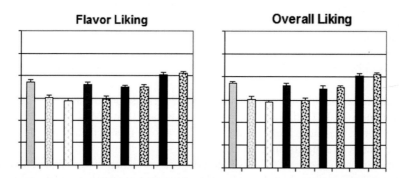

Figure 20.5. A comparison of the overall liking and flavor liking scores (ordinates) for the nine bread samples in study #3. From left to right the breads are: hard red refined, hard red whole wheat, hard red whole wheat plus sodium stearyl lactylate, hard white refined, hard white whole wheat, Kids Choice[TM], the best selling local refined wheat bread, Sara Lee[TM] 100% whole wheat—the best selling local whole wheat bread, Breadsmith[TM] refined, and Breadsmith[TM] 100% whole wheat. Each bar represents the mean score from all 89 participants.

Summary

Both questionnaire and taste test data generally show that white bread is preferred to whole wheat bread, especially by young people. Our results suggest that the liking of these breads is more strongly influenced by their flavor than by their texture or appearance. In spite of this general preference, sizable proportions of people find both types of bread equally acceptable or actually prefer the whole wheat bread. Bread made from 100% whole wheat can be modified so people who say they prefer whole wheat breads like it equally as well as white breads.

We need more research on the acceptability of breads over their shelf lives and under different usage conditions (e.g. plain, in sandwiches with specific fillings, as toast with specific toppings, etc.). We also need more research on the acceptability of breads for children and the acceptability and healthiness of whole wheat breads modified to increase their acceptability to children.

Acknowledgements

We thank Betsy Brenny and Samantha Tucker for their technical help conducting these studies. This research has been supported in part by the Minnesota Agricultural Experiment Station and the Sensory Center in the Department of Food Science and Nutrition at the University of Minnesota.

References

Berg, C., Jonsson, I., Conner, M., and Lissner, L. (2003) Perceptions and reasons for choice of fat- and fibre-Containing Foods by Swedish schoolchildren. *Appetite* 40, 61–67.

Cardello, A.V., and Maller, O. (1982) Relationships between food preferences and food acceptance ratings. *J. Food Sci.* 47, 1553–1557, 1561, 1982.

King, F.B., Coleman, D.A., and LeClerc, J.A. (1937) Report of the U.S. Department of Agriculture Bread Flavor Committee. *Cereal Chem* 14, 49–58.

Mialon, V.S., Clark, M.R., Leppard, P.I., and Cox, D.N. (2002) The effect of dietary fibre information on consumer responses to breads and "English" muffins: A cross-cultural study. *Food Quality and Preference* 13, 1–12.

Peryam, D.R. (1960) Food preferences of men in the U.S. Armed Forces (Chicago: Dept. of the Army, Quartermaster Research and Engineering Command, Quartermaster Food and Container Institute for the Armed Forces).

Schutz, H.G., and Cardello, A.V. (2001) A labeled affective magnitude (L.A.M.) scale for assessing food liking/disliking. *J. Sens. Stud.* 16, 117–160.

Vickers, Z., Nielsen, S.S., and Theologides, A. (1981) Food preferences of patients with cancer. *Journal of the American Dietetic Association* 79, 441–445.

21 The Whole Grain Stamp Program

Jeff Dahlberg, K. Dun Gifford, and Cynthia W. Harriman

An Urgent Consumer Need Spawns a Universal Packaging Symbol

When the legendary Ancel Keys (1959) wrote *Eat Well, Stay Well*, nutritionists were just beginning to suspect that whole grains might offer health advantages over enriched flour. Keys wrote,

> Enriched flours have added thiamine as well as riboflavin, niacin, and iron, approaching whole-wheat flour in these respects. But other ingredients are removed from the wheat when it is refined; possibly enriched white flour is not actually the full nutritional equivalent of the natural grain.

Yet over the next four decades, even as the evidence for eating whole grains was solidly documented by nutrition scientists, consumers made only miniscule increases toward eating more whole grains. According to U.S. Department of Agriculture disappearance data (2004), whole grains constituted 0.5% of our calorie intake in 1972, and 1.4% of intake in 1999.

Knowledgeable experts attributed this, in large part, to consumers' difficulty in identifying whole grain products. Even those who were convinced of the benefits of whole grains found themselves confused and overwhelmed by misleading packaging claims in the bread and cereal aisles and throughout supermarkets.

Formation of the Whole Grains Council and Initial Goals

In April of 2002, Oldways Preservation Trust, a non-profit organization known for its effective work in translating nutrition science into consumer-friendly health-promotion tools, held a Whole Grains Summit in San Diego, California. At this event, Oldways issued a whole grains challenge to consumers: "For one week, eat whole grains each morning, as cereal, as toast or as a roll" and then "notice whether you still crave your mid-morning coffee-break snack."

Also at this conference, scientists, chefs, and industry leaders joined together to explore the idea of helping consumers more readily identify whole grains through a universal packaging symbol. This call was echoed a year later in the *Proceedings of the Nutrition Society* by leading grain researchers collaborating in an article entitled "Whole Grain Health Claims in the U.S.A. and Other Efforts to Increase Whole Grain Consumption." According to Marquart et al. (2003), the authors stated,

> There is a need to develop a "consumer-friendly" whole grain definition so that consumers can easily identify what is a whole grain product. In addition, a universal on-package whole grain identifier would be useful, such as a seal, logo, or insignia to readily signify whole grain products. It cannot be hoped to successfully educate, market, and increase whole grain consumption until consumers can identify whole grain foods.

By mid-summer of 2003, Oldways had organized a consortium called the Whole Grains Council (W.G.C.) to carry on the work started at the San Diego summit. The group held its first formal meeting that July and, in the course of the following twelve months, assembled a strong group of twenty-five founding members—large companies and small ones, ingredient suppliers and packaged-goods producers, private corporations and commodity associations. These twenty-five industry pioneers were:

American Institute of Baking
Arrowhead Mills
Barbara's Bakery
Bob's Red Mill
Campbell Soup
Farmer Direct Foods
Fleischmann's Yeast
Frito-Lay
General Mills
Hodgson Mill
King Arthur Flour
Lesaffre Yeast
Lotus Foods
Montana Flour & Grains/Kamut Assn.
National Grain Sorghum Producers
Natural Ovens
Nature's Path
Oldways Preservation Trust
Panera Bread
Roman Meal Company
Rudi's Organic Bakery
Snyder's of Hanover
Sorghum Partners
Sunnyland Mills
U.S.A. Rice Federation

Consensus on a Consumer-Friendly Definition of Whole Grains

The Whole Grains Council set as its first two goals (1) establishing a consumer-friendly consensus definition of whole grains, and (2) creating a universal packaging symbol for foods delivering a significant dietary level of whole grains. Neither goal could exist without the other; it is impossible to denote foods containing whole grains without defining "whole grains," and it is an empty gesture to define whole grains but then provide no mechanism for consumers to take action in finding them.

Through a careful process of industry collaboration, the Council crafted a whole grains definition based on the American Association of Cereal Chemist's (A.A.C.C.) widely-accepted definition, but adapted it to be understandable to consumers rather than scientists alone; in short, to meet the goal of being consumer-friendly. The end result (W.G.C. 2004), which was posted for feedback on the A.A.C.C. Web site and later endorsed at a Whole Grains Council meeting in Chicago in May 2004, reads:

> Whole grains or foods made from them contain all the essential parts and naturally-occurring nutrients of the entire grain seed. If the grain has been processed (e.g., cracked, crushed, rolled, extruded, lightly pearled and/or cooked), the food product should deliver approximately the same rich balance of nutrients that are found in the original grain seed.
>
> Examples of generally accepted whole grain foods and flours are: Amaranth, Barley (lightly pearled), Brown and Colored Rice, Buckwheat, Bulgur, Corn and Whole Cornmeal, Emmer, Farro, Grano (lightly pearled wheat), Kamut^{TM} grain, Millet, Oatmeal and Whole Oats, Popcorn, Quinoa, Sorghum, Spelt, Triticale, Whole Rye, Whole or Cracked Wheat, Wheat Berries, and Wild Rice.

The Need for a Whole Grains Packaging Symbol

While work was going forward on the definition, the council forged ahead in creating the whole grains packaging symbol so urgently needed by consumers. Aware that the final result would need widespread support across all segments of the industry and from government to be successful, the Whole Grains Council explored a wide range of options.

After consultation and discussion, the council determined that the packaging symbol should have these attributes:

1. It should identify products with significant dietary levels of whole grains, while differentiating between various levels of whole grain content, to help consumers make a gradual transition to the nuttier, fuller taste of whole grains.
2. It should clearly say "whole grain" with its graphics—even to those not familiar with the symbol—and be simple but eye-catching.
3. It should be easy for manufacturers to put on packaging—economical to print, and reproducible through all common printing methods.

The first point was especially important. Although the U.S. Food and Drug Administration (F.D.A.) had already authorized whole grain health claims for foods, these packaging claims have several limitations: To be eligible for the claims, foods must contain at least 51% whole grain ingredients by weight. Because moisture is factored into total weight, foods such as bread—which averages 40% moisture—can only reach this standard with great difficulty. Eligibility is determined by a "fiber proxy." Only foods containing 11% fiber, the amount found in wheat, can use the claim.

This means that a bag of brown rice cannot carry the whole grains health claim, because rice contains only 3.5% fiber by weight. Other whole grains, such as millet (8.5% fiber), quinoa (5.9% fiber), and whole cornmeal (7.3% fiber) also would not qualify. Finally, a words-only health claim, without a graphic symbol, is not easy for consumers to recognize as they rush down cluttered grocery aisles.

The Whole Grains Council felt strongly that increased consumption of whole grains would happen only if packaging could highlight foods in all food categories, made from all varieties of whole grains. It also was important to the council that its symbol encourage "transition foods"—foods that may not be made entirely with whole grains but that nonetheless contribute significantly to consumers' diets. Just as consumers moved gradually from whole milk to skim milk by choosing 2% and 1% milk in turn, most consumers can best start their transition from refined grains to whole grains by having clear choices for foods that are made in part—but not entirely—with whole grains. In doing so, however, they need to be assured that their choices contain meaningful amounts of whole grains.

Consumer, Industry, and Government Input

The Whole Grains Council spent a year, beginning in October 2003, mocking up rough graphics to refine a successful system of content levels. Portland-based Koopman-Ostbo Inc. offered early graphic support, and once a system was adopted by the members, in October 2004, graphic artist Susan Godel translated the council's concept into a finished, professional design.

Early concepts (Figure 21.1) featured percents, stars, and gauges to differentiate between levels of whole grain content. Several options were explored before the Council settled on the best approach.

In January and February of 2004, the Council carried out consumer interviews in three geographic areas of the country (New Hampshire, Minnesota, and California) to get broad-based input on what would constitute a successful seal. In almost 500 interviews with supermarket shoppers, the majority reacted positively to mockups of the symbol on a cracker box, with comments such as these:

> The symbol looks like it is official so I would trust it.

> I've been eating a lot of whole grains lately so this product would catch my attention.

> I don't really know much about whole grains but the crackers look good so I just might try it.

> It looks like a good product and the label makes me think the crackers are healthy foods.

> I'd be more likely to buy that—I've been trying to eat whole grains. They're better for my heart.

> A logo would be a faster way to find whole grain products.

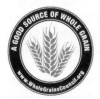 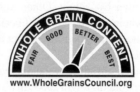 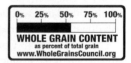

Figure 21.1. Early concepts for a universal whole grain packaging symbol took many different approaches, before the "stamp" design was finally chosen.

This research indicated that an attractive, easy-to-understand symbol would attract both current consumers of whole grains and those who were not yet eating whole grains. With this largely-positive feedback from "the trenches," the council continued to work with members to fine-tune the development of its whole grain packaging symbol.

At this point, one important element was missing in the symbol's development. Although the council had firm direction from consumers and from its members, it did not yet have guidance from the U.S. government. At the January meeting of the Dietary Guidelines Advisory Committee (D.G.A.C.), in Washington, D.C., Joanne Slavin, Ph.D., a scientific advisor to the Whole Grains Council, testified on the health benefits of whole grains and on the need for a consistent and universal whole grain packaging seal. A transcript of the meeting (D.G.A.C. 2005) reports, "Dr. Slavin stressed that it is important to help consumers understand what whole grains are and where they can be found. The best way to find whole grain products is to read the ingredients label. A whole grains seal or a whole grain health claim on the package can be helpful, but different companies use them in different ways."

In May 2004, General Mills, which had recently joined the Whole Grains Council to further the group's efforts, filed a Citizen's Petition with the F.D.A. to establish descriptor claims for whole grains. This petition (F.D.A. Docket 2004P-0223) proposed an industry standardization of packaging descriptors for whole grain content as follows:

> Excellent source of whole grain: The terms "excellent," "rich in," or "high in" whole grain(s) may be used on the label and in labeling of foods provided that the food contains 16g or more of whole grain per labeled serving.

> Good source of whole grain: The terms "good source," "contains," or "provides" whole grain(s) may be used on the label and on the labeling of foods provided that the food contains 8g to 15g of whole grain per labeled serving.

> Made with whole grain: The term "made with" whole grain(s) may be used on the label and on the labeling of foods provided that the food contains at least 8g of whole grain per labeled serving.

The filing of this petition codified a de facto industry standard that would complement the existing whole grain health claims with consumer-friendly descriptor claims. The Whole Grains Council leadership conferred with its members and decided to align itself with this potential standard, as long as this standard was in line with government guidance that was expected soon.

A few months after the filing of the General Mills Citizen's Petition, in August of 2004, the Dietary Guidelines Advisory Committee released its report summarizing the science that would be used to formulate the 2005 Dietary Guidelines. The report's conclusion on the subject of whole grains (D.G.A.C. 2005) was:

> Consuming at least three servings of whole grains per day can reduce the risk of diabetes and coronary heart disease and may help with weight maintenance. Thus, daily intake of three or more servings of whole grains per day is recommended, preferably by substituting whole grains for refined grains.

Previously, the U.S.D.A. had defined a "grain serving" as "the grams of grain product containing 16 grams of flour" (Pyramid Servings Database). Therefore, a recommendation for three servings or more of whole grains would mean consumption of 48g or more of whole grain content. In addition to setting "three or more whole grains a day" as the goal for most Americans, the Dietary Guidelines Advisory Committee report also endorsed the importance of recognizing consumption of "transition foods"—those containing both whole and enriched grains.

According to the D.G.A.C. (2005), "In practice, when a person selects a mixed grain bread or cereal, he gets both a whole grain portion and an enriched grain portion. Because of the desirable baking properties of enriched flour, these mixed grain products are often appealing to consumers who do not choose to eat 100% whole grains. . . . While many are not entirely whole grains, they provide some whole grains in the diets of those who might not otherwise select any. The proposed Pyramid food patterns suggest that half of all grain servings be whole grains. This approach allows these mixed products to fit readily into a person's food choices."

Now that the U.S.D.A. had clearly indicated its goals for whole grain consumption, the Whole Grains Council was able to confirm that the descriptors outlined by General Mills' Citizen's Petition would support and complement U.S.D.A. efforts and definitions. The council finalized its decision to create a symbol identifying foods containing a half serving (8g) and a full serving (16g) of whole grains.

On November 14, 2004, the Council previewed the actual graphics of the Whole Grain stamp to the public and the press at the "Whole Grains Go Mainstream" conference in New Orleans, Louisiana, organized by Oldways Preservation Trust, the Council's parent organization. That same day, the council's board of directors met with Dr. Eric Hentges, director of U.S.D.A.'s Center for Nutrition Policy and Promotion. In his capacity as manager of the Dietary Guidelines update process, Dr. Hentges expressed his support for a symbol that could be an important tool in helping consumers increase consumption of whole grains. He reviewed the Whole Grain stamp and urged the Council to make clear to consumers that any food bearing the 100% stamp must also provide a full serving of whole grain ("Excellent Source"). The following day, the council's members formally approved the new stamp program.

The Whole Grain Stamp is Unveiled, with Three Versions

The 2005 Dietary Guidelines for Americans were released on January 12. The guidelines, as widely expected in the wake of the Advisory Committee Report, called for all Americans to "consume three or more ounce-equivalents of whole grain products per day, with the rest of the recommended grains coming from enriched or whole grain products. In general, at least half the grains should come from whole grains."

U.S. Code, Title 7, Section 5341 requires that the Dietary Guidelines "shall be promoted by each Federal agency in carrying out any Federal food, nutrition, or health program" (U.S. Code). A week after the guidelines' introduction—with the knowledge that official govern-

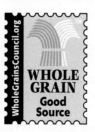

Figure 21.2. **Good Source:** A half serving of whole grains; at least 8 grams of whole grain per labeled serving.

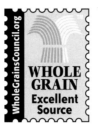

Figure 21.3. **Excellent Source:** A full serving of whole grains; at least 16 grams of whole grain per labeled serving.

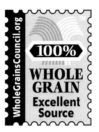

Figure 21.4. **100% Excellent Source:** A full serving of whole grains; at least 16 grams of whole grains per labeled serving AND no refined grain.

ment policy now required a many-fold increase in whole grains consumption—the Whole Grains Council unveiled its Whole Grain Stamp program to the public and authorized its members to begin the process of placing the Stamps on qualifying foods.

The Whole Grain Stamp (Figures 21.2, 21.3, and 21.4), as originally introduced, had three levels:

The three levels of the stamp made it easy for consumers to translate the Dietary Guidelines into action: Eat three foods labeled "Excellent Source" or six foods labeled "Good Source" to reach the minimum of three whole grain servings a day—or a total of 48g of whole grain content. The 100% Excellent Stamp offered the added option of eating only foods where all the grain is whole grain, a choice that is important to selected consumers. With the Whole Grain Stamps, all Americans could find the type of whole grain foods that met their needs.

Within six weeks, two members of the Council—Great Harvest Bread Company and Bruegger's Bagels—began using the Whole Grain Stamp at their bakery-cafés across the country. Because the two chains together had more than 450 locations, with sites in almost every state of the union, the stamp quickly caught consumers' attention. By springtime, the stamp began appearing on packaged goods from early adopters such as Bob's Red Mill and Kashi cereals.

As word of the Whole Grain Stamps spread through the grain-foods industry, membership in the Whole Grains Council rose steeply. The group grew from thirty-three members at the time of the stamp program's introduction in late January to fifty-four by the end of March, then to seventy-eight by July 1. At the end of the summer of 2005, membership included ninety-three of America's leading companies and grain organizations. By this time, more than half of these companies were already using the stamps, and they had collectively registered more than 400 products with the council's compliance system. Consumers were beginning to notice the stamp in supermarkets around the country, and the Whole Grains Council was carrying out an aggressive education campaign to explain the significance of the Whole Grain Stamps.

This media campaign began with newspaper articles in early spring, with extensive coverage of the Stamp program in publications including *USA Today*, the *Washington Post*, the *San Jose* (California) *Mercury News,* the *Dallas* (Texas) *Morning News,* and the *San Francisco* (California) *Chronicle*. In March, the Whole Grain Stamps were featured on the Today show, and in early May, an hour-long segment of the Oprah Winfrey show explained the importance of whole grains and fiber and praised the introduction of the stamps, advising viewers, "If you still aren't sure which of your favorite foods are really made with whole grains, look soon for these stamps on products. They're going to help take out the guesswork." As the year wore on, information about the Whole Grain Stamp program also appeared in leading magazines including *Cooking Light*, *Prevention,* and *Time*.

Good Source and Excellent Source Become an Industry Standard

At the same time that the logo of the Whole Grain Stamp was becoming widely established in 2005, several other companies augmented and complemented this growing standard by tagging their products as "Good Source of Whole Grains" (for products with 8 grams or more of whole grains per serving) and "Excellent Source of Whole Grains" (for products with 16 grams of whole grains per serving), but using their own brand-oriented graphics. General Mills cereals, Kraft cookies and crackers (under the Nabisco brand) and cereals (under the Post brand), and Pepperidge Farm crackers were among the many products reinforcing and supporting the prevailing Good Source/Excellent Source standard in this way.

This significant and virtually unprecedented industry cooperation ensured that consumers would receive a clear message about whole grains, in stark contrast to the confusion that existed before the food industry closed ranks around a common standard.

Enhanced Whole Grain Stamp Gives More Information

The Whole Grains Council launched the second phase of its stamp program in June 2006 to give consumers even more information about the whole grain content of different prod-

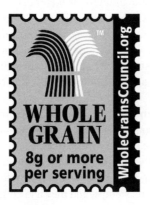

Figure 21.5.

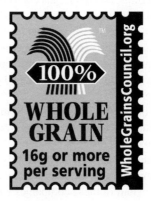

Figure 21.6.

ucts. The same familiar black-and-gold graphic was retained, but the words "Good Source" and "Excellent Source" were replaced with language detailing the number of grams of whole grain per serving, as illustrated in Figures 21.5 and 21.6. The message "Eat 48g or more of whole grain daily" was added to help consumers understand these numbers in the context of their daily needs.

Although the wording changed, the qualifications for the new stamp remained the same: foods must contain at least 8 grams (half a serving) of whole grain in each standard serving to use the stamp. Products using the 100% stamp must contain a full serving—16 grams or more—of whole grain. Manufacturers appreciated the newfound ability to spotlight healthy foods exceeding these minimums, and packages soon appeared saying "36g or more of whole grain per serving," "43g or more of whole grain per serving," or any of a wide range of values. At the same time, consumers benefited from a more sophisticated tool for making wise choices.

Through the efforts of the Whole Grains Council and its stamp program, consumers find it much easier to increase their consumption of whole grains.

References

2005 Dietary Guidelines, at www.healthierus.gov/dietaryguidelines/.

Dietary Guidelines Advisory Committee Report 2005. Appendix G2, page 16–17.

Dietary Guidelines Advisory Committee Report, Part D. 2005. (Science Base), Section 5 (Carbohydrates) available at www.health.gov/dietaryguidelines/dga2005/report/PDF/D5_Carbs.pdf.

Keys, A. and Keys, M. 1959. *Eat Well and Stay Well* Doubleday & Co.

Food Consumption U.S.D.A./E.R.S. Disappearance Data, Jacobs - as reported by Julie Miller Jones at the Whole Grains Go Mainstream conference, November 2004.

Marquart, L.; Wiemer, K.; Jones, J.; and Jacob, B. 2003. *Proceedings of the Nutrition Society* 62, 151–160.

Pyramid Servings Database, 3.2.2.1 (page 3–13) available at www.ba.ars.usda.gov/cnrg/services/section2.pdf.

U.S. Code, Title 7, Section 5341 is available at http://uscode.house.gov.

www.cfsan.fda.gov/~dms/flgrain2.html

www.fda.gov/ohrms/dockets/dockets/04p0223/04p0223.htm

www.health.gov/dietaryguidelines/dga2005/minutes01_2829_2004.htm.

www.wholegrainscouncil.org/ConsumerDef.html.

22   Whole Grains and Consumers

Mary Ann Johnson, Teri Burgess-Champoux,
Mark A. Kantor, and Marla Reicks

Introduction

National dietary intake data show that whole grain intake is lower than recommended for most population subgroups; however, intake by some are lower than others (Kantor et al. 2001). Specific barriers to intake may differ by subgroup; for example, the financial constraints of purchasing whole grain foods may be greater for limited-income groups than for more affluent groups. Therefore, different promotion and education strategies may be particularly applicable for specific groups. For example, modifying school menus may be useful for school-aged children because many children eat school meals.

Interventions based on different strategies have been developed and tested for particular target groups of consumers (older adults, children, Cooperative Extension Service audiences). Needs assessment studies also have been conducted with educators working with specific audiences, including low-income women with children. Each subsection of this chapter describes research conducted with a particular audience, identifying specific needs and barriers as well as opportunities to apply the findings to further research and practice.

Older Adults

Through at least the middle of this century, about 1 million Americans will turn 65 each year (U.S. Census Bureau 2004). Currently there are more than 35 million older Americans, of whom nearly 3 million receive community-based nutrition services such as congregate meals, home delivered meals, and nutrition and health education programs through Older Americans Act Nutrition Programs (O.A.A.N.P., Wellman and Kamp 2004). Whole grain foods may be particularly beneficial to this subgroup of the older adult population, because they are at high risk for poor nutritional status and have a high prevalence of chronic diseases that have been associated with low whole grain intakes. In a national survey of O.A.A.N.P. congregate meal recipients, 18% had diabetes, 28% had heart disease, 13% had cancer, and 41% reported at least three coexisting chronic health conditions (Ponza et al. 1996).

Programs such as congregate meals and home-delivered meals must follow the Dietary Reference Intakes and the Dietary Guidelines for meal planning when they receive federal or state funding (Wellman and Kamp 2004). In some states, such as Georgia, these meal programs did not require that whole grain foods be included until 2005. Prior to this requirement, this population in Georgia generally were not served whole grain foods with the congregate meal nor did they voluntarily consume whole grains at other meals. Therefore, a study was conducted to examine the intakes and behaviors related to whole grain foods, as well as the effects of an educational intervention on the voluntary consumption of whole grain foods by congregate meal recipients in Georgia (Ellis et al. 2005).

Methods

A convenience sample of older adults was recruited from nine senior centers in seven counties in northern Georgia (Ellis et al. 2005). The only exclusion criterion was the inability to answer the questions and participate in the education activities. Procedures were approved by the Institutional Review Boards of the Georgia Department of Human Resources and The University of Georgia, and all participants provided informed consent.

Pre-tests, post-tests, and an educational intervention were developed, implemented, and evaluated as previously described (Ellis et al. 2005). For the pre- and post-tests, trained interviewers read the questions to the participants and recorded their responses. A food frequency questionnaire asked about the intake of specific whole and non-whole grain foods. Serving sizes were not estimated, because it was determined that the frequency of intake was more important than the serving sizes to gauge exposure of this population to whole grain foods.

The non-whole grain and whole grain foods that were estimated were white bread, brown bread, whole grain bread, whole grain cereal, whole grain crackers, oatmeal, brown rice, popcorn, whole grain pasta or noodles, whole grain English muffins, whole grain granola bars, whole grain bagels, and other products using whole wheat flour. Participants also were asked about their current or past disease conditions (heart disease, cancer, diabetes, hypertension, blood cholesterol, and bowel troubles, e.g. constipation, diverticulosis, and diverticulitis); health beliefs about the associations between whole grains and chronic disease; knowledge and attitudes toward whole grain foods using recall, yes/no, and true/false formats; and specific barriers to whole grain consumption.

The nutrition education intervention entitled "Whole Grains and Your Health Program" was implemented after the pre-test questionnaires were completed. The conceptual framework for the intervention was based on the health belief model (Strecher and Rosenstock 1997), including perceived susceptibility and severity (e.g. health conditions in older people that are associated with low intake of whole grains), perceived benefits (e.g. decreasing the risk of health conditions), perceived barriers (e.g. information about labeling of whole grain foods), cues to action (e.g. "how-to" information on including whole grain foods at various meals), and self-efficacy (e.g. food demonstrations and tips on ways to consume whole grain foods).

The intervention consisted of five lessons, and each lesson was given one time at each senior center. Each lesson had a lesson plan and handouts including tips on how to increase whole grain consumption. The curriculum is available for download at NOAHnet: Nutrition for Older Adults' Health (http://www.arches.uga.edu/~noahnet/planswg.html). Each lesson emphasized three messages: how to identify a whole grain food, whole grains protect against diseases, and three are key.

The first lesson, "Getting the Whole Grain Story," covered the definition of a whole grain, how to identify whole grain foods, and the health benefits gained from whole grain consumption. The second lesson, "The Whole Truth about Whole Grain Bread," identified ways to identify whole grain breads and compared the nutritional benefits of eating whole grain bread to those of white bread. The third lesson, "The Great Whole Grain Cereal and Oatmeal Chapter," addressed how to identify whole grain cereals and creative ways to include them in meals. The fourth lesson, "The Brown Rice Bonus," focused on how to cook and store brown rice. The fifth lesson, "The Final Chapter—Don't Forget those Grains," covered snacking ideas using whole grain foods and identified some less common grains. One to two lessons were provided each month over a period of five to six months. The post-test was administered one to three months after the last lesson to allow participants time to make behavior changes.

The data were analyzed using the Statistical Analysis System Software (Version 8, S.A.S. Institute, Cary, North Carolina). Descriptive statistics, including frequencies, means, standard deviations, and Spearman correlation coefficients, were calculated. Data from the pre-test and post-test were compared using the Signed Rank Test, paired T-tests, and Chi-square analyses to identify changes that were statistically significant ($P \leq 0.05$). Partial Spearman correlation coefficients for associations of changes in whole grain intake with other behaviors or diseases were calculated (Ellis et al. 2005).

Results

Ninety-five people enrolled and completed the pre-test and eighty-four individuals completed the post-test. These eighty-four participants had a mean age of 77 years (SD $\pm$ 7, 40% $\geq$ 80 years), 88% were female, 76% were Caucasian, 24% were African American, and 30% were obese (body mass index $\geq$ 30 kg/m^2). The self-reported history of diseases included cancer (23%), heart disease (32%), high blood cholesterol (49%), diabetes (32%), high blood pressure (67%), and bowel disorders (37%). At the pre-test, completers and non-completers did not differ in age, gender, ethnicity, nor mean intakes of whole grain foods. Therefore, further analyses include only the data for the eighty-four participants who completed both the pre-test and post-test.

After the intervention there was a significant increase in the total intake of whole grain bread, whole grain cereal, and whole wheat crackers (Table 22.1); these were the three whole grain foods with the largest increase in intake. However, there was no significant change in the total intake of the eleven whole grain foods examined. Less than 15% of the participants consumed whole grain foods three or more times daily before or after the intervention.

There were no statistically significant changes between the pre-test and the post-test in the percentage of people who thought that eating more whole grains would reduce their risk of cancer, heart disease, type 2 diabetes, or bowel disorders (range was 65% to 86% at the two time points). There was a trend for an increase in the percentage of participants who knew that three servings of whole grain foods should be eaten daily (Table 22.1).

Participants were asked to suggest ways to identify whole grain foods and the interviewers recorded their responses (Table 22.1). There were significant increases from the pre-test to the post-test in suggesting "first ingredient is whole grain," providing one or more correct suggestions, and in the mean number of correct answers (0.5 vs. 0.8, $P \leq 0.05$). After participants finished suggesting possible ways to identify whole grain foods, they were asked a series of true/false questions. Following the intervention, there was an increase in the percentage of participants who answered "true" to "all 100% whole wheat bread is whole grain," but there were no improvements in correctly answering any of the other identification questions (Table 22.1). After the intervention, at least 75% of the participants indicated that they tried to follow a healthier diet, ate more whole grain foods because they thought they were good for them, and/or felt more strongly than before that eating whole grain foods will reduce the risk of chronic disease.

Age, gender, ethnicity, cognition, and body mass index were not significantly associated with whole grain intake at the pre-test or post-test, nor with changes in whole grain intake. However, at the pre-test, intake of whole grains was positively correlated with self-report of

Table 22.1. Intake and knowledge of labeling of whole grain foods: Eighty-four adults in the Georgia Older Americans Act Nutrition Program.

	Pre-test	Post-test	P-values
Intake	Mean ± SD (%≥once/week)	Mean ± SD (%≥once/week)	
Intake of 11 whole grain foods	10.5 ± 6.2 (74)	11.7 ± 6.9 (77)	NS
Intake of three whole grain foods with the largest increases after the intervention (whole grain bread, whole grain cereal, and whole wheat crackers)	5.8 ± 4.4 (50)	6.9 ± 4.8 (54)	0.05*
	Frequency Correct (%)	Frequency Correct (%)	
Consumed 3 or more whole grain foods daily	10	14	NS
Knowledge			
Three whole grains are recommended daily	38	52	NS (P = 0.06)
Participants' suggestions on ways to identify whole grain foods			
First ingredient is whole grain (correct)	5	14	0.05*
Whole grain health claim is on the package (correct)	5	8	NS
Whole grain logo is on the package (correct)	20	32	NS (P = 0.08)
100% whole wheat or 100% whole grain is in the name (correct)	20	20	1.0
By brown color (incorrect)	24	18	NS
Wheat is in the name (incorrect)	4	5	NS
Multi-grain is in the name (incorrect)	0	1	NS
Stone ground is in the name (incorrect)	0	0	—
One or more correct suggestions	45	62	0.05*
Participants' knowledge of labeling			
All 100% whole wheat bread is whole grain (true)	65	82	0.01*
A food is whole grain if the whole grain logo is on the package (true)	65	75	NS
Bread is always whole grain if it is brown in color (false)	56	48	NS
All wheat bread is whole grain (false)	45	48	NS
All multi-grain bread is whole grain (false)	36	40	NS
All stone ground bread is whole grain (false)	31	39	NS
A food is whole grain if the first ingredient is a whole grain, such as whole wheat, whole rye, or whole oats (true)	69	70	NS
White bread is whole grain (false)	80	83	NS

*Indicates a P-value ≤ 0.05
NS is not significantly different.

diabetes, liking the taste of whole grain foods, knowledge of whole grain labeling, knowledge of recommended whole grain intake, and thinking that eating more whole grains would reduce the risk of cancer and heart disease, but was negatively correlated with tobacco use and self-report of cancer, and preferring the taste of white bread to whole grain bread ($P \leq 0.05$, Ellis et al. 2005). Changes in whole grain intake were significantly and positively correlated with increases in thinking that eating more whole grains would reduce the risk of bowel disorders ($rho = 0.28$, $P \leq 0.05$) and feeling more strongly at the post-test that whole grain foods will reduce the risk of disease ($rho = 0.31$, $P \leq 0.01$).

Discussion

Consumption of whole grains foods is one of several dietary habits that are beneficial for older people (Johnson 2004), but there is little information available on successful ways to increase whole grain consumption in various subgroups of older adults. Based on a review of the literature, this is the first reported study of an intervention designed to increase the voluntary intake of whole grain foods in congregate meal participants (Ellis et al. 2005). This educational intervention was associated with participants feeling more strongly that whole grains would reduce the risk of chronic disease, as well as increased recognition of whole grain foods and increased intakes of whole grain bread, whole grain cereal, and whole wheat crackers.

Prior to the educational intervention, 61% to 85% of the participants already knew about the positive benefits of whole grain foods for decreasing the risk of chronic diseases, liked the taste of whole grain foods, and preferred the taste of whole grain bread to white bread. However, many participants had a low knowledge of ways to identify whole grain foods and thought that whole grain bread was more expensive than white bread. Therefore, barriers to increasing consumption are more likely to include cost and identification problems rather than taste or knowledge about the health benefits of whole grain foods.

It is not surprising that this sample of congregate meal participants had a high awareness of the health benefits of whole grains. The foods and nutrition department at the University of Georgia has been providing nutrition and health education to this population since 1997. Also, the 1999 "Shopping for Health" survey found that older adults (ages 54 and over) were more likely than younger shoppers to want information on fiber (52% vs. 39%) and whole grains (28% vs. 18%) (Prevention Magazine/Food Marketing Institute 1999).

Recognizing the many ways whole grain foods are labeled may be a barrier to improving consumption, as was seen in this study of congregate meal participants (Ellis et al. 2005). Older people may have difficulties identifying these foods, finding them in the grocery store, and knowing that some of the foods are marketed in both refined grain forms and whole grain forms (e.g. bagels, English muffins, whole wheat flour, etc.). Some foods, such as brown rice or whole wheat pasta, may be somewhat easy to identify because they generally only come in the whole grain or the refined/white forms. Products with multiple ingredients such as breads, crackers, and other baked goods may be difficult to identify and may be labeled as "multigrain," "nine-grain," or "made with whole grain."

At the pre-test, most congregate meal participants incorrectly answered the questions about ways to identify whole grain foods. Therefore, more effort should be focused on educating consumers about how to identify whole grains. In the present education intervention, several messages were used to help improve label identification. As a result of these messages (at post-test), there were significant increases in the number of participants who knew that "all 100% whole wheat bread is whole grain" (by 17 percentage points) and were able to suggest that a food is whole grain if "the first ingredient is a whole grain" (by 15 percentage points).

Other barriers to consumption may include unfamiliar taste, lack of preparation time, lack of monetary resources, higher cost of some whole grain foods compared to their non-whole grain counterparts, unfamiliarity with whole grain foods, and a lack of knowledge of the health benefits of whole grains. Also, behavior change may require a longer intervention period and follow-up time than was provided for these participants.

Taste and preference are important predictors of food selection and consumption. Before the intervention was introduced, 85% of the congregate meal participants indicated that they liked the taste of whole grain foods and 60% said they preferred whole grain bread to white bread. This suggests that including whole grain foods in congregate meals should be acceptable to many participants. Further study is needed to determine what types of whole grain foods would be accepted by older adults in congregate meal programs.

Another opportunity for promoting whole grain foods, especially non-breakfast cereal foods, is to improve the micronutrient profile by fortifying with folic acid, vitamin B_{12}, and/or vitamin D. While whole grain cereals may be fortified with 25% to 100% of the Daily Value for many vitamins and minerals, whole grain breads typically are not heavily fortified and, unlike white bread, might not even include folic acid as a fortificant. Folic acid has many health benefits such as decreasing homocysteine, which is a risk factor for cardiovascular and possibly neurological disease (Lökk 2003). Moreover, congregate meal participants may be at high risk for vitamin B_{12} deficiency and hyperhomocysteinemia (Johnson et al. 2003) and most do not use a vitamin D-containing supplement (Cheong et al. 2003) that is needed to optimize vitamin D status in older adults (U.S. Department of Health and Human Services and U.S. Department of Agriculture 2005). Thus, improving the micronutrient profile of whole grain breads may improve nutritional status in older adults.

In agreement with Marquart et al. (2003), it is suggested that behavioral interventions, as well as focus groups and surveys, will be necessary to identify messages and campaigns to increase whole grain intake. Interventions must emphasize familiar foods such as breads and cereals at both the community (e.g. grocery store) and individual level to assist consumers in identifying and purchasing whole grain food products. These findings of modest increases in whole grain food intake and improved recognition of some aspects of product labeling suggest that increasing consumption of whole grain foods is possible, even among a population with a high prevalence of low income and low literacy skills.

Additional research is needed to assess the feasibility and acceptability of including whole grain foods in the congregate and home-delivered meals, with consideration of the cost of the meal and the taste preferences of the recipients. The positive outcomes of this study add to the growing body of evidence that congregate meal program participants can benefit from nutrition and health education programs that address the prevention of chronic diseases (Cheong et al. 2003, McCamey et al. 2003).

School-age Children

Increased intake of whole grain foods by children represents a positive dietary change. However, current intake of whole grains among U.S. children and adolescents is low, with just 9% of those 2 to 19 years of age consuming three or more servings on a daily basis (Cleveland et al. 2000). Ready-to-eat cereals (30.9%), corn and other chips (21.7%), and yeast breads (18.1%) were the major food sources, accounting for approximately 71% of the whole grain intake for this age group (Harnack et al. 2003).

Developing healthy eating habits during childhood is the basis for healthy adult eating behaviors and reduced risk of chronic disease. School-based health promotion programs have an immense potential to reach a wide audience including students, parents, administrators, and members of the community. Overseen by the U.S. Department of Agriculture (U.S.D.A.), the National School Meals Program provides school breakfast to approximately 8 million children and school lunch to 28.3 million children on a daily basis (Food and Nutrition Service, U.S.D.A.). School-based interventions have been successful in increasing the fruit and vegetable intake of children; however, based on a review of the literature, no intervention study has had a major focus on whole grains. Therefore, the purpose of this study was to pilot test a school-based intervention aimed to increase whole grain consumption by fourth- and fifth-grade students.

Methods

A convenience sample of children was recruited from two schools in one school district in the Twin Cities metropolitan area of Minnesota. Assignment of schools to intervention and control was done on the basis of the school district recommendation regarding the ease of incorporating whole grain foods into the school menu. Schools were matched by demographic characteristics, size, and the number of fourth- and fifth-grade students at baseline. Similar lunch menus were served at each school during the intervention. Parent-child pairs were recruited via a letter sent home from school. Informed consent was obtained from the parents and assent from the children. The study was approved by the University of Minnesota Human Subjects Protection Committee and the Hopkins School District Research Committee.

Social cognitive theory (S.C.T.) provided the theoretical foundation for this behaviorally-based nutrition intervention. It explains human behavior in terms of a triadic, dynamic, and reciprocal relationship in which personal factors, behavior, and environmental factors interact (Baranowski et al. 2002). The three main components of the intervention model were (1) a classroom educational program to address personal factors, (2) school cafeteria changes in the food environment, and (3) family involvement to impact both environmental and behavioral factors.

"The Power of 3: Get Healthy with Whole Grains" was a five-lesson educational program taught on a weekly basis by two nutrition graduate students at the intervention school. The overall aim of the program was to improve instrumental knowledge to identify whole grain foods, enhance self-efficacy through tasting experiences, promote menu planning and goal setting, and encourage advocacy for peers and family members to increase whole grain intake. Learning objectives for each lesson were based on S.C.T. and previous focus group discussions. Activities included grain identification, hand milling grains, reading labels, preparing snacks, and sampling whole grain foods.

Intervention staff worked with the district nutritionist and foodservice director to modify the existing school menu in the intervention school. This resulted in the incorporation of whole or partial whole grain products to replace refined grain counterparts on a daily basis in the school cafeteria throughout the intervention period. Selected whole grain products were donated by ConAgra, Inc., and others were purchased from local vendors.

Plate waste measurements of various red and white whole wheat products were completed before, during, and after the intervention to assess acceptability. Trained research staff followed a standardized protocol for collecting the data. Lunch meal observations were conducted before and after the intervention with students in the intervention and control groups to estimate whole grain intake from the noon meal. Compared to other dietary assessment methods, direct meal observation is frequently considered optimal because the method is practical, economical, and avoids recall bias (Baglio et al. 2004, Simons-Morton et al. 1992).

The intervention staff received ten hours of didactic and practicum training regarding the standardized protocol, portion size estimation, and completion of the data collection forms. The amount of food consumed by each child was determined by combining the amount recorded as consumed by the observer and the measured amounts remaining on the tray and subtracting from the initial quantity served. Interobserver reliability assessments were completed at baseline and throughout the intervention to ensure consistency between the different observers. There was 91% overall mean agreement across the five observers.

The family component of the intervention included weekly parent newsletters, parent/child bakery and grocery store tours, and a "Whole Grain Day" event at a local milling museum (http://www.millcitymuseum.org). Five parent newsletters containing interactive parent/child activities that reinforced the classroom curriculum were developed based on previous focus group discussions with parents and S.C.T. constructs. The overall aim was to increase the availability of whole grain foods in the home environment and encourage parents to demonstrate greater frequency of role modeling consumption of whole grain foods. "Whole Grain Day" for children and their families included a Quiz Bowl event for children to demonstrate their acquired knowledge and skills, a scavenger hunt throughout the museum, and whole grain food demonstrations with sampling and complementary whole grain products for home.

Children and parents in both the intervention and control groups completed separate survey instruments before and after the intervention to assess changes in knowledge, availability, and self-efficacy. Survey items were developed based on existing instruments tested and validated regarding intake of other foods (i.e. fruits and vegetables) and used a multiple choice, yes/no, and three- to five-point scale format. Trained intervention staff administered the questionnaire to children in the classroom, whereas the parent survey was self-administered at home and returned to school. The instruments were assessed for content validity by experts in nutrition and pilot tested for reliability with fifth-grade students and their parents from a third school within the school district and revised as needed.

Survey evaluation data were entered into an Excel file prior to analysis using S.A.S. (The S.A.S. Institute, Inc; Version 9.1 for Windows). Descriptive statistics were used to describe demographic characteristics and survey responses. Paired t-tests were used to determine whether there were differences between pre- and post-test measures in participants in both the intervention and control groups. Analysis of variance was used to detect significant changes in difference values between the intervention and control group. The significance level was set at $p < 0.05$.

Results

Sixty-eight parent/child pairs from the intervention school and eighty-three parent/child pairs from the control school participated in this pilot study. The mean age of the children was 10 years with 45% male and 55% female. Although the schools were selected based on similar demographic characteristics and percentage of free and/or reduced lunch participants at baseline, the intervention school was more ethnically diverse than the control school, with 52% non-white versus 24% non-white respectively. The mean age of the parents was 40 years. The majority were female, white, and well-educated, and approximately half were employed full-time.

Whole grain intake increased by 1 serving in the lunch meal, refined grain intake decreased by 1 serving, and whole grain foods were more available for children in the intervention school compared to the control school post-intervention based on meal observations. Mean percentage plate waste for products made with red and white whole wheat flour indicated that children in the intervention school for grades one through six accepted whole grain products. However, acceptance was variable depending on attributes of the products such as product type, size, color, and accompanying menu items.

There were trends toward increased whole grain knowledge (p = 0.06) and reported home availability of whole grain foods (p = 0.07) by children in the intervention school increased significantly compared with the control school. No differences in self-efficacy or intention to choose whole grain foods over refined grain foods were observed for children. Three parenting scales were developed as a result of factor analysis of seventeen items from the parent survey instrument: whole grain adequacy (i.e. buy whole grain foods, encourage child to eat whole grain foods), whole grain behaviors (i.e. use whole grain bread for sandwiches, eat whole grain pasta), and perceptions of health benefits. Pre/post changes in whole grain adequacy scores were significantly greater for the intervention compared to the control school (p < 0.009), while changes in the whole grain behaviors score approached significance (p = 0.08). No differences in the changes in health benefits score were observed for parents. Regarding the weekly newsletters, the majority of parents (78%) reported receiving most/all of the newsletters and greater than half (69%) reported reading most/all of them. Forty percent of parents reported completing the weekly newsletter activities with their child at home. Overall participation in the family activities (i.e. bakery and grocery store tours) was approximately 25%.

Discussion

The results of this study suggest that a multi-component school-based intervention can be effective in increasing the availability of whole grain foods in the school environment, enhance acceptance of whole grain products that replace refined grain counterparts, and increase knowledge regarding whole grain foods by preadolescent children. The school cafeteria represents a powerful vehicle for increasing acceptance and intake of whole grain foods by children through sampling and repeated exposures to new foods. Whole grain foods that are both affordable and acceptable to children are needed to increase the incorporation of these foods into school menus on a daily basis.

Eating behaviors and health beliefs of children are strongly influenced by their parents, who are considered to be influential role models in addition to peers (Patrick and Nicklas 2005). Previous nutrition interventions have experienced limited success in increasing family involvement (Harrington et al. 2005). Therefore, development and testing of effective strategies for engaging parents in the change process is needed.

Limitations to this pilot study include a small sample size representing only one age cohort and short duration of the intervention. Design and implementation of additional school-based intervention research on a broader scale is needed to increase the whole grain consumption of children to recommended levels. Changes brought about by this program are expected to contribute to the overall improvement in eating habits and long-term health of children as well as promote positive parenting practices. Educators can use these findings to develop whole grain nutrition education programs for children.

Extension Audiences

Advice to increase whole grain consumption is becoming an integral part of mainstream nutrition guidance. The multiple health benefits of whole grain foods, coupled with low dietary intakes, underscore the need for education programs to urge increased consumption. A pilot study was conducted to investigate consumers' knowledge of health benefits attributed to whole grain foods; the ability to identify whole grain foods from a list of food items; attitudes about whole grains regarding taste, purchasing, convenience, and preparation; frequency of consumption of selected grain foods; and self-efficacy (self-confidence) regarding the capacity to eat more or new whole grain foods.

The purpose of this study was to identify potential barriers that may prevent consumers from eating whole grain foods and to determine whether providing printed educational materials on whole grains would positively change attitudes. Through this research the investigators hoped to improve their understanding of why consumers avoid purchasing and consuming whole grain foods, and to develop insights into motivating consumers to eat more whole grains.

Methods

The sampling frame consisted of individuals who previously participated or expressed interest in programs conducted by Maryland Cooperative Extension (M.C.E.) in three Maryland counties. Databases were pooled and 300 names were randomly selected using a random numbers generator.

The survey instrument contained a total of seven items that addressed knowledge (three items), attitudes (two items), and behaviors (two items) with respect to whole grains. The instrument, which took about fifteen minutes to fill out, underwent face validation by University of Maryland faculty members and was pilot tested with fifteen subjects to assess comprehension and clarity. After modification, the survey was mailed in December 2003 along with a consent form and cover letter explaining the purpose and significance of the study. Approval to perform this study was obtained from the Institutional Review Board of the University of Maryland. A total of 125 subjects returned their completed baseline surveys and consent forms.

In June 2004, the sample subjects were mailed a packet of nutrition education materials containing excerpts from the Dietary Guidelines for Americans (2000 edition) and Food Guide Pyramid, a nutrition newsletter (written by cooperative extension specialists from the University of Rhode Island and the University of Connecticut) featuring whole grain recipes and preparation tips, a brochure entitled *Get on the Grain Train* (Home & Garden Bull. 267-2, U.S.D.A., Center for Nutrition Policy Promotion, 2002) which discussed the structure and health benefits of whole grains, and a handout from the Bell Institute (General Mills, Minneapolis, Minnesota) on whole grain food labels and health claims. A cover letter requested that participants read the materials and try some of the recipes.

In September 2004, about twelve weeks after the educational materials were mailed, a follow-up (post-intervention) survey similar to the baseline survey was mailed to subjects. This survey was designed to evaluate perceptions of the educational materials and to assess changes in attitudes toward whole grain consumption. The subjects were asked to return the completed surveys by October 2004.

Data were analyzed using S.A.S., version 8.2. Frequencies were determined for all categorical variables. Differences in attitude measurements between baseline values and the twelve-week post intervention values were analyzed using Generalized Estimating Equations. Differences and associations were considered statistically significant for values of $p < 0.05$.

Results

The sample (n = 125) was predominantly female (90%), white (91%), and older (mean age = 59 years, range 20 to 84 years). About 56% of the subjects were older than 60 years of age. Half of the subjects had a bachelor's degree or higher.

Knowledge and consumption of whole grain foods were assessed with the baseline survey. On a forced-choice survey item which addressed the recommended daily number of whole grain servings, only 44% answered "two to three" servings/day, which was the correct answer at the time of the survey, while 21% chose "six to eleven" servings/day, the number recommended for all grain foods. The rest of the subjects chose either "one" (7%) or "four to five" (29%) servings/day.

When asked to select from a list of diseases for which risks could be lowered by consuming whole grains, 71% of the subjects properly identified heart disease, but only 17% correctly indicated that the risk of diabetes also could be lowered by eating whole grains. More than 60% of the respondents incorrectly answered that the risk of cataracts and Alzheimer's disease could be reduced by whole grain consumption.

Subjects were presented with a list of fourteen grain foods and asked to indicate which items they thought were whole grains. The foods most likely to be correctly identified as whole grain foods were whole wheat bread, oatmeal, and brown rice. Less than two-thirds of the subjects thought that bulgur and popcorn were whole grains, and a majority did not think that tabouli salad, which is typically made with bulgur, was a whole grain food. Nearly two-thirds of the subjects thought that multi-grain bread, seven-grain bread, and stone ground wheat bread were whole grain foods, although typically these foods do not meet the definition of whole grain bread because the first ingredient is not a whole grain. The term "enriched" seemed to be confusing to the subjects; 80% reported not knowing if enriched white rice was a whole grain food and 64% did not know if enriched wheat flour was a whole grain.

Subjects were asked about their frequency of consumption of various whole grain and non-whole grain products. As expected, products such as white bread and white rice were consumed more frequently than whole wheat bread and brown rice. Bulgur was hardly eaten at all. The one whole grain product that was eaten relatively frequently was oatmeal; 38% of the subjects reported eating this food either several times a week or almost daily. A health claim for oats has existed since 1997, which may have contributed to the popularity of oatmeal in this sample.

Attitudes about whole grains with respect to taste, cost, preparation, convenience, availability in stores, and eating more whole grain foods were assessed before (baseline) and after the mail intervention. Subjects in this study initially had positive attitudes about whole grains. At baseline, most subjects agreed either "a lot" or "a little" that whole grain foods taste good (91% agreement), are convenient to eat (84%), and that their family would want to eat more whole grains (58%). Similarly, a majority of subjects disagreed either "a lot" or "a little" that whole grain foods are difficult to prepare or are difficult to find at the store (66% and 56% disagreement, respectively).

Positive attitudes about whole grains with respect to taste, availability in stores, and willingness of family members to eat all improved even further after the intervention (p < 0.05). Several measures of self-efficacy, which also were high to begin with, also improved after the intervention (Table 22.2).

Table 22.2. Consumer self-efficacy (% of responses) concerning whole grain consumption before and after receiving educational materials in the mail.

	Percent "sure" or "somewhat sure"		
How sure are you that you can:	Baseline	Post mail-intervention	p
Eat 1 serving of whole grain food each day?	95	100	
Eat 2-3 servings of a whole grain food each day?	83	90	*
Eat whole grain bread instead of white bread?	95	96	
Choose a whole grain cereal when you eat cereal?	92	99	*
Try a whole grain food you never ate before?	84	95	*
Prepare a whole grain food that is new to you?	87	93	*

Note: Subjects (n = 125, 90% female, 91% white, mean age = 59 years) were randomly selected from Maryland Cooperative Extension mailing lists from three counties in Maryland. * signifies $p < 0.05$

Most of the subjects indicated on the follow-up survey that the educational materials they received were either "very useful" or "somewhat useful."

Discussion

The mail intervention seemed to be effective in positively changing attitudes toward whole grains. Therefore, nutrition researchers may want to consider using written materials (including recipes and newsletters) in nutrition education efforts, because interventions involving personal contact with consumers are time-consuming and expensive. However, because this was a small pilot study using initially motivated subjects who previously were exposed to M.C.E. nutrition education programs, the results cannot be extrapolated to other populations.

Several barriers to whole grain consumption were identified in this study, including a lack of knowledge about health benefits, an inability to identify whole grain foods, and uncertainty about finding whole grain foods in stores.

What can nutrition educators do? Cooperative extension consumer education programs, which are administered through the nation's land grant universities, are open to all individuals. Extension audiences, however, are often comprised of older adults, as seen in this study. According to a framework proposed by Sahyoun et al. (2004), effective nutrition education programs or interventions that target older adults should be based on sound behavioral theories (such as the Health Belief Model) and consider issues of motivation and self-efficacy. People who perceive themselves at greater risk of developing a chronic disease may be more likely to positively change their eating behaviors, especially if their self-efficacy to implement changes is high (Gordon 2002).

Nutrition education efforts should follow established principles of communication. Successful outcomes are more likely to occur if educational messages are short, simple, flexible, and have a positive tone. Nutrition educators should use a behaviorally focused approach and tailor their messages to accommodate individual preferences and life styles (Jones et al. 2004).

Messages should focus on taste and health. Because the most important determinant of food intake is taste, it is essential to emphasize that whole grains have a pleasurable taste and favorable sensory attributes, and to dispel any preconceived notion that one must sacrifice taste when eating nutritious foods.

Although nutrition is an important predictor of food choices, it is probably less significant than taste, convenience, and cost. However, past experience demonstrates that when consumers are repeatedly exposed to advertising campaigns (e.g. for Kellogg's All Bran[TM] cereal and celebrities wearing "milk moustaches") they can positively alter their perceptions of foods as well as their eating habits. It is plausible that some consumers could be motivated to eat more whole grains if educators address the link between whole grains and weight control.

It is also important that educators consider whole grains in the context of the total diet and not minimize the contribution of other foods. Messages about whole grains that also include fruits and vegetables will seem more believable to consumers and may help to avert confusion or cynicism arising from conflicting messages about diet and health. In educating the public about whole grains, nutrition professionals should strive to "help consumers understand the principles of a healthful diet, and empower them to achieve it" (Freeland-Graves and Nitzke 2002).

What can the food industry do? It is essential that food companies make it easy for consumers to identify whole grain foods when shopping (Marquart et al. 2003). This could be done by implementing an easily recognizable logo or seal, perhaps analogous to the seal and labeling guidelines established in 2002 for foods through the National Organic Program (U.S.D.A./Agricultural Marketing Service) or by adopting models proposed by the Whole Grains Council (2005).

Companies also should agree to make ingredient lists uniform and unambiguous, because labeling standards for whole grain foods remains problematic (Kantor et al. 2001). Different whole wheat breads currently on the market list as the first ingredient "whole wheat flour," "whole wheat," or "100% stone ground 'whole of the wheat' flour." Potentially misleading terms such as "stone ground" could be removed from package labels. Furthermore, companies should not be tempted to add trivial amounts of whole grain ingredients to various food products (such as donuts) and then promote these foods as being a whole grain source.

Although we found that consumers had positive attitudes about whole grains, it is unlikely they will substantially increase their consumption until whole grain foods become more convenient and available. Just as the marketing of pre-washed and packaged ready-to-eat baby carrots and salad greens resulted in increased consumption of raw vegetables, new ways to market whole grains should be considered. Perhaps new pre-cooked and frozen whole grain products could be developed that simply need to be heated in a microwave oven prior to consumption. For people living alone or for older individuals, companies could market whole grains in convenient sized packages that are easy to open. Some manufacturers already have launched new whole grain products, and this trend is expected to continue (Buzby et al. 2005).

What can grocery stores and restaurants do? Grocery stores should strive to increase the variety of whole grain products they carry, especially in areas of the country where choices may be limited. Grocery stores could assist with consumer education efforts by holding special promotions and providing samples during the day (e.g. to target older shoppers) of products that may not be familiar to consumers, such as tabouli salad served with whole grain crackers or pita. Supermarkets also could publicize that many whole grain products are similar in price to their conventional (refined) counterparts. Because consumers eat so many meals away from home, encouraging restaurants (especially fast food chains) to offer whole grain breads and rolls would be an important step toward increasing whole grain consumption.

More research is needed to understand barriers that prevent consumers from eating whole grains, especially the rejection of whole grains by children (Jones et al. 2002). In recent years there has been considerable misinformation about grains and other carbohydrates, and consumers remain confused about nutrition. The declining popularity of low-carbohydrate diets offers an ideal opportunity to publicize the desirable attributes of grains in general and whole grains in particular. Furthermore, the release of the Dietary Guidelines for Americans and MyPyramid by the federal government in 2005 provides a solid scientific framework for educating the public about whole grains and healthy diets. Consumer education programs that address serving sizes are especially needed.

To be effective in changing behavior, health messages about whole grains should be perceived by consumers as being endorsed by mainstream government and health agencies, rather than emanating primarily from the food industry. Consumers prefer health claims that are expressed in brief, simple language. They are skeptical of health claims made by food companies unless it is clear that the claims have government approval (Williams 2005). The F.D.A. should maintain rigorous scientific standards for health claims and reconsider using qualified health claims (International Food and Information Council 2005).

Effective communication depends on understanding the knowledge, attitudes, and beliefs of the target audience, but nutrition educators need to recognize that there is often a gap between what people say they believe and what they actually do. Further research is needed on ways to frame positive messages about whole grains that broadly appeal to all age groups, and that counter negative stereotypes sometimes associated with healthful foods.

There is a need for nutrition and food science professionals to collaborate on a variety of fronts to encourage the increased consumption of whole grains. Consumer education programs are more likely to be more successful if they include examples of foods and activities that reflect the target audience's lifestyle, preferences, and culture. Behavioral change is difficult to achieve, but is more likely to occur if food and nutrition professionals can speak with one voice about the benefits of eating whole grain foods as an integral part of an overall healthy diet.

W.I.C. Professionals

Nutrition educators can play an important role in promoting an increased intake of whole grain foods for low-income mothers and young children participating in the W.I.C. Program (Special Supplemental Nutrition Program for Women, Infants, and Children). Participants in food assistance programs may face greater constraints related to cost and availability compared to more affluent population groups. A survey of attitudes and practices related to the promotion of whole grain foods by W.I.C. educators was conducted to assess needs for the development of educational materials to promote increased intake for low income women with children. A random national sample of W.I.C. educators completed a mailed survey. The study was approved by the University of Minnesota Human Subjects Protection Committee.

Methods

Initial survey items were based on a review of the literature regarding health professionals' attitudes and practices regarding whole grain foods and results of a previous survey of registered dietitians (Chase et al. 2003a). A small convenience sample of W.I.C. educators in Minnesota provided feedback regarding survey items for appropriateness, clarity, understanding of specific terms, best response strategies, and format. The survey items were reviewed by several university nutrition professors and nutrition professionals from the National W.I.C. Association and the Bell Institute of Nutrition and Health at General Mills, and revised prior to mailing.

Names and mailing addresses of all local W.I.C. agency directors were obtained from the National W.I.C. Association. The names of 500 directors were randomly selected from the mailing list. Letters were mailed to the directors requesting that they ask an educator who regularly interacts with clients to complete the survey. A packet for the educator contained a consent form, the survey, and a postage-paid return envelope. A gift of fifty books for children was provided in return for participation.

Survey data were entered into an Excel file prior to analysis using S.A.S. (The S.A.S. Institute, Inc., Version 8e, Cary, North Carolina). Descriptive statistics were used to describe demographic characteristics and attitudinal beliefs and practices encouraging clients to eat whole grain foods. The Chi-square test was used to determine if there were significant differences between responses to items based on demographic items. The significance level was set at $p < 0.05$.

Results

A total of 306 surveys were returned, resulting in a response rate of 61%. About 60% and 30% had baccalaureate or master's degrees, respectively, with about 70% reporting that they had more than five years of experience as a W.I.C. educator. Almost all (97%) were women. About half (47%) indicated that they worked in a city setting, 19% in a metropolitan area including urban and suburban, and 18% indicated that they worked in a rural setting. The racial/ethnic background of clients was estimated to be about 60% white and about 15% each for African American and Hispanic groups.

A majority of educators (63%) reported that they spent 50% or more of their time on nutrition education. Of the time spent on nutrition education, many reported that half or more of this time was spent working one-on-one with clients (78%) and less than one-fourth of this time was spent conducting group sessions (83%). Those educators who worked primarily in metropolitan and city areas were more likely to conduct group sessions than educators working in more rural areas ($p < 0.05$).

The majority (60%) of respondents rated their level of exposure to new information about whole grain foods as fairly high, while about 75% rated their comfort level regarding teaching clients about whole grain foods as moderate to high. Exposure to new information and comfort level were greater as the level of education increased ($p < 0.05$). About 65% indicated that they placed a fairly high level of priority on encouraging clients to eat whole grain foods.

The majority indicated that they used the criteria of fiber content and whether the first ingredient on the ingredient list was whole grain to identify whole grain foods. More than half reported that they recommended more than three daily servings of whole grain foods to their clients. Attitudes toward the benefits of whole grains were very positive, with most indicating that they recommended whole grain foods to their clients to maintain normal bowel function; control weight; and prevent heart disease, cancer, and diabetes.

More than half of the educators felt that barriers to consumption of whole grain foods were that parents do not like these foods and do not model the behavior to children, children won't eat whole grain foods, and these foods are costly. Other important barriers included difficulty in identifying whole grain foods, and a possible lack of compelling reasons to increase intake of whole grain foods. Educators felt that clients would react favorably to whole

Table 22.3. Difficulty helping clients with concepts/practices related to whole grain foods

	Mean ± SD
Identify a whole grain food	3.5 ± 1.3
Determine what portion of a food constitutes a whole grain serving	3.3 ± 1.4
Find whole grain foods that are culturally appropriate	3.1 ± 1.3
Find whole grain foods the client likes	2.8 ± 1.1
Provide whole grain foods to their child	2.7 ± 1.1
Overcome barriers like cost and taste	2.2 ± 1.0

Values represent the mean ± SD, scaled from 1 = very difficult and 6 = very easy.

grain foods that are tasty and flavorful, have more nutrients and are healthier, keep one regular, prevent disease, and help children learn healthy eating habits.

More than half of those who indicated that they regularly encourage clients to eat whole grain foods reported that they did so because of the overall healthfulness, fiber content, and usefulness for maintaining regularity and preventing disease. Relatively few respondents indicated that they did not regularly encourage consumption of whole grain foods. Reasons for not regularly encouraging consumption of whole grain foods included preferring to focus on fiber (15%), feeling that other dietary changes are more important (21%), not having enough time (18%), limited educational materials to use to encourage consumption by clients (22%), and not having enough current information (11%).

The educational concepts that were identified most often as being difficult to convey to clients were overcoming barriers such as cost and taste, finding whole grain foods that clients like, and providing whole grain foods for children (Table 22.3). Many educators also felt that it was difficult to help clients identify a whole grain food and to determine what portion of a food constitutes a whole grain serving.

When asked about the likelihood of using various education resources/materials to teach about whole grain foods, educators indicated they were likely to use handouts (97%), interactive displays (59%), take-home activities (47%), audiovisual materials (34%), and group discussion modules (26%). The majority reported that they prefer to learn to use new educational materials via a self-teaching manual (77%), while others also preferred a group-learning situation (44%) or computer-based tutorial (45%). Many educators reported that within the past year, they had provided handouts to clients about whole grain foods (71%), provided a brief explanation about whole grain foods during regular sessions (84%), or displayed information about whole grain foods (44%).

Discussion

W.I.C. professionals were very positive about the benefits of whole grain foods for mothers and children and regularly promoted intake of these foods. Educational materials for clients should focus on barriers that most educators thought were important for their clients, such as helping mothers find whole grain foods that children like. Previous focus group and other qualitative research have identified that parents perceive that children do not like whole grain foods and that their children prefer white bread and sweetened cereals (Chase et al. 2003b, Burgess-Champoux et al. 2006). Helping clients identify whole grain foods was found to be problematic for W.I.C. professionals and dietitians (Chase et al. 2003a). The use of various terms on food packages to describe grain products has contributed to the confusion. Focusing on general rules to identify whole grain products may be helpful as educational materials are developed and used with clients.

In the current study, educators preferred to use fairly non-intensive approaches involving handouts and displays to educate clients about whole grain foods. Because many factors affect dietary intake (Wetter et al. 2001), some clients may need more in-depth educational sessions involving skills training to foster shopping and food preparation habits that can improve consumption of whole grain foods among families.

As the marketplace continues to offer more whole grain food choices, cost and accessibility of these foods may improve so that these issues are not significant barriers for low-income W.I.C. mothers (Kantor et al. 2001). W.I.C. educators can play an important role in helping clients learn about new whole grain versions of traditional favorite cereals, breads, crackers, and other processed food products.

Conclusion

In this chapter, nutrition education intervention strategies to increase intake of whole grain foods were described for older adults participating in congregate meal programs, school-aged children, extension audiences, and low-income women in the W.I.C. program. Based on these studies, several common barriers were identified, including lack of knowledge about health benefits, unfamiliar taste, difficulty identifying whole grain foods, lack of monetary resources, unfamiliarity with whole grain foods, and uncertainty about finding whole grain foods in stores. For W.I.C. mothers, educators also were concerned about their ability to help mothers find whole grain foods that children like. Strategies varied for how interventions addressed needs based on audience characteristics and opportunities to deliver messages or alter the environment for the group.

The interventions that were described were implemented through a series of lessons and applied activities, mailed materials, and environmental changes. In all cases, positive outcomes were observed regarding whole grain knowledge, attitudes, or behavior. While positive changes were realized, the authors suggest that further behavioral interventions need to focus on general rules for identifying whole grain products, incorporating whole grain foods into the school cafeteria and congregate dining programs, and emphasizing familiar foods at both the community and individual levels to help consumers purchase and consume more whole grain food products.

References

Baglio ML, Domel Baxter S, Gunn CH, Thompson WO, Schaffer NM, Frye FHA. Assessment of interobserver reliability in nutrition studies that use direct observation of school meals. *Journal of the American Dietetic Association* 2004;104:1385–1392.

Baranowski T, Perry CL, Parcel GS. How individuals, environments, and health behavior interact: Social cognitive theory. In: Glanz K, Lewis FM, Rimer BK, eds. *Health Behavior and Health Education: Theory, Research, and Practice*. San Francisco: Jossey-Bass, 2002;165–184.

Burgess-Champoux T, Marquart L, Vickers Z, Reicks, M. Perceptions of children, parents and teachers regarding whole grain foods and implications for a school-based intervention. *Journal of Nutrition Education and Behavior*; 2006;38:230–237.

Buzby J, Farah H, Vocke G. Will 2005 be the year of the whole grain? *Amber Waves* 2005;3(3):13–17.

Chase K, Reicks M, Miller-Jones J. Applying the theory of planned behavior to promotion of whole grain foods by dietitians. *Journal of the American Dietetic Association* 2003a;103:1639–1642.

Chase K, Reicks M, Smith C, Henry H, Reimer K. Factors influencing purchase of bread and cereals by low-income African American women and implications for whole grain education. *Journal of the American Dietetic Association* 2003b;103:501–504.

Cheong JMK, Johnson MA, Lewis RD, Fischer JG, Johnson JT. Reduction in modifiable osteoporosis-related risk factors among adults in the Older Americans Nutrition Program. *Family Economics and Nutrition Review* 2003;15(1):83–91. http://www.cnpp.usda.gov/FENR/FENRv15n1/fenrv15n1p83.pdf.

Cleveland LE, Moshfegh AJ, Albertson AM, Goldman JD. Dietary intake of whole grains. *Journal of the American College of Nutrition* 2000; 19:331S–338S.

Ellis J, Johnson MA, Fischer JG, Hargrove JL. Nutrition and health education intervention for whole grain foods in the Georgia Older Americans Nutrition Program. *Journal of Nutrition for the Elderly* 2005;24(3):67–83.

Food and Nutrition Service, United States Department of Agriculture. National School Lunch Program: Participation and lunches served. http://www.fns.usda.gov/pd/slsummar.htm [Accessed Dec. 22, 2003].

Freeland-Graves J, Nitzke S. Position of the American Dietetic Association: Total diet approach to communicating food and nutrition information. *Journal of the American Dietetic Association* 2002;102(1):100–108.

Gordon JC. Beyond knowledge: Guidelines for effective health promotion messages. *Journal of Extension* 2002;40(6) (online at http://www.joe.org/joe/2002december/a7.shtml).

Harnack L, Walters SA, Jacobs DR. Dietary intake and food sources of whole grains among U.S. children and adolescents: data from the 1994–1996 Continuing Survey of Food Intakes by Individuals. *Journal of the American Dietetic Association* 2003;103:1015–1019.

Harrington KF, Franklin FA, Davies SL, Shewchuk RM, Brown Binns M. Implementation of a family intervention to increase fruit and vegetable intake: the Hi5+ experience. *Health Promotion and Practice* 2005; 6:180–189.

International Food and Information Council. 2005. Qualified health claims consumer research project executive summary http://www.ific.org/research/qualhealthclaimsres.cfm Accessed Aug. 14, 2005.

Johnson MA. Hype and hope about foods and supplements for healthy aging. *Generations* 2004;28(3):45–53.

Johnson MA, Hawthorne NA, Brackett WR, Fischer JG, Gunter EW, Allen RH, Stabler SP. Hyperhomocysteinemia and vitamin B-12 deficiency in elderly using Title IIIc nutrition services. *American Journal of Clinical Nutrition* 2003;77(1):211–220.

Jones JM, Reicks M, Adams J, Fulcher G, Weaver G, Kanter M, Marquart L. The importance of promoting a whole grain foods message. *Journal of the American College of Nutrition* 2002;21(4):293–297.

Jones JM, Reicks M, Adams J, Fulcher G, Marquart L. Becoming proactive with the whole-grains message. *Nutrition Today.* 2004;39(1):10–17.

Kantor LS, Variyam JN, Allshouse JE, Putnam JJ, Lin B-H. Choose a variety of grains daily, especially whole grains: A challenge for consumers. *Journal of Nutrition* 2001;131:473S–486S.

Lökk J. News and views on folate and elderly persons. *Journal of Gerontology Series A: Biological Sciences and Medical Sciences* 2003;58(4):354–61.

Marquart L, Wiemer K, Jones JM, Jacob B. Whole grain health claims in the U.S.A. and other efforts to increase whole-grain consumption. *Proceedings of the Nutrition Society* 2003;62(1):151–160.

McCamey MA, Hawthorne NA, Reddy S, Lombardo M, Cress ME, Johnson MA. A Statewide educational intervention to improve older Americans' nutrition and physical activity. *Family Economics and Nutrition Review* 2003;15(1):56–66. http://www.usda.gov/cnpp/FENR/FENRv15n1/fenrv15n1p47.pdf.

Patrick H, Nicklas TA. A review of family and social determinants of children's eating patterns and diet quality. *Journal of the American College of Nutrition* 2005;24:83–92.

Ponza M, Ohls JC, Millen BE, McCool AM, Needels KE, Rosenberg L, Chu D, Daly C, Quatromonic, PA. Serving elders at risk. The Older Americans Act Nutrition Programs—National evaluation of the Elderly Nutrition Program, 1993–1995. 1996; http://www.aoa.gov/prof/aoaprog/nutrition/program_eval/eval_report.asp.

Prevention Magazine/Food Marketing Institute. Shopping for health. Emmaus, Penn.: Rodale Press. 1999.

Sahyoun NR, Pratt CA, Anderson A. Evaluation of nutrition education interventions for older adults: A proposed framework. *Journal of the American Dietetic Association* 2004;104(1):58–69.

Simons-Morton BG, Forthofer R, Wei Huang I, Baranowski T, Reed DB, Fleishman R. Reliability of direct observation of schoolchildren's consumption of bag lunches. *Journal of the American Dietetic Association* 1992; 92:219–221.

Strecher VJ, Rosenstock IM. The health belief model. Chapter 3, In *Health Behavior and Health Education: Theory, Research and Practice,* Eds. Glanz K, Lewis FM, Rimer BK, 1997. pp. 41–59. San Francisco, CA: Jossey-Bass.

U.S. Census Bureau. U.S. Interim projection by age, sex, race, and Hispanic origin. 2004. http://www.census.gov/ipc/www/usinterimproj/.

U.S.D.A./A.M.S. The National Organic Program. http://www.ams.usda.gov/nop/indexNet.htm. Accessed Aug. 14 2005.

U.S. Department of Health and Human Services and U.S. Department of Agriculture. Dietary Guidelines for Americans. 2005. http://www.health.gov/dietaryguidelines/dga2005/document/pdf/DGA2005.pdf.

Wellman NS, Kamp B. Federal food and nutrition assistance programs for older people. *Generations* 2004; 28(3):78–85.

Wetter AC, Goldberg JP, King AC, Sigman-Grant M, Baer R, Crayton E, Devine C, Drewnowski A, Dunn A, Johnson G, Pronk N, Saelens B, Snyder D, Novelli P, Walsh K, Warland R. How and why do individuals make food and physical activity choices? *Nutrition Reviews* 2001;59(3 Pt 2):S11–20; S57–65.

Williams P. Consumer understanding and use of health claims for foods. *Nutrition Reviews* 2005;63(7):256–264.

23 The Industry's Commitment to Whole Grains Education

Judi Adams

The Grain Foods Foundation (G.F.F.) was formed in 2004 to help the public understand the importance of both enriched/fortified grains and whole grains in the diet. The foundation is voluntarily funded by the milling and baking industries, including allied companies and associations. It is directed by an elected board of trustees, a staff of one, and a public relations agency. The foundation strongly backs the government's recommendation to make at least three—or half—of one's grains whole grains.

The Effects of the Low-Carb Diets

Low-carbohydrate diets, which became popular in the late 1990s and peaked in 2004, had wreaked havoc on industry sales, not to mention the potential harm to the health of Americans. The industry decided to become engaged in the media rhetoric because the nutritional value of grain-based foods was rarely discussed and accurate information about the negative effects of low-carb diets were also being ignored. Hence, the foundation was organized by the millers and bakers.

At the same time that the sales of white bread and rolls, pasta, and breakfast cereals were decreasing, whole grain products actually increased in sales. White bread had lost 7.0% of sales in 2004, while whole wheat breads had increased 13.8% and total multigrain bread had increased 15.6% (Figure 23.1).

Various grain-based food companies completed their own research on consumer attitudes about whole grains to determine whether joining the council would be appropriate. A study conducted by ConAgra Food Ingredients in December, 2004, showed that three-fourths of Americans believe ". . . eating whole grains is important for good health" (ConAgra Food Ingredients 2004) (Figure 23.2).

However, the same survey showed that an equal number of consumers will not give up taste for nutrition (ConAgra Food Ingredients 2004). It is, therefore, imperative that the industry develop good-tasting whole grain products, which is currently being accomplished.

Educating Consumers

The Grain Foods Foundation launched its consumer education program February 1, 2005, in New York City and Washington, D.C. These cities were chosen because of the opportunity to reach the majority of national media outlets and legislators.

The Reuter's Jumbotron in Times Square displayed foundation messages and artwork throughout the day, along with interactive photos of shoppers on the street with their favorite loaf of bread (Figure 23.3). People dressed as huge loaves of bread distributed nutrition materials and health clubs displayed posters and distributed nutritional flyers to their clients. Buses, bus stops, subway stations and huge wallscapes also told the grains story.

Market Trends – Fresh Bread Category

52 Week Trends – Fresh Bread

Unit Sales

	Latest 52 Weeks Ending Dec 26, 2003	Latest 52 Weeks Ending Dec 26, 2004	% Change
Total Fresh Bread	3,558,807,372	3,454,341,517	-2.94%
Total White Bread	1,626,115,263	1,512,876,836	-6.96%
Total Whole Wheat Breads	271,775,833	309,305,928	13.81%
Total Wheat Breads	604,535,831	605,225,575	0.11%
Total Multigrain Bread	139,563,439	161,293,550	15.57%
Total Other Breads	916,817,007	865,639,628	-5.58%

Figure 23.1. The sales trends for various categories of breads in 2004.

The message on all of the materials was focused on bread. In the future, the foundation will expand its message to include all grain-based foods. The message was consistent: "Bread is delicious." "Filled with healthy grains and makes life better." "Bread. It's Essential." The creative posters, postcards, and "take-ones" highlighted the health benefits of grains in a light-hearted, fun manner.

Positive Attitudes On Whole Grains

Three out of four consumers believe that eating whole grains is important for good health.

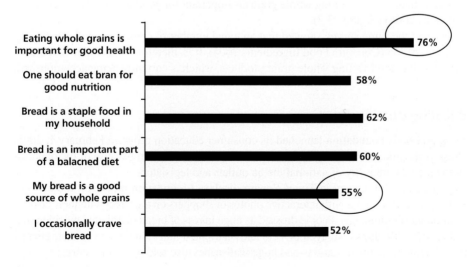

Figure 23.2. ConAgra surveyed consumers in 2004 about their attitudes toward whole grains.

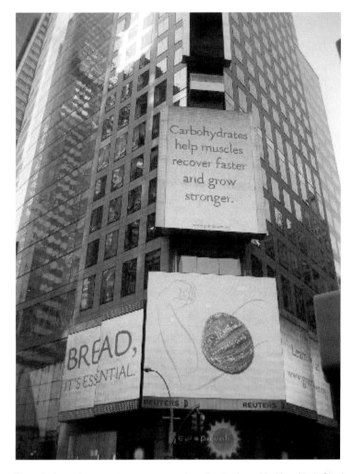

Figure 23.3. The whole grains message was prominently displayed in New York City in early 2005.

The Foundation launch ran through April, although several of the giant wallscapes were up longer because the space had not been resold.

A satellite media tour resulted in a pick-up of fifty-five television stations across the country. After totaling all print and broadcast media, the launch accumulated an "ad equivalency" (if all of the stories were paid for as advertisements) of more than $31.5 million—considerably greater than the total foundation budget of $4 million.

The Kroger Company's Atlanta division displayed the foundation's materials in their stores the last quarter of 2004 as a pilot study for future in-store promotions (Figure 23.4). Sales rose considerably over the fourth quarter of the previous year, which inspired Flowers Foods, which produces a number of baked goods under a variety of names, to extend this program to other divisions.

Grupo Bimbo, with headquarters in Mexico City, also extended the foundation's messages by putting up 115 bus stop signs and a giant billboard in Los Angeles, California. They used the foundation's creative work, but tied it to their own brand (Figure 23.5).

The Grain Foods Foundation's messages are all based on science and approved by an advisory board of thirteen dietitians, exercise physiologists, and medical doctors. These scientists

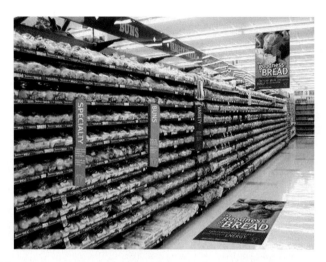

Figure 23.4. The Atlanta division of the Kroger Company successfully displayed Grain Foods Foundation materials.

reviewed the scientific journal articles in the four years preceding the start-up of the foundation and decided which messages could be scientifically approved.

One way the industry has helped overcome the public's dislike of whole grains is by using a class of hard white wheat which is milled into fine whole wheat flour with the taste and texture of white flour and the nutrients of whole wheat. Several G.F.F. members, including the five largest millers—ConAgra, Archer Daniels Midland (A.D.M.), General Mills, Inc., Horizon Milling, and Cereal Food Processors—as well as some smaller ones, are providing this product to a variety of bakers throughout the U.S.

Improvements in Products and Labeling

Shortly after the release of the 2005 Dietary Guidelines, General Mills, Inc. announced that they had consumer tested and developed new whole grain cereal formulas for all of their non-whole grains breakfast cereals. While some only contain enough whole grains to be labeled "made with whole grains," many are "good sources" and "excellent sources" of whole grains. This covert action ensures that many Americans who might never consume whole grains will now be getting at least some whole grains in their diet, similar to the health initiatives of fortifying milk with vitamin D and fortifying enriched grains with folic acid.

The largest and smallest bakers in the U.S. are all adding whole grain products to their bread and bun lines. Whole grain pasta is becoming more readily available in supermarkets and super centers throughout the U.S., as are whole grain tortillas.

The Whole Grains Council (underwritten by Oldways Preservation Trust) has developed two stamps to go on whole grain products). Several surveys and focus groups have shown that not only consumers but also health professionals have trouble identifying whole grain foods (Chase et al. 2003, Warber et al. 1996, U.S.D.A. 2004). The stamps will assist the consumer at the point of purchase in identifying whole grain foods in the supermarket (see stamps in Chapter 21).

The U.S. grain foods industry is committed to helping consumers recognize, purchase and consume more delicious whole grains products with a goal of at least three a day, up from the current level of less than one serving per day.

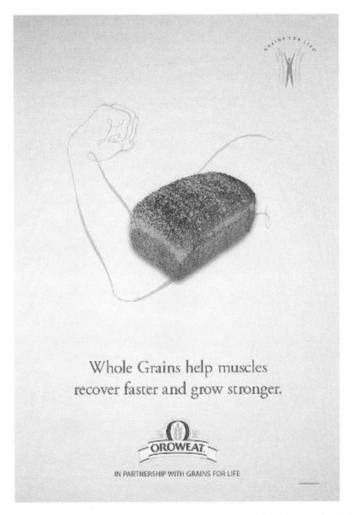

Figure 23.5. A Mexican company tied Grain Foods Foundation materials into an advertising campaign for their own bread in Los Angeles, California.

References

2005 Dietary Guidelines for Americans. www.cnpp.usda.gov/DG2005/index/html. Accessed Jan. 12, 2005

Chase K, Reicks M, Jones JM. Applying the theory of planned behavior to promotion of whole-grain foods by dietitians. *J.A.D.A.* 2003. 103 (12):1639–1642.

ConAgra Food Ingredients. Proprietary survey. Omaha, Neb. Dec. 2004.

U.S. Department of Agriculture, Center for Nutrition Policy Promotion. Consumer Food Guide Pyramid Study, May 27, 2004.

U.S. Department of Agriculture. MyPyramid. www.mypyramid.org Accessed Apr. 19, 2005.

Warber JP, Haddad RD, Hodgkin GF, Lee JW. Foodservice specialists exhibit lack of knowledge in identifying whole-grain products. *J.A.D.A.* 1996. 96 (8):796–798.

WWW.wholegrainscounil.org/WholeGrainStamp.html

24 Industry Initiatives in Whole Grain Education

Trish Griffiths

There is now a substantial and growing body of evidence from scientific studies to suggest that grains—especially whole grains—are well placed to satisfy the demands of health-conscious consumers. This information is embedded in public health recommendations, and Australian dietary guidelines encourage adults, children, and adolescents to "Eat plenty of cereals (including breads, rice, pasta, and noodles), preferably whole grain" (National Health and Medical Research Council 2003).

These guidelines represent the consensus of current scientific evidence, but the grains industry knows it cannot afford to become complacent. Competition for consumer's "share of mind" and "share of stomach" in the modern day marketplace is fierce, and grain-based foods face many challenges. Targeted strategies that communicate clear, consistent messages about grains, nutrition, and health are essential if grain foods are to maintain this healthy positioning with consumers.

The Challenge for Grains

Health and convenience have traditionally been recognized as key factors driving consumer food choice, and the concept of "wellness" is becoming increasingly important. People are living longer and are motivated to prolong their quality of life. More people are reading the information on food labels (a recent global study found 93% of Australians refer to the nutritional labeling on products) (A.C. Nielsen 2005) and the market for foods that deliver a health benefit beyond normal nutrition ("functional foods") is growing.

In the overall context of consumer interest in health, the benefits of foods such as breads and breakfast cereals are not well understood (Go Grains 2004a). This has been made worse over recent years by widespread media misinformation propagated in regard to "low-carb" diets for weight reduction. Glycemic index (G.I.), emerging as the next fad to take over from low carb, also is unfavorable for many grain products.

Low-carb

The low-carb phenomenon in its purest form discourages consumption of all healthy, high-carbohydrate foods such as bread, breakfast cereals, rice, and pasta. Ultimately, however, followers rebel against a life without "carbs," and various versions of the diet—such as the South Beach Diet—have evolved to accommodate "low-G.I." carbs such as mixed grain bread and other whole grain foods. Ironically, the end result could be an increased interest in whole grain foods, although it is unlikely that whole grains will ever substitute for total grain food consumption.

Research conducted in 2004 (Go Grains 2004b) revealed that around 2.5 million Australians (nearly one in five) had tried or intended to try a low-carbohydrate diet. The research revealed confusion surrounding the identity and recommended amount of carbohydrate foods in a balanced diet. Only one-third of Australians knew that confectionary and soft drinks were carbohydrates. Seven in ten Australians were not aware of the amount of carbohydrate-based foods—such as bread, breakfast cereal, rice, and pasta—recommended for a healthy diet.

The connection between carbohydrates and grains is not well understood by Australian consumers. Between 2002 and 2004 there was an 8% increase in people agreeing with the statement that "carbohydrates are fattening" (Figure 24.1), while about two-thirds of people believed "regular consumption of grain foods can help in weight loss and weight control" (Figure 24.2) (Go Grains 2004a). This would indicate that carbohydrates are not directly linked to grains in consumer's minds.

The disconnect between carbohydrates and grains may, in fact, be beneficial in helping people to understand that there are some high-carbohydrate foods such as pastries, pizza, and soft drinks that do not have a daily place in a healthy diet, while grain foods such as bread, breakfast cereals, and pasta (preferably whole grain) should be eaten on a daily basis.

Glycemic Index

Australians have embraced the G.I. concept, with all its limitations. G.I. is a measure of the rate at which carbohydrates are digested. Awareness of G.I. increased from 28% in 2002 to 86% in 2005 (Glycemic Index Ltd. 2005), driven largely by media interest, a G.I. symbol on food products, and regular consumer-targeted book launches by Australian scientists in the field. Eighty-four percent of Australians say that they would be "very likely" or somewhat likely" to use the G.I. rating when choosing food (up from 71% in 2002).

The G.I. concept encourages consumption of whole grain foods that contain intact grains, but not those that contain milled grains nor refined grains. Milling increases G.I. by increasing the accessibility of starch to digestive enzymes. The fundamental issue in translating the science of G.I. into practice is the tendency for high-G.I. foods (G.I. greater than 70) to be

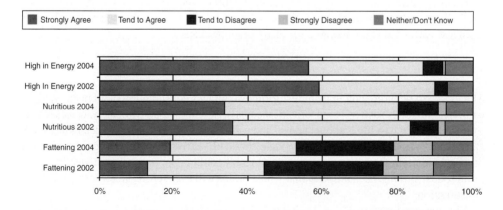

Source: Go Grains Tracking Study. Sept 2004. Conducted by Newspoll.

Figure 24.1. Newspoll conducted a survey to learn more about the attitudes of Australians about whole grains.

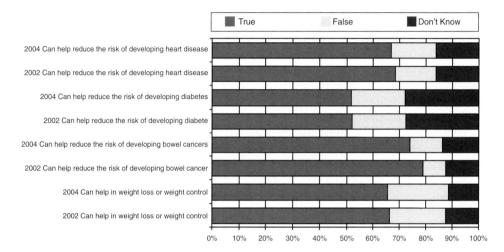

Source: Go Grains Tracking Study. Sept 2004. Conducted by Newspoll.

Figure 24.2. Australians were surveyed to determine their knowledge about whole grains.

classified as less healthy than their low-G.I. (G.I. less than 55) counterparts. In reality, there are many high-G.I. foods that are very nutritious—including whole grain foods such as whole meal breads and many breakfast cereals made from milled grains—and many other low-G.I. foods that are much less nutritious, such as chocolate and sausages.

Misunderstanding of the G.I. concept potentially poses a threat to consumption of grain-based foods that have a high-G.I, and this is unlikely to be resolved until there is better understanding that G.I. should not be used to rate the nutritional value of a food.

The Definition of Whole Grain

Australian food regulations define whole grain as: "the unmilled products of a single cereal or mixture of cereals" (Australia New Zealand Food Authority 1987). Few foods contain an appreciable amount of unmilled grains, so this definition limits the ability to communicate messages about whole grains and health on food labels and in advertising. An application to change this definition is currently under consideration by Food Standards Australia New Zealand (F.S.A.N.Z.). The proposed new definition is "whole grain is intact, dehulled, ground, cracked, or flaked grains where the components—endosperm, germ, and bran—are present in substantially the same proportions as they exist in the intact grain."

This proposed definition is consistent with international practice and with the intent of public health documents such as the Dietary Guidelines for Australian Adults that recommend "Eat plenty of cereals (including breads, rice, pasta, and noodles), preferably whole grain"(N.H.& M.R.C. 2003).

Broadening the definition would pave the way for developing criteria to define a "source" (proposed as 25% whole grain ingredients) or a "good source" (proposed as more than 50% whole grain ingredients) to be used on food labels.

The extensive body of data that now supports a role for whole grains in reducing the risk of heart disease (Truswell 2002), diabetes (Venn 2004), and some cancers (McIntosh 2001) provides an outstanding opportunity for the grains industry to promote consumption of grain-based foods.

Go Grains, an initiative of B.R.I. Australia Ltd. (an independent grains research organization) and the Grains Research and Development Corporation, was established in 1998 to promote the nutrition and health benefits of grain-based foods.

The work of Go Grains is directed by an advisory committee comprised of a coalition of major grain food manufacturers, research organizations, and public health interests. Industry members are serious competitors in the marketplace, but unite as Go Grains for the common purpose of communicating positive messages (Figure 24.3) about grains and health and addressing industry-wide nutrition-related issues such as "low carb" and Glycemic Index. Advisory committee members provide input to strategy development, contribute to outputs, and provide Go Grains with valuable access to networks and resources.

Over its seven years in existence, Go Grains has built brand recognition with health professionals, educators, journalists, and the food industry. These target groups are engaged to disseminate information and teaching resources through their students, clients, patients, and customers. More than 430,000 pieces of information have been distributed through these networks and millions more people have been reached through media activity.

The success of Go Grains, and its support from industry, is due largely to its independent and authoritative positioning, and to the fact that it is able to address important issues in a way that food manufacturers cannot. Credibility, based on sound science, provides the foundation for positive messages about grains and health and allows Go Grains to counter misinformation with integrity.

Communications are based on scientific reviews of the international literature and address issues identified in consumer research. Literature reviews have been commissioned on topics including heart disease, cancer, diabetes, cereal grain hypersensitivity, and weight control. Authors are encouraged to submit reviews to peer-reviewed journals for publication. The findings of these reviews provide the basis for targeted public relations activities and printed resource materials and provide the opportunity to engage health professionals and teachers to promote grains.

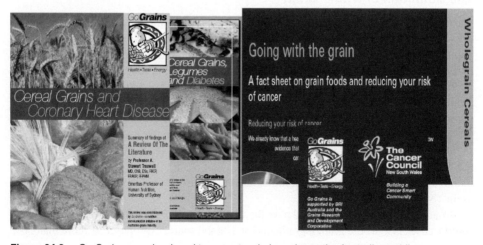

Figure 24.3. Go Grains was developed to promote whole grains to the Australian public.

Communications are managed by a professional communications agency. Media releases typically achieve national coverage across all media—print, radio, TV, and the Web. Key Go Grains messages focus on the health benefits of eating more grain foods, with an emphasis on whole grains. Reduced risk of heart disease (around 30%), diabetes (20% to 40%) and some cancers (30% to 40%) are particularly relevant in an environment where heart disease remains the leading cause of death (Australian Institute of Health and Welfare 2004) and the incidence of obesity and diabetes is increasing dramatically (Cameron 2003, Catford 2003, Dunstan 2001).

A major Go Grains initiative in 2004-05 addressed the potential threat to grain food consumption posed by the increasing interest in low-carb diets. Two major bursts of media activity were conducted over a twelve-month period. The first promoted the findings of a review of the literature titled "De-bunking the myths about carbohydrates and weight control." The second publicized the findings of a consumer Newspoll survey that investigated the understanding of Australian consumers about carbohydrates and their intention to follow a low-carb diet. The findings of the survey were launched at a media function attended by journalists, health professionals, and key opinion leaders in the food industry. In the period between the two bursts of media activity, the feature article "De-bunking the myths about carbohydrates and weight control" was placed in a popular women's magazine (circulation 2.5 million) and copies of this article were subsequently used as a consumer resource (around 47,000 copies have been distributed to date).

Overview of Go Grains Activities

Go Grains uses a variety of strategies to communicate its messages to target groups:

Consumer education materials are direct-mailed to teachers, dietitians, and other relevant audiences (this varies with the topic) through their respective professional associations. Follow-up requests for bulk orders of resources are fulfilled through a mailing house.

Curriculum-based teaching resources for schools are developed in conjunction with education professionals and promoted through school and teacher networks.

Public relations activities use independent expert spokespeople and where possible, link with other non-government organizations such as the Heart Foundation, Diabetes Australia, or Cancer Council New South Wales to enhance credibility and to increase the reach of communications.

A monthly E-newsletter keeps subscribers up to date with the latest research and news about grains, nutrition, and health. It is accessible through and archived on the Go Grains Web site.

The actively maintained Web site is a source of information about nutrition, health, and grains, and includes recipes, media releases, consumer publications, and links to other organizations.

Conference presentations and articles contribute reach and frequency to the communication strategy.

References

A.C. Nielsen. 2005. Online Consumer Opinion Survey. http://www.acnielsen.com.au/news.asp?newsID=299

Australia New Zealand Food Authority. 1987. Australia New Zealand Food Standards Code. 2005. Anstat. Pty. Ltd. A.C.N. 005446748.

Australian Institute of Health and Welfare. 2004. Australia's Health 2004.

Cameron AJ, et al. 2003. Overweight and obesity in Australia: the 1999-2000 Australian Diabetes, Obesity and Lifestyle Study. *M.J.A.* Vol 178.

Catford J, Caterson I. 2003. Snowballing obesity: Australians will get run over if they just sit there. *M.J.A.*; 179(11/12):577–579.

Dunstan D, Zimmet P, Welborn T, et al. 2001. Diabesity and associated disorders in Australia. Final report of the Australian diabetes, obesity and lifestyle study. International Diabetes Institute. http://www.aihw.gov.au/riskfactors/overweight.cfm

Glycemic Index Ltd. 2005. Glycemic Index Symbol Program Consumer Research. University of Sydney. Australia. (unpublished). (http://www.gisymbol.com.au/pages/index.asp)

Go Grains. 2004a. Newspoll Consumer Tracking Study. Sydney. (unpublished).

Go Grains. 2004b. Newspoll Diet and Carbohydrates study. Sydney. (unpublished).

McIntosh GH. Cereal foods, fibres and the prevention of cancers. *Aust. J. Nutr. Diet.* (2001) 58 Suppl 2.

National Health and Medical Research Center. 2003. Food for Health. Dietary Guidelines for Australian Adults. Dept of Health & Ageing. Commonwealth of Australia.

Truswell A. Cereal grains and coronary heart disease. *Eur. J. Clin. Nutr.* (2002) 56, 1–15.

Venn BJ, Mann JI. Cereal grains, legumes and diabetes. *Eur. J. Clin. Nutr.* (2004) 58, 1443–1461.

25 Communicating with Consumers: Whole Grain Messaging

Mindy Hermann

Introduction

Health professionals should view themselves as having two different types of jobs. The first is their primary position, be it in research, industry, or academia. The second is a position as a communicator. Communicators translate scientific or industry findings and materials into language that the consumer can understand and act upon. Communications are successful when they reach the desired consumer, as well as when the consumer takes the desired action, for example, eating more whole grain foods.

Of the two measures of success, reaching consumers and seeing positive action, reaching consumers with new information that increases consumer knowledge is far easier than motivating actions. Consumers are willing to listen; they are less willing to change their behavior. Surveys repeatedly show that a large number of consumers know about nutrition and healthful eating. A much smaller number say that they take action to improve their eating habits.

Nutrition messages can be confusing to consumers. In today's world, study results are widely communicated, reaching the consumer through the media and the Internet. Conflicting findings, complex scientific explanations, and even an abundance of information on nutrients, how they work, and where they are found often are overwhelming to the average consumer. In contrast, simple messages that present the health benefits of eating a particular food—for example, eating a diet rich in whole grains to lower heart disease risk—help convince consumers that simple steps are worthwhile.

Solely providing information is not enough. Consumers need strategies for changing their behavior (International Food and Information Council 2004). Certainly this holds true for motivating consumers to eat whole grains. As shown in this brief article, media coverage of the topic of whole grains can help guide consumer behavior.

Forming a partnership with the media allows health professionals to effectively reach large numbers of consumers. The media are a powerful ally for getting Americans to change their eating behaviors (Goldberg 1997) because hundreds, thousands, even millions of consumers can hear, watch, or read nutrition messages.

The Importance of Timing

Timing the release of a message through the media requires careful thought. The message could be communicated as a free-standing message. The communication of new study findings at the same time that they appear in a medical journal, for example, creates news. Alternately, study findings can be communicated to media when they can be part of a bigger story. The creation of the 2005 Dietary Guidelines was a bigger story on which whole grain messages could be piggybacked.

Jumping onto an existing story is far easier than creating news. Details, a new angle, an expert opinion, or a service angle (how consumers can apply the news to their own lives) enhance a story and bring it closer to the consumer. Consumers also may be more likely to "hear" the message because the topic already is familiar to them.

Crafting the Message

Transforming scientific or industry information into material for the media is an art that can be learned. The first step is to think about what the consumer wants or needs. The next is to make a list of important facts or product features (Hudnall 1994). The initial list can be long; ultimately it will be whittled down into three key points or product features. Pair each point or feature with at least one consumer benefit. Those that do not have an obvious consumer benefit should be crossed off the list. Decide what the consumer needs to know to take action: In the case of whole grains, the universal goals are to get consumers to try them, like them, and include adequate amounts in their diets every day. Finally, pick three main points or features that are likely to induce consumers to change their behavior and turn those three points into material for the media.

Language should be easy for consumers to understand. Write in consumer-friendly terms, unless writing for the business or scientific press. Make sure that all points are clear, easy to understand, and actionable. Keep messages simple and tell the truth.

The Perfect Storm: Dietary Guidelines for Americans, 2005

The 2005 Dietary Guidelines for Americans provided, and continue to provide, a perfect opportunity to communicate whole grain messages. Strongly emphasizing the importance of including whole grains in the diet opens the door for researchers, academia, health professionals, and food companies to provide the media with news and practical advice on whole grains.

An informal survey of Google News between April 15 and May 15, 2005, generated more than 1,500 whole grains news stories. This number represented U.S. publications only and included newspapers, general news Web sites, and medical news Web sites. Articles were classified into several broad categories.

"What" stories described whole grains. They primarily offered information without practical advice on how to take action. This type of article leaves the consumer needing additional information to motivate behavior change. For consumers who already are seeking out a variety of whole grains, the list of whole grains included in many articles—whole wheat, corn, cornmeal, brown rice, whole oats—might validate their food choices and assure them that their eating behavior is desirable.

"Why" stories can motivate consumers by explaining the health rationale for including whole grains. Commonly, stories listed a suggested number of daily servings—at least three—and the diseases against which whole grains may be protective, namely heart disease, type 2 diabetes, and some cancers.

Stories that present the "where" of whole grains help consumers find whole grains. Information can be general, focusing on supermarket aisles (bread, pasta, cereal) that are likely to contain whole grains. Articles on business pages or in business publications tend to provide more specific information on new whole grain products being introduced by major companies.

Related to "where" articles were those with information on "how" to find whole grains. Numerous articles referred to the industry's Whole Grain Stamp as a starting point. Information about the Whole Grain Stamp provided a news angle because the stamp is new to many consumers. Whole Grain Stamp articles also offered a service angle, helping consumers take action by providing specific information on how to use the stamp to find whole grain foods. Also popular were articles with information on using the ingredient list to find whole grains.

Less common were "who" articles naming celebrities who cook with or eat whole grains. Celebrity chef Bobby Flay, who hosts national cooking shows and has written several cookbooks, was quoted in several articles regarding his interest in eating more whole grains. In conjunction with his new cookbook, Flay offered whole grain recipes to the media.

Numerous articles aimed to take the "fear factor" out of whole grains by discussing the ease with which whole grains can be added to a person's daily diet. This type of article calls attention to everyday foods that consumers may not realize are whole grain foods, such as whole wheat bread, popcorn, and oatmeal. Pointing out how easy it is to eat whole grains, and bringing in the surprise element with mention of fun foods like popcorn, can help break down consumer barriers to eating more whole grains.

The post-low-carbohydrate diet era offered numerous opportunities for articles on how to add back grains and whole grains to the diet. Piggybacking onto the diet book movement from no-carb to "good carb," articles highlighted whole grains as carbohydrates that should be included in the diet.

Articles aiming to reduce consumer confusion regarding whole grains discussed the difference between whole grain foods and whole grain-sounding foods. This type of article pointed out potentially confusing terms, such as multigrain and stone-ground, and offered tips to consumers on differentiating between whole grain imposters and true whole grains. Few articles tackled the challenge of differentiating between whole grain and high fiber.

Conclusion

The media, including magazines, newspapers, and other traditional outlets, as well as the Internet, blogs, and other news media, is a highly useful tool for communicating messages about whole grains. The challenge is to create and communicate messages that catch the attention of the media, are broadly distributed, and motivate consumers to take action.

References

Goldberg, JP, Hellwig JP. Nutrition research in the media: The challenge facing scientists. *J Am Coll Nutr* 1997; 16–544–50.

Hudnall, M. News releases, advertising copy, and brochures. In Chernoff, R (ed.). *Communicating as Professionals*, Second Edition. Chicago: American Dietetic Association, 1994.

International Food and Information Council Foundation. Fitting carbohydrates into a healthful diet: A consumer point-of-view—Qualitative Research Findings. September 3, 2004. Accessed on-line at http://www.ific.org/research/upload/Fitting_Carbohydrates_into_a_Healthful_Diet.pdf

26 Global Regulation, Labeling, Claims and Seals: Perspectives and Guidelines

Kristen Schmitz, Nils-Georg Asp, David Richardson, and Len Marquart

Introduction

With the incidence of obesity and being overweight increasing at alarming rates in the United States and in other developed and developing countries, diseases directly related to being obese and overweight will also increase (World Health Organization, 2003). A report by the Centers for Disease Control and Prevention in 2005 (C.D.C. 2005b) estimates the cost of heart disease and stroke in the United States for 2005 to be $394 billion (the estimate covers health care expenditures and lost productivity from death and disability).

More than 927,000 Americans die of cardiovascular disease (C.V.D.) annually and more than 70 million people live with C.V.D., greater than one-fourth the population (C.D.C. 2005a). Although C.V.D. is most common among people over the age of 65, the incidence is increasing among those aged 15 to 34. Therefore, decreasing annual C.V.D. cases has immediate implications for the medical and economic health throughout the world.

Considerable research indicates that whole grain foods, as commonly consumed in the U.S. and Europe, may help to reduce the risk for coronary heart disease (Jacobs et al. 1998, Liu et al. 1999, Anderson et al. 2000, Fung et al. 2002, Truswell 2002), certain cancers (Jacobs et al. 1998, Chatenoud et al. 1998), diabetes (Meyer et al. 2000, Liu et al. 2000, Montonen et al. 2003, Venn and Mann 2004), and all-cause mortality (Jacobs et al. 1999, Jacobs et al. 2000, Liu et al. 2003). It is well recognized that whole grains contain biologically active compounds, beyond dietary fiber, such as antioxidants (phenolics, tocotrienols, and phytoestrogens) that may elicit health benefits either individually, in combination, and/or synergistically.

The United States forged the path for whole grain health claims with the 1999 approval of the first whole grain health claim for both heart disease and cancer. Subsequently, the United Kingdom Joint Health Claims Initiative (J.H.C.I.) published an authoritative endorsement for whole grain foods in 2002 followed by the 2003 Swedish Code whole grain health claim. Previous works outlined the whole grain health claims in the United States (Marquart et al. 2003) and the similarities and differences between whole grain health claims in the United States, United Kingdom, and Sweden (Marquart et al. 2004). This chapter specifically examines the current health claims in these three countries, the recent whole grains petition to the U.S. Food and Drug Administration (F.D.A.), and the use of whole grain seals in the United States, and provides an update on the developments in Europe, especially regarding the scientific substantiation of health claims on foods.

Codex

The Codex Alimentarius Commission, created in 1963 by the Food and Agriculture Organization (F.A.O.) and World Health Organization (W.H.O.), serves to develop food standards and guidelines under the Joint F.A.O./W.H.O. Food Standards Program. The primary objectives of the Food Standards Program are to protect the health of consumers, ensure fair food trade practices, and promote coordination of all food standards work. There are three different types of health claims under Codex guidelines: nutrient function claims, other function claims, and reduction of disease risk claims (C.A.C. 2004). Aside from the health claims, Codex has not accepted a definition of whole grains as an official standard and should work to develop an internationally accepted definition.

Whole Grain Regulations in the United States

In January 2005 the U.S. Department of Agriculture (U.S.D.A.) released the 2005 Dietary Guidelines for Americans recommending at least three daily servings of whole grain (3 oz). Mypyramid.gov recommends that at least three servings from grains be whole grain (U.S.D.A./H.H.S. 2005a, b). Additionally, Healthy People 2010 aims to get at least 50% of the population older than the age of 2 to consume three daily servings of whole grains by 2010 (D.H.H.S. 2000).

Given the substantial evidence supporting disease prevention with whole grain consumption, and recommendations to consume three servings or more per day, estimates suggest average daily whole grain consumption is less than one serving per day (Cleveland et al. 2000). The lack of whole grain consumption in part stems from consumer confusion in identifying products containing whole grains. There is no official definition of whole grain foods and no identifiable universal symbol. The Whole Grains Council currently endorses usage of the Whole Grain Stamp (see Chapter 21) to create awareness and help the general population to more easily identify whole grain food products.

The Nutrition Labeling and Education Act of 1990 introduced health claims for food to educate consumers and encourage consumption of healthful foods. In 1993 the F.D.A. passed the first seven health claims based on scientific consensus from results of epidemiological, animal, and clinical research studies. After passing the first seven health claims, the F.D.A. established a process to petition for new health claims that addressed substance/disease relationships. To establish a new claim, the petitioner must provide sufficient scientific support and meet the F.D.A.'s specific regulatory requirements. Since the initial seven health claims were approved in 1993, six more have been approved—the first was soluble fiber from whole oats and risk of coronary heart disease (F.D.A. 1997).

Although health claims can make a major contribution toward improving health, the standard procedure for approval can take more than a year. This is attributed to the scientific review, publication of a proposed rule, and time for public comments, which are all mandated under the F.D.A.'s 1993 Nutrition Labeling Education Act (N.L.E.A.) food labeling rules for health claims. Therefore, the F.D.A. approved the Food and Drug Administration Modernization Act (F.D.A.M.A.) of 1997 (F.D.A. 1997), providing a method to accelerate review and regulation of health claims for foods.

Health claims are approved faster through the F.D.A.M.A. process than the standard process. The whole grain health claim was the first to be allowed through the F.D.A.M.A. process in July 1999 (F.D.A. 1999). The claim, "Diets rich in whole grain foods and other plant foods and low in total fat, saturated fat, and cholesterol may reduce the risk of heart disease and some cancers," is allowed on any product that contains 51% whole grain per reference amount customarily consumed (R.A.C.C.). While 51% whole grain is easily achieved for dry foods such as breakfast cereal, it is hard to attain for foods with a higher moisture content, such as bread.

After substantial review of a health claim petition submitted by The National Barley Foods Council, the F.D.A. provided a final rule extending the health claim on the relationship between oat β-glucan soluble fiber and the reduced risk of coronary heart disease to include products made with dehulled and hull-less whole grain barley and other specific dry milled barley products (F.D.A. 2006). The F.D.A. concluded that β-glucan soluble fiber from barley is analytically the same substance as β-glucan soluble fiber from oat sources. Manufacturers are permitted to immediately use the health claim for barley and the reduced risk of coronary heart disease.

To qualify for the health claim, the barley-containing foods must provide at least 0.75 grams of soluble fiber per serving. This is a tremendous opportunity for barley to elicit health benefits through commonly consumed food products due to its excellent product functionality and naturally rich nutrient and phytochemical content. The health claim reads: "Soluble fiber from foods such as (name of food), as part of a diet low in saturated fat and cholesterol, may reduce the risk of heart disease. A serving of (name of food) supplies (X) grams of the soluble fiber necessary per day to have this effect."

Recent F.D.A. Position on Labeling Whole Grains

General Mills, Inc. submitted a petition on May 11, 2004, requesting definitions for whole grain content descriptors: "excellent source," "good source," and "made with." The assumptions made in the petition were that whole grain is a substance, not a broad category of food, and that the descriptors are neither nutrient content nor health claims. For each of the descriptors, the level of whole grains per serving would be 16 grams or more, 8 grams to 15 grams, and at least 8 grams, respectively. In November, 2005 the F.D.A. denied the petition on the basis that they do not know how to classify whole grains (i.e., food category, food ingredient, nutrient, or other).

These particular descriptors are typically used for nutrient content claims on nutrients with established reference daily intakes (R.D.I.); however, "whole grain" does not have an R.D.I. and thus cannot be classified as a nutrient. Although General Mills, Inc. recommended usage of the fiber content as a marker for whole grains, the F.D.A. felt the use of the descriptors would imply a nutrient content claim for fiber and not necessarily whole grain. The F.D.A. denied the petition because they need to carefully consider a definition of whole grain and how the term should be classified. However, the F.D.A. acknowledges a need for action to resolve the myriad questions, especially because the 2005 Dietary Guidelines for Americans recommend consumption of whole grains.

The Whole Grains Council (W.G.C.) has designed a set of stamps that food manufacturers, bakeries, and grocers that are members of the group can use to indicate the number of grams of whole grains per serving. This effort has enhanced consumers' ability to identify whole grain foods in retail outlets.

Whole Grain Regulations in the United Kingdom

The final ruling on the whole grain health claim by the United Kingdom Joint Health Claims Initiative (J.H.C.I.) came in 2002. The official claim reads, "People with a healthy heart tend to eat more whole grain foods as part of a healthy lifestyle," and may be applied to foods deemed appropriate by the committee. The claim is allowed based on the following six conditions as determined in the final report of the Expert Committee to the J.H.C.I. Council (J.H.C.I. 2002):

1. The health impact of a diet containing whole grain foods depends on the rest of the diet as well as other lifestyle factors such as exercise. The claim must be set within this context.
2. The evidence supports an association between a healthy heart and whole grain consumption but is insufficient to demonstrate cause and effect.
3. The evidence is insufficient to support claims targeted specifically at men.
4. The claim relates to foods containing 51% or more whole grain ingredients by weight per serving. The term "whole grain" refers to the major cereal grains including wheat, rice, maize, and oats. The structure for all grains is similar and the grain is made up of three components: the endosperm, the germ, and the bran.
5. The J.H.C.I. strongly recommends that companies seek advice from the Secretariat before using this claim to help ensure that the food product is consistent with good nutrition principles and complies with the J.H.C.I. Code of Practice for Health Claims on Food.
6. The wording of the claim has been carefully formulated to reflect the evidence on which the claim has been approved. Wording may be altered, in consultation with the J.H.C.I., as long as the claim does not imply health benefits beyond the scope of the evidence, change the meaning of the claim, or confuse consumers.

Whole Grain Regulations in Sweden

The Swedish Code, entitled "Health Claims in the Labeling and Marketing of Food Products, The Food Industry's Rules (Self-Regulating Programme)," was developed by national organizations representing primary production, the food industry, and major retail organizations, in close collaboration with relevant authorities (Asp and Trossing 2001). The Swedish Nutrition Foundation (S.N.F.) participated in the development of the Swedish Code and has an advisory and coordinating role.

The original Swedish Code allowed generic claims in two steps concerning eight different, generally recognized diet-health relationships, closely related to the official nutrition recommendations. In June 2003 the whole grain claim was adopted as the ninth generic claim: "A healthy lifestyle and a balanced diet rich in whole grain products reduces the risk for (coronary) heart disease. Product (X) is a good source of whole grain (contains (Y)% whole grain)." Aside from the product showing a substantial effect on the composition of the entire diet, the percentage of whole grain must be at least 50% on a dry weight basis, which also is realistic for soft bread. Furthermore, there are restrictions regarding fat, sugar, and salt content. The latest revision of the Swedish Code (http://www.hp-info.nu/SweCode_2004_1.pdf) is applicable from September 2004 (Asp and Bryngelsson 2004).

Recognizing the extensive research showing the physiological effects of specific foods, the Swedish Code implemented "product-specific physiological claims" in 2001 (Asp and Trossing 2001). These product-specific claims require human intervention studies to show that the product, under normal consumption conditions, caused the claimed physiological effect. The scientific substantiation is subject to premarketing expert evaluation. So far, six products have been approved with expert statements available (http://www.snf.ideon.se/snf/en/rh/PFP.htm). Recently a number of low-glycemic index products were approved after a simplified expert evaluation.

Health Claims in Europe

Awaiting a European Union regulation (expected in 2006), health claims in Europe have primarily been country specific. However, the European Commission supported the Functional Foods Science in Europe (F.U.F.O.S.E.) project in 1995, which established a scientific approach to the development of functional food products (Diplock et al. 1999). Scientific substantiation of claims is one of the most important aspects of approving health claims to provide truthful information to consumers, satisfy regulatory requirements, and allow fair market competition.

Accordingly, the European Commission recently concluded a four-year project called "Process for the Assessment of Scientific Support for Claims on Foods (P.A.S.S.C.L.A.I.M.)." As with F.U.F.O.S.E., the project was organized by the International Life Sciences Institute of Europe to produce a generic tool for assessing the scientific support for health claims on food. Almost 200 scientists representing academia, industry, research institutes, public interest groups, and the regulatory environment provided input for defining criteria for scientific substantiation of claims, which was the final facet of P.A.S.S.C.L.A.I.M. The criteria for scientific substantiation, developed in the consensus document (Aggett et al. 2005), are:

1. The food or food component to which the claimed effect is attributed should be characterized.
2. Substantiation of a claim should be based on human data, primarily from intervention studies, the design of which should include the following considerations:
   a. Study groups that are representative of the target group.
   b. Appropriate controls.
   c. An adequate duration of exposure and follow-up to demonstrate the intended effect.
   d. Characterization of the study groups' background diets and other relevant aspects of lifestyle.
   e. An amount of the food or food component consistent with its intended pattern of consumption.
   f. The influence of the food matrix and dietary context on the functional effect of the component.
   g. Monitoring of subjects' compliance concerning intake of food or food component under test.
   h. The statistical power to test the hypothesis.
3. When the true endpoint of a claimed benefit cannot be measured directly, studies should use markers.
4. Markers should be:
   a. Biologically valid in that they have a known relationship to the final outcome and their variability within the target population is known.
   b. Methodologically valid with respect to their analytical characteristics.
5. Within a study the target variable should change in a statistically significant way and the change should be biologically meaningful for the target group, consistent with the claim to be supported.
6. A claim should be scientifically substantiated by taking into account the totality of the available data and by weighing of the evidence.

The criteria describe the standards by which the quality and relevance of the scientific evidence should be judged and the extent to which a claim based on them can be said to be scientifically valid. The substantiation of a claim is heavily weighted toward intervention studies that provide extensive evidence toward a food or food component and function and/or disease relationship. The end result of P.A.S.S.C.L.A.I.M. is to bolster consumer confidence in the claims being made so consumers may make well-informed healthy lifestyle choices.

Future Direction

There are two crucial issues facing the successful introduction of whole grain foods into the food supply. One is a salient and working definition for both a whole grain ingredient and a whole grain food. Within the past year the American Association of Cereal Chemists International (A.A.C.C.) and the W.G.C., a consortium of industry, scientists, chefs, and the Oldways Preservation Trust, worked together to formulate a consumer-friendly definition for whole grains and whole grain foods. The entire food industry would benefit from Codex adopting this definition as an official standard followed by implementation to country-specific food law. Another key issue is to identify the nutrients and other bioactive components in whole grains that confer health benefits through well-designed human intervention studies. A major new European Commission-supported project is addressing these issues (http://www.healthgrain.org/pub/).

In Europe, the United Kingdom and Sweden are currently the only countries with whole grain health claims. Once a European Union regulation on health claims is in place there will be formal possibilities to extend into other European countries. International harmonization of health claims and regulatory efforts for greater whole grain consumption would be ideal. Suggested actions for setting international regulatory and policy standards for whole grains include:

1. Creating one international definition and symbol of identification for whole grains by committee involvement.
2. Building international whole grain food labeling standards and eliminating confusing terminology.
3. Exploring fortification of whole grains with nutrients low or deficient in the population, e.g. folic acid and phytonutrients.
4. Educating the public about what constitutes whole grain foods and where to find them in the marketplace.
5. Creating meaningful and easy-to-understand portion size descriptors.

Additionally, A.A.C.C. has developed a task force on whole grains and health dedicated to exploring four areas: bioactive components, health claims, the whole grain barley definition, and the whole grain corn definition. The objective of this task force is to encompass whole grain ingredients and whole grain food definitions involving all major sectors from an international perspective.

Conclusion

Whole grain health claims can benefit consumers, government, industry, and academia. From a public health standpoint, a whole grains claim can help government agencies and consumers achieve diet- and health-related goals, and potentially contribute to the overall reduction of chronic disease risk. Increased visibility and promotion of a whole grains claim offers consumers the opportunity to identify whole grain foods, learn about their health benefits, and explore ways to increase consumption. Industry can benefit from additional incentives to develop and promote whole grain products, along with increased product demand.

However, the health claim also has highlighted the need for research on whole grains, primarily from an academic perspective with additional interest from the governmental scientific community. Identification of the active substances and principles will establish the basis for further development of nutritious whole grain raw materials and products. Additional consumer education, scientific research, and government policy are needed to reinforce and expand the effectiveness of whole grain health claims.

References

Aggett, P.J.; Antoine, J.-M.; Asp, N.-G.; Bellisle, F.; Contor, L.; Cummings, J.H.; Howlett, J.; Müller, D.J.G.; Persin, C.; Pijls, L.T.J.; Rechkemmer, G.; Tuijtelaars, S.; and Verhagen, H. 2005. P.A.S.S.C.L.A.I.M., Process for the Assessment of Scientific Support for Claims on Foods. *European Journal of Nutrition*. 44:S1–31.

Asp, N.-G. and Bryngelsson, S. 2004. The Swedish Code on health claims for foods—Revised version in action. September 2004. *Scandinavian Journal of Nutrition*. 48:188–189.

Asp, N.-G. and Trossing, M. 2001. The Swedish Code on health-related claims in action—extended to product-specific physiological claims. *Scandinavian Journal of Nutrition*. 45:189–192.

Centers for Disease Control and Prevention. 2005a. Death:Preliminary data for 2003. *National Vital Statistics Reports*. 53:1–48.

Centers for Disease Control and Prevention. 2005b. Preventing heart disease and stroke: Addressing the nation's leading killers. United States Department of Health and Human Services. Atlanta, GA.

Chatenoud, L.; Tavani, A.; LaVecchia, C.; Jacobs, D.; Negri, E.; Levis, F.; and Franceschi, S. 1998. Wholes grain food intake and cancer risk. *International Journal of Cancer*. 77:24–28.

Cleveland, L.E.; Moshfegh, A.U.J.; Albertson, A.M.; and Goldman, J.D. 2000. Dietary intake of whole grains. *Journal of the American College of Nutrition*. 19:331S–338S.

Codex Alimentarius Commission. 2004. Guidelines for use of nutrition and health claims. Guideline 23–1997. Revised 1-2004.

Diplock, A.T.; Aggett, P.J.; Ashwell, M.; Bornet, F.; Fern, E.B.; and Roberfroid, M.B. 1999. Scientific concepts of functional foods in Europe: Concensus document. *British Journal of Nutrition*. 81:S(1–27).

Food and Drug Administration. 1997. Food and Drug Administartion Modernization Act of 1997. Washington, D.C. http://www.fda.gov/cder/guidance/105-115.htm#sec.%20303.

Food and Drug Administration. 1999. Whole-Grain Authoritative Statement Claim Notification. Food and Drug Administration. Docket 99P–2209, Washington, D.C. http://www.fda.gov/ohrms/dockets/dailys/070899/070899.htm

Jacobs, D.; Meyer, K.; Kushi, L.; and Folsom, A. 1998. Whole-grain intake may reduce the risk of ischemic heart disease death in postmenopausal women: The Iowa Women's Health Study. *American Journal of Clinical Nutrition*. 68:248–257.

Jacobs, D.; Meyer, K.; Kushi, L.; and Folsom, A. 1999. Is whole grain intake associated with reduced total and cause-specific death rates in older women? The Iowa Women's Health Study. *American Journal of Public Health*. 89:322–329.

Jacobs, D.R.; Meyer, H.E.; and Solvoll, K. 2000. Reduced mortality among whole grain eaters in men and women in the Norwegian County Study. *European Journal of Clinical Nutrition*. 55:137–143.

Jacobs, D.R.; Marquart, L; Slavin, J.; and Kushi, L.H. 1998. Whole grain intake and cancer: An expanded review and meta-analysis. *Nutrition and Cancer*. 30:85–96.

Joint Health Claims Initiative. 2002. Generic Claims Assessment. www.jgci.co.uk.

Liu, S.; Manson, J.E.; Stampfer, M.J.; Hu, F.B.; Giovannucci, E.; Colditz, G.A.; Hennekens, C.H.; and Willett, W.C. 2000. A prospective study of whole grain intake and risk of type 2 diabetes mellitus in U.S. women. *American Journal of Public Health*. 90:1409–1415.

Liu, S.; Sesso, H.D.; Manson, J.E.; Willett, W.C. and Buring, J.E. 2003. Is intake of breakfast cereals related to total and cause-specific mortality in men? *American Journal of Clinical Nutrition*. 77:594–599.

Marquart, L.; Wiemer, K.L.; Jones, J.M.; and Jacob, B. 2003. Whole grain health claims in the U.S.A. and other efforts to increase consumption. Proceedings of the Nutrition Socitey. 62:151–160.

Marquart, L.; Asp, A.G.; and Richardson, D.P. 2004. Whole grain health claims in the United States, United Kingdom and Sweden. In *Dietary Fibre bioactive carbohydrates for food and feed.* Eds. Van der Kamp, J.W.; Asp, N.G.; Miller Jones, J.; Schaafsma, G. Wageningen Academic Publishers. Netherlands. p 39–57.

Montonen, J.; Knekt, P.; Jarvinen, R.; Aromaa, A.; and Reunanen, A. 2003. Whole-grain and fiber intake and the incidence of type 2 diabetes. *American Journal of Clinical Nutrition.* 77:622–629.

U.S. Department of Agriculture, Department of Health and Human Services. 2005. Dietary Guidelines for Americans. U.S. Govt. Printing Office. Washington, D.C.

U.S. Department of Health and Human Services. 2000. Healthy People 2010. (Conference Edition in Two Volumes. U.S. Govt. Printing Office. Washington, D.C.

U.S. Food and Drug Association. 2005. Food labeling: health claims; soluble dietary fiber from certain foods and coronary heart disease. *Federal Register.* May 22, 2006. Docket #2004P-0512

Venn, B.J. and Mann, J.I. 2004. Cereal grains, legumes and diabetes. *European Journal of Clinical Nutrition* 58: 1443–1461.

World Health Organization. 2003. Diet, nutrition and the prevention of chronic diseases. W.H.O. Technical Report Series 916, Geneva 2003, pp. 1–160.

Index